Genetic Variation in Hormone Systems

Volume I

Editor

John G. M. Shire

Senior Lecturer
Department of Genetics
University of Glasgow
Glasgow, Scotland

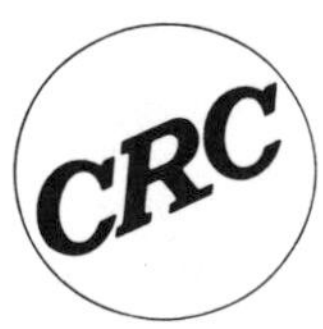

CRC Press, Inc.
Boca Raton, Florida 33431

Library of Congress Cataloging in Publication Data

Main entry under title:

Genetic variation in hormone systems.

Bibliography: v. p.
Includes index.
1. Endocrine genetics. 2. Variation (Biology)
I. Shire, J. G. M.
QP187.5.G46 574.1'4 78-11400
ISBN 0-8493-5283-5 (Volume I)
ISBN 0-8493-5284-5 (Volume II)

International Standard Book Number 0-8493-5283-5 (Volume I)
International Standard Book Number 0-8493-5284-3 (Volume II)

Library of Congress Card Number 78-11400

Printed in the United States

PREFACE

Genetics and endocrinology are both branches of biology that are concerned with the regulation of metabolism in multicellular organisms. This book shows how the two are related, at least in the eyes of 15 individual biologists. The different contributions represent both pure and applied aspects, and consider both variation within the range of normality and variation with pathological consequences.

I should like to thank the contributors for their chapters, which have taught me a great deal about both organisms and their organization. I am indebted to the late Dr. S. G. Spickett who introduced me to the field of endocrine genetics, and to Professor J. M. Thoday, F. R. S., for his encouragement of the subject over the years.

As both contributor and editor I am very grateful to Mrs. I. Wood for the excellence of her typing.

J. Shire
Bar Harbor, Maine
July 1978

THE EDITOR

DR. JOHN G. M. SHIRE is Senior Lecturer in the Department of Genetics, University of Glasgow, Glasgow, Scotland.

Dr. Shire received his B. A. and Ph. D. from the University of Cambridge, England. In 1969 he joined the Department of Psychiatry at Stanford University, Palo Alto, California as Research Associate. In 1971 he went to the University of Glasgow, Scotland, as University Lecturer. In 1976 he became a Senior Lecturer in the Department of Genetics at the University of Glasgow.

Dr. Shire has had over 30 articles published in various journals in the fields of Genetics and Endocrinology. In 1976 he was appointed Honorary Treasurer of the British Genetical Society, and has been a member of the British Society for Endocrinology for several years.

His field of research is physiological genetics, and its relations with developmental biology, behavior, and quantitative and population genetics.

CONTRIBUTORS

Michael Ashburner, Ph.D.
University Lecturer
Department of Genetics
University of Cambridge
Cambridge, England

Fouad M. Badr, Ph.D.
Professor and Head
Zoology Department
University of Kuwait
Kuwait City, Kuwait

Andrzej Bartke, Ph.D.
Associate Professor
Department of Obstetrics and Gynecology
University of Texas
Health Science Center
San Antonio, Texas

Leslie P. Bullock, D.V.M.
Senior Research Associate
Department of Medicine
Associate Professor
Department of Comparative Medicine
Milton S. Hershey Medical Center
Hershey, Pennsylvania

Wilfrid R. Carr, C. Chem. F.R.I.C.
Biochemist, Principal Scientific Officer
Department of Physiological Genetics
A.R.C. Animal Breeding Research Organization
Edinburgh, United Kingdom

Roland D. Ciaranello, M.D.
Assistant Professor of Psychiatry and Behavioral Sciences
Stanford University Medical Center
Stanford, California

Herman J. Degenhart, Ph.D.
Assistant Professor
Department of Pediatrics
Erasmus University
Rotterdam, Netherlands

Michael D. Gale, Ph.D.
Developmental Geneticist
Plant Breeding Institute
Trumpington, Cambridge, England

Roger B. Land, Ph.D.
Principal Scientific Officer
A.R.C. Animal Breeding Research Organization
Edinburgh, United Kingdom

Zvi Laron, M.D.
Professor of Pediatric Endocrinology
Director
Institute of Pediatric and Adolescent Endocrinology and Israel Counselling Center for Juvenile Diabetics
Bellinson Medical Center
Petah Tikva, Israel

Robert Lindsay, Ph.D.
Head of Human Pharmacology
Beecham Research
Walton Oaks
Tadworth, Surrey, England

John G. M. Shire, Ph.D.
Senior Lecturer
Department of Genetics
University of Glasgow
Glasgow, Scotland

Roger Smith, Ph.D., M.D.
Consultant Physician in Metabolic Medicine
Radcliffe Infirmary
Oxford and Nuffield Orthopedic Center
Clinical Lecturer in Medicine
University of Oxford
Oxford, England

Alistair D. Stewart, Ph.D.
Lecturer in Genetics
University of Lancaster
Lancaster, England

John C. Woodrow, M.D.
Reader in Medicine
Consultant Physician
Department of Medicine
University of Liverpool
Liverpool, England

TABLE OF CONTENTS

Volume I

TABLE OF CONTENTS

Volume II

Chapter 1

THE USES AND CONSEQUENCES OF GENETIC VARIATION IN HORMONE SYSTEMS

J. G. M. Shire

TABLE OF CONTENTS

I. INTRODUCTION

Endocrinology is the study of the coordination processes within living organisms that are mediated by chemical messengers. Genetics is concerned with the diversity of form and function found within and between species. The aim of this first chapter is to show some of the relationships between these two branches of biology and to introduce the succeeding chapters. Twelve of these are concerned with the major endocrine systems of vertebrates, while the last two discuss those of plants and insects. As befits a book dealing with genetic variation, the interests and approaches of the authors are varied. The contributors include practicing clinicians, a qualified veterinarian, and a plant breeder. Some chapters are written by zoologists and biochemists who later became geneticists, while others are by geneticists who have acquired expertise in other areas of biology. What they have in common is an interest in the regulation of metabolism, and the ways this differs from one individual to the next.

II. WHAT KINDS OF VARIATION ARE THERE?

Each and every step shown in Figure 1 is subject to genetic variation. The following chapters give specific examples for many endocrine systems, although variants affecting every step for every hormone have not yet been demonstrated. In the case of polypeptide hormones, the prohormone is transcribed from a specific DNA sequence. The

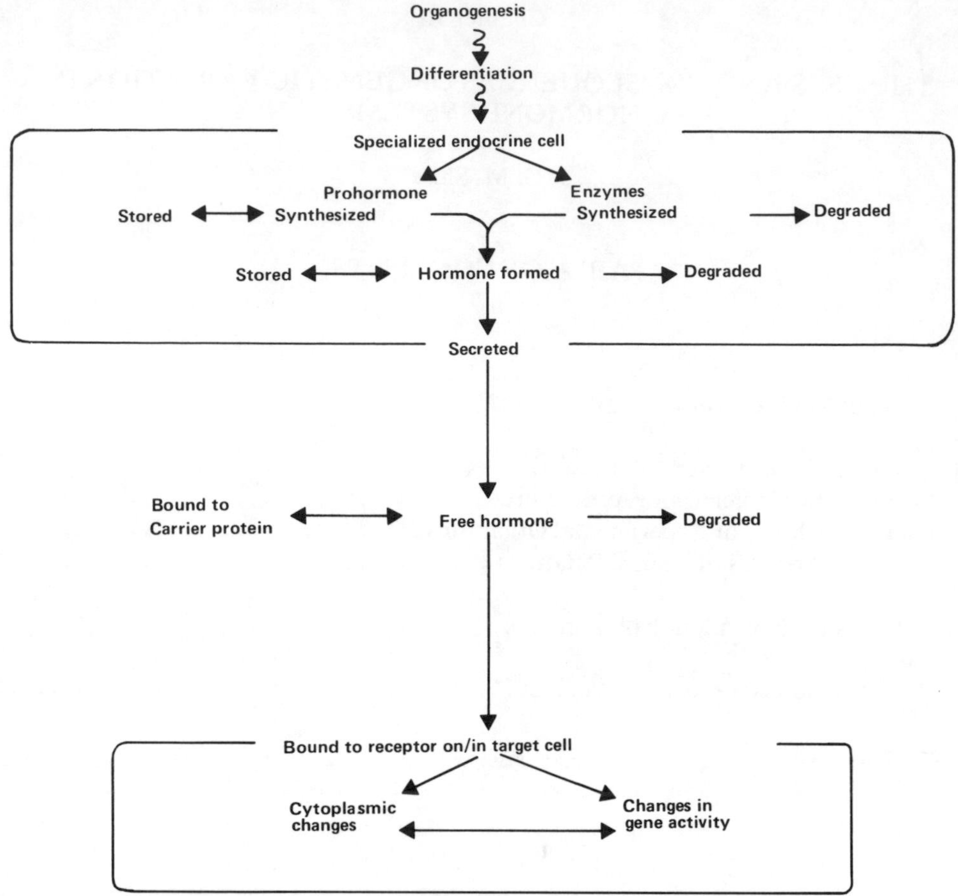

FIGURE 1. A generalized scheme of hormone synthesis and action.

structure of the prohormone may vary genetically in ways that affect its qualities as a substrate for the modification enzymes, leading to differences in the amount or structure of the hormone formed. Many hormones of low molecular weight, such as steroids,[1] are made from substrates, such as cholesterol, which are produced by the general metabolism of the endocrine cell, or by cells elsewhere in the organism. Thyroid hormones can be thought of as being synthesized from a stored polypeptide prohormone, thyroglobulin, which is extensively modified by a network of enzymes.[2] In some systems hormone formation occurs during transport, as with the generation of angiotensin in plasma,[3] or even within the target organ itself, as with the formation of 5-dihydrotestosterone.[4]

Catabolism and interactions with carrier proteins during transport or diffusion may modulate the signal reaching the target tissues. The receptors for some hormones, such as steroids[3,4] and vitamin D,[5] are cytoplasmic and, when combined with hormone, interact with the nuclear genetic material.[6,7] Receptors for other hormones, including most peptides, reside in the cell surface and bring about their effects by activating nucleotide cyclases[5,8] and altering the levels of cAMP or cGMP.[9,10] In some hormone systems, particularly in insects[11] and plants,[12] receptor proteins that initiate the responses of target tissues have yet to be identified. Genetic variation can also affect the trophic stimuli and feedback systems that control hormone levels.

The variants that people choose to study are far from a random sample. In man, clinical considerations result in most studies being on genetic variants with pathological effects. These include deficiencies of growth hormone,[13] parathyroid hormone,[5] and thyroxine,[2] and also diabetes, both mellitus[14] and insipidus.[8] In experimental biology[3,15] and agriculture,[11,12,16] more attention tends to be given to differences between normal individuals, though many mutants of considerable usefulness do exist, in plants,[12] insects,[11] and rodents.[3,4,8,15,17]

When a geneticist looks at an endocrine system, he or she tends to ask about the kinds and numbers of genes present. Sometimes only a single, easily identifiable mutant is involved, but often the variation is quantitative or of variable penetrance and expression. Quantitative differences may be due to the combined effects of many genes or caused by relatively few genetic determinants interacting with each other and with environmental factors. In some such situations individual genetic factors can be revealed by specific environmental manipulation[12] or by defining the observed phenotype more exactly.[18,19] In other cases procedures like cloning or progeny testing[20] are necessary to isolate and identify the genes involved. For a particular genetic variant a geneticist will want to know whether it is a structural gene controlling the amino acid sequence of a protein like growth hormone[21] or vasopressin,[8] or a gene that controls the concentration of a particular protein, such as an enzyme in the pathway of catecholamine biosynthesis.[22] There are various kinds of such regulatory genes, with different genetic and biochemical properties.[23]

Apart from metamorphosis in amphibians,[2] very little is known about the endocrine genetics of lower vertebrates or of invetebrates other than insects. Even among mammals, despite great phenotypic variation, very little is known of the extent of genetic variation in the hormone systems of horses[24] and dogs, except for the pituitary and thyroid of the latter species.[2,25] Some endocrine systems, such as the APUD (amine-uptake and decarboxylating) cells, particularly in the gut,[26] and insect protein hormones have received little attention. The effects of hormones on and in the central nervous system, and their relation to conventional neurotransmitters, is becoming an important field. Already the recently discovered endorphin-enkephalin system shows signs of differing between genotypes.[27] The development and differentiation of the immune system seems to be controlled by pituitary hormones,[15,28] steroids, and thymosin.[29] These control mechanisms are being analyzed by using inbred strains,[29] segregating hybrids,[25] major mutants,[15,30] and somatic cells in culture.[3,31] Interpretation of immune functions like antibody production, histocompatibility, and T and B cell interactions in endocrinological terms could prove rewarding.

III. USEFULNESS OF GENETIC VARIATION

A. In Medicine and Agriculture

Knowledge of the genetics of certain endocrine diseases allows predictions of the risk to individuals. Genetic counseling in man and selective breeding in domestic animals can lead to lower frequencies of affected individuals in succeeding generations, particularly if screening tests for heterozygous carriers can be devised.[1] Differences in susceptibility to certain diseases can be established by phenotypic screening either for predisposing metabolic states[5] or for associated marker genes, like HLA in diabetes mellitus.[14] Studies on animal models of genetic diseases such as dwarfism,[13,15] testicular feminization,[4] and diabetes insipidus[8] throw light on pathological mechanisms and allow tests of possible therapies. Replacement therapy with an active hormone should be effective when a nonfunctional protein is being made, as in some cases of human dwarfism,[13] but would be expected to induce an antibody response in genotypes in which the protein is completely missing. The repair of defective cellular receptors for hormones by the addition of components,[32] or the genes coding for them, will depend strongly on studies of the endocrine genetics of cells in culture.[3,10,31]

In agriculture, commercially important characteristics are being improved by selecting directly for genetic variation affecting the underlying physiological and developmental processes and their endocrine control. Exploitation of favorable variation has already produced gibberellin-resistant grain,[12] increased the reproduction rate of sheep,[16] and improved the suitability of silkworms for sericulture.[11] Knowledge of endocrine genetics has increased the resistance of farm stock to the diseases of stress[3] and offers the prospect of eliminating stress-sensitive pigs[3] and riboflavin-dependent chickens.[33] The genetics of resistance to hormone-analog insecticides[11] and herbicides[12] is of increasing importance in agriculture.

B. Choice of Experimental Organisms

The existence of genetic variation affecting experimental organisms can either be ignored or turned to advantage. Mutants can be used to provide individuals lacking particular hormones, such as dwarf mice[15] and Brattleboro rats,[8] or insensitive to such hormones as testosterone,[4] ecdysone,[11] and plant hormones.[12] In these cases, appropriate crosses will generate the required individuals without the necessity for surgery and with the provision of normal sibs as controls. Organisms with an optimal phenotype can also be chosen from among the various strains and breeds that are available. In studies on the isolation of the pregnancy-blocking pheromone of mice, inbred strains with high and low rates of production were compared.[34] Soay sheep, in which the onset of breeding is strongly dependent on photoperiod, were chosen for studies on the control of seasonal breeding.[35] Horses, donkeys, and their reciprocal hybrids were used to study the roles of mother and fetus in the control of PMSG (pregnant mare serum gonadotropin).[36]

Stocks with appropriate mean value and slope of the dose-response curve[37] should be chosen for bioassays. Variability can be reduced, and the precision of the assay increased, in two ways: by choosing an inbred stock with a well-stabilized development, or by using F1 hybrids. Repeatability, both within and between laboratories, can be improved by the use of individuals of defined genotype. In rats and mice these should include not only the strain, but the subline as well, for there can be marked differences between sublines in endocrine characters.[22,37,38]

C. Analysis of Causal Relations

Many situations in biology can be reduced to the following general form: variation in A causes (is accompanied by) variation in B. Such situations come in a wide range of forms. The variation can be continuous or qualitative, and B may be a single metric or a set of phenotypic characteristics. It is important to be sure that such "pedigrees of causes" are well-founded, and are not based on mere assertion. The range of possible and postulated causal relations is shown by the following examples. Are all the correlated responses in endocrine function found when lines are selected for emotional reactivity,[2,3] or caries resistance,[39,40] causally related to the character studied, or have some of them been fixed in the selected lines by chance? C57 Black mice do not respond to goitrogens[2] or neonatal castration[41] with endocrine neoplasia as most mice do. They also differ from most strains of mice in their prolonged adrenocortical response to stress,[3] their pituitary gonadotropin content,[15] and the relative unimportance of many androgen-dependent functions.[42,43,44] Are many of these peculiarities the consequence of a single hypothalamic difference, or are they caused by a number of independent differences?[45] Are the paradoxical responses to gibberellin of hormone-insensitive dwarf wheats[12] due to pleiotropic effects of the *Gai* mutant, or to closely linked genes? The spontaneous hypertension of SHR rats has been considered to be entirely due to differences in thyroid[2], adrenal,[3] or prostaglandin[9] metabolism. In one investigation, all the differences found between commercially hypophysectomized rats of one strain and intact laboratory-reared rats of another were attributed to the absence of the pituitary. All the differences between rats of one strain, homozygous for diabetes insipidus, and normal rats of another strain were attributed to the mutation,[46] without considering the possibility of differences between normal rats of the two strains.

The existence of genetic variation affecting these systems allows the causality of the observed correlations to be tested. Studies on mutants must include observations on families in which the gene is segregating, for only then can its effects be separated from those of the genetic background. This applies even when congenic strains are being compared,[47] even though they should only differ by a small chromosomal segment.

When dealing with differences that are not known to be due to single, fully penetrant factors, studies on hybrids between the strains are essential. Sometimes, because of differences in dominance relations or sex-linkage, correlations will break down when the F1 hybrids are measured.[37] More often, studies on segregating generations are necessary. Studies on F2 hybrids upheld the positive correlation found between pituitary acidophilia and thymus weight of parental basset hounds and bulldogs.[25] Studies on backcross mice supported coordinate regulation of the enzymes of catecholamine synthesis,[22] but showed that the correlation found between β-glucuronidase activity and the number of pituitary gonadotrophs for C57BL and DBA/2 was not a causal one.[45] Causal analysis can be extended to characters such as dose-response relations, which cannot be measured in individuals if the organism can be cloned or if homozygous stocks can be derived from segregating generations. Recombinant-inbred strains provide such material for studies on mice.[3,48] The finding of similar pleiotropic patterns in different species, as with the correlation between lack of hair and absence of thymus found in both *nude* rats and mice,[17] strengthens the possibility that the two characters form part of the same "pedigree of causes".

Experiments with variant, often neoplastic lines of cells in culture have certain advantages, but also pose some special problems. At present it is often impossible to be sure that a variant phenotype is caused by a change in DNA sequence rather than by a modification of the state of activation of the cell's DNA. Some analysis by mitotic segregation, involving the loss of whole chromosomes, can be done.[49] The possibility of combining the usefulness of studies on cultured cells with meiotic segregation analysis has been opened up by the successful incorporation of cells into the germ lines of chimeric mice[50,51] and flies.[52]

Confirmation of the pathway by which A causes B requires the production of phenocopies. In these the phenotype of one genotype is made to resemble that of another. With pathological variation this may be by repairing the mutant, as in the treatment of pituitary dwarfs with growth hormone,[15] or by altering the wild type, in this case by hypophysectomy. Studies on individuals containing tissues of two functional genotypes can reveal in which tissues a particular gene is autonomously active and in which its phenotypic effects are indirect. Such mosaic individuals can be made by grafting,[15] by fusing embryos,[3] or by genetic means. These include enhanced non-disjunction[53] and the use of X-linked genes in mammals.[4,54]

Apparently identical phenotypes can mask genotypic diversity. Mice of the AKR and DBA strains both have lipid-depleted adrenals, but half of the backcross mice had adrenals of normal appearance.[3] The existence of mimic genes, such as those for dwarfism in man,[13] mouse,[15] and higher plants,[12] not only shows that certain processes have multiple steps, but also provides the material for their investigation.

IV. GENES DO NOT ACT IN ISOLATION

During development, an organism's genome interacts with its immediate environment to produce the fully differentiated adult. The products of one gene often act to control the activity of other genes during differentiation. Hormones control many developmental processes, such as sexual differentiation,[4] puberty,[16] metamorphosis,[2,11] and the initiation of flowering.[12] The regulation of transcription of specific loci by ecdysone in insects[6] can be observed directly.

The effect of substituting one allele for another at a particular locus often depends on which alleles are present elsewhere in the genome. The *db* and *ob* mutants produce acute severe disturbances of carbohydrate metabolism on the C57BL/KsJ background, but only mild chronic changes on the C57BL/6J genetic background.[55] The diabetes mutant itself seems to be a modifier of the susceptibility of mice to virus infection.[56] Similarly, the immunocompetence of dwarf mice[15] and the severity of testicular feminization[4] and nephrogenic diabetes insipidus[8] all depend on which modifying genes are present in the affected individual.

The phenotype of an individual depends on the particular environmental influences to which it has been exposed, as well as on its genotype. However, the effect of an environmental factor often depends strongly on the genotype of the exposed individual. Much genetic variation in susceptibility to disease is of this kind, determining whether an individual mouse will show endocrine neoplasia after castration,[41] or which men[14] and mice[57] will develop diabetes after a virus infection. Stress precipitates hypertension in rats of some, but not all, genotypes.[3] Genetic differences affect the susceptibility of individuals to endocrine disturbances caused by dietary alterations involving calcium and vitamin D,[5] iodine,[2] fats,[3,58] and carbohydrates.[14,58] Natural and synthetic hormone analogs produce very different effects on different genotypes, whether used as drugs,[2-5,8,13,16,59] teratogens,[3] pesticides,[11,12] or as a defense against insect attack.[11]

V. POPULATION ASPECTS

The study of frequencies of genes affecting endocrine systems in natural populations is in its infancy, though there are some interesting observations on neoteny in amphibia,[2] stress-susceptibility in pigs,[3] and eclosion in marine insects.[11] In human populations there is evidence that some of the variation in risk of developing mammary cancer acts through endocrine differences.[15,60] Progress in population studies requires variants that affect protein structure, and unequivocal tests for heterozygotes,[1] as many endocrine metrics are likely to be affected by the individual's unknown prior history.

In natural populations the balance of advantage will lie with different genotypes in different environmental situations and will change as conditions change. Knowledge not only of the forms that genetic variation takes, but also of the way that the genome is organized, will be important for understanding ecological and evolutionary changes. It seems reasonable that inbred strains and natural populations should have evolved coadapted sets of genes.[8,61] In DBA mice, for example, a low rate of corticosteroid production is balanced by a low rate of hormone catabolism.[3] Coadapted complexes may sometimes be held together by close linkage.[20] The chromosomal region containing the major histocompatibility complex is associated with genetic factors determining susceptibility to diabetes mellitus[14] and thyroiditis,[2] and apparently also with responsiveness to androgens *(Slp, Hom-1)*[17] and corticosteroids.[3] Mimic genes may sometimes be the result of duplications, which seem to have provided the raw material for the diversification of function during the evolution of the vertebrate hormones, such as growth hormone and prolactin,[62] gonadotropins and thyrotropin,[62] pituitary octapeptides,[8] and, perhaps, steroid receptors.[3,4] Knowledge of genetic organization can suggest where particular genes might be located.[63] Duplicate dwarfing genes may be sought in homologous chromosomes,[12] and genes that are sex-linked in one vertebrate, like plasma hormone-binding globulins[2,3] and testicular feminization,[4] may be sex-linked in another.[64]

Many endocrine situations involve the interaction of two or more individuals, which will often be of different genotypes in natural populations. Such situations include the endocrine effects of social and behavioral events,[22] whether mediated by pheromones[34] or not, and the complex endocrine interactions between mother and fetus.[3,16,36] Studies of the maternal and social inheritance of endocrine variables have hardly begun.[3] These situations may well be complex, as is the interplay between viral and host genomes that controls the endocrine events that accompany mammary cancer in mice.[15,65] Interspecies interactions involving endocrine functions are not restricted to those between host and microbial pathogen.[12] They will also occur between host and parasite, in both vetebrates and invertebrates,[11] and in symbiotic relations, such as the coordinated endocrine control of reproduction and development in the figwasp-fig complex.[66]

I hope that the study of specialized laboratory and farm stocks will help us to understand the way in which genetic and hormonal regulatory systems interact in natural polymorphic populations.

REFERENCES

1. **Degenhart, H. J.,** Normal and abnormal adrenal steroidogenesis in man, in *Genetic Variation in Hormone Systems,* Vol. 1, Shire, J. G. M., Ed., CRC Press, Boca Raton, Fla., 1979, chap. 2.
2. **Shire, J. G. M.,** The thyroid gland and thyroid hormones, in *Genetic Variation in Hormone Systems,* Vol. 2, Shire, J. G. M., Ed., CRC Press, Boca Raton, Fla., 1979, chap. 1.
3. **Shire, J. G. M.,** Corticosteroids and adrenocortical function in animals, in *Genetic Variation in Hormone Systems,* Vol. 1, Shire, J. G. M., Ed., CRC Press, Boca Raton, Fla., 1979, chap. 3.
4. **Bullock, L. P.,** Genetic variations in sexual differentiation and sexsteroid action, in *Genetic Variation in Hormone Systems,* Vol. 1, Shire, J. G. M., Ed., CRC Press, Boca Raton, Fla., 1979, chap. 4.
5. **Lindsay, R. and Smith, R.,** The genetics of hormonally mediated disorders of calcium metabolism, in *Genetic Variation in Hormone Systems,* Vol. 2, Shire, J. G. M., Ed., CRC Press, Boca Raton, Fla., 1979, chap. 2.
6. **Ashburner, M. and Richards, G.,** The role of ecdysone in the control of gene activity in the polytene chromosomes of *Drosophila,* in *Insect Development,* Lawrence, P. A., Ed., Blackwell Scientific, Oxford, 1976, 203.
7. **Buller, R. E. and O'Malley, B. W.,** The biology and mechanism of steroid hormone receptor interaction with the eukaryotic nucleus, *Biochem. Pharmacol.,* 25, 1, 1976.
8. **Stewart, A. D.,** Genetic variation in the endocrine system of the neurohypophysis, in *Genetic Variation in Hormone Systems,* Vol. 1, Shire, J. G. M., Ed., CRC Press, Boca Raton, Fla., 1979, chap. 8.
9. **Badr, F. M.,** Genetic variation in prostaglandins, in *Genetic Variation in Hormone Systems,* Vol. 2, Shire, J. G. M., Ed., CRC Press, Boca Raton, Fla., 1979, chap. 3.
10. **Coffino, P., Bourne, H. R., Friedrich, U., Hochman, J., Insel, P. A., Lemaine, I., Melmon, K., and Tomkins, G. M.,** Molecular mechanisms of cyclic AMP action: a genetic approach, *Recent Prog. Horm. Res.,* 32, 669, 1976.
11. **Ashburner, M.,** Genetic variation in insect endocrine systems, in *Genetic Variation in Hormone Systems,* Vol. 2, Shire, J. G. M., Ed., CRC Press, Boca Raton, Fla., 1979, chap. 6.
12. **Gale, M. D.,** Plant hormones and plant breeding, in *Genetic Variation in Hormone Systems,* Vol. 2, Shire, J. G. M., Ed., CRC Press, Boca Raton, Fla., 1979, chap. 7.
13. **Laron, Z.,** Human growth hormone, in *Genetic Variation in Hormone Systems,* Vol. 1, Shire, J. G. M., Ed., CRC Press, Boca Raton, Fla., 1979, chap. 7.
14. **Woodrow, J. C.,** Genetics of diabetes mellitus, in *Genetic Variation in Hormone Systems,* Vol. 2, Shire, J. G. M., Ed., CRC Press, Boca Raton, Fla., 1979, chap. 5.
15. **Bartke, A.,** Genetic models in the study of anterior pituitary hormones, in *Genetic Variation in Hormone Systems,* Vol. 1, Shire, J. G. M., Ed., CRC Press, Boca Raton, Fla., 1979, chap. 6.

16. **Land, R. B. and Carr, W. R.**, Reproduction in domestic mammals, in *Genetic Variation in Hormone Systems*, Vol. 1, Shire, J. G. M., Ed., CRC Press, Boca Raton, Fla., 1979, chap. 5.
17. **Shire, J. G. M.**, Appendix: mutations affecting the hormone systems of rodents, in *Genetic Variation in Hormone Systems*, Vol. 2, Shire, J. G. M., Ed., CRC Press, Boca Raton, Fla., 1979.
18. **Spickett, S. G., Shire, J. G. M., and Stewart, J.**, Genetic variation in adrenal and renal structure and function, *Mem. Soc. Endocrinol.*, 15, 271, 1967.
19. **Thompson , J. N.**, Quantitative variation and gene number, *Nature (London)*, 258, 665, 1975.
20. **Thoday, J. M.**, Uses of genetics in physiological studies, *Mem. Soc. Endocrinol.*, 15, 297, 1967.
21. **Seavey, B. K., Singh, R. U. P., Lewis, U. J., and Geschwind, I. I.**, Bovine growth hormone: evidence for two allelic forms, *Biochem. Biophys. Res. Commun.*, 43, 189, 1971.
22. **Ciaranello, R. D.**, Genetic regulation of the catecholamine synthesizing enzymes, in *Genetic Variation in Hormone Systems*, Vol. 2, Shire, J. G. M., Ed., CRC Press, Boca Raton, Fla., 1979, chap. 4.
23. **Sutcliffe, R. G., Carritt, B., and Wilson, R. H. W.**, Genes, proteins and the control of gene expression, in *Human Biochemical Genetics*, 2nd ed., Brock, D. J. H. and Mayo, O., Eds., Academic Press, London, 1978, chap. 2.
24. **Walton, A. and Hammond, J.**, The maternal effects on growth and conformation in Shire horse-Shetland pony crosses, *Proc. R. Soc. London Ser. B.*, 125, 311, 1938.
25. **Stockard, C. R.**, The genetic and endocrinic basis for differences in form and behavior, *Am. Anat. Mem.*, 19, 1, 1941.
26. **Polak, J. M., Pearse, A. G. E., Grimelius, L., and Marks, V.**, Gastrointestinal apudosis in obese hyperglycemic mice, *Virchows Arch. B.*, 19, 135, 1975.
27. **Trabucchi, M., Spano, P. F., Racagni, G., and Oliverio, A.**, Genotype-dependent sensitivity to morphine: dopamine involvement in morphine-induced running in the mouse, *Brain Res.*, 114, 536, 1976.
28. **Pierpaoli, W., Kopp, H. G., and Bianchi, E.**, Interdependence of thymic and neuroendocrine factors in ontogeny, *Clin. Exp. Immunol.*, 24, 501, 1976.
29. **Bach, M. A. and Niaudet, P.**, Regulatory influence of a circulating thymic factor on antibody production against PVP in NZB mice, *J. Immunol.*, 117, 760, 1976.
30. **Pantelouris, E. M.**, Athymic development in the mouse, *Differentiation*, 1, 437, 1973.
31. **Yamamoto, K. R., Gehring, U., Stampfer, M. R., and Sibley, C. H.**, Genetic approaches to steroid hormone action, *Recent Prog. Horm. Res.*, 32, 3, 1976.
32. **Orly, J. and Schramm, M.**, Coupling of catecholamine receptor from one cell with adenylate cyclase from another cell by cell fusion, *Proc. Natl. Acad. Sci., U.S.A.*, 73, 4410, 1976.
33. **Hammer, C. H., Buss, E. G., and Clagett, C. O.**, Avian riboflavinuria. IX. Qualitative action of a mutant gene in chicken on riboflavin-binding protein synthesis, *Genetics*, 82, 467, 1976.
34. **Hoppe, P. C.**, Genetic and endocrine studies of the pregnancy-blocking pheromone of mice, *J. Reprod. Fertil.*, 45, 109, 1975.
35. **Lincoln, G. A. and Peet, M. J.**, Photoperiodic control of gonadotrophin secretion in the ram, *J. Endocrinol.*, 74, 355, 1977.
36. **Stewart, F., Allen, W. R., and Moor, R. M.**, Influence of foetal genotype on the follicle-stimulating hormone: luteinizing hormone ratio of pregnant mare serum gonadotropin, *J. Endocrinol.*, 73, 419, 1977.
37. **Shire, J. G. M.**, The forms, uses and significance of genetic variation in endocrine systems, *Biol. Rev.*, 51, 105, 1976.
38. **Bartke, A. and Shire, J. G. M.**, Differences between mouse strains in testicular cholesterol levels and androgen target organs, *J. Endocrinol.*, 55, 173, 1972.
39. **Sreebny, L. M., Rosen, S., Bachem, E., Hunt, H. R., and Hoppert, C. A.**, The effect of castration on the submaxillary gland of Hunt-Hoppert caries-resistant and caries-susceptible rats, *J. Dent. Res.*, 38, 67, 1959.
40. **Mullen, R. J. and Hoornbeek, F. K.**, Genetic aspects of fertility and endocrine organ size in rats, *Genet. Res.*, 16, 251, 1971.
41. **Woolley, G. W.**, Experimental endocrine tumors with special reference to the adrenal cortex, *Recent Prog. Horm. Res.*, 5, 383, 1950.
42. **Wilson, C. M., Erdos, E. G., Dunn, J. F., and Wilson, J. D.**, Genetic control of renin activity in the submaxillary gland of the mouse, *Proc. Natl. Acad. Sci., U.S.A.*, 74, 1185, 1977.
43. **Shire, J. G. M. and Bartke, A.**, Strain differences in testicular weight and spermatogenesis with special reference to C57Bl/10J and DBA/2J mice, *J. Endocrinol.*, 55, 163, 1972.
44. **McGill, T. E. and Manning, A.**, Genotype and retention of the ejaculatory reflex in castrated male mice, *Anim. Behav.*, 24, 507, 1976.
45. **Håkansson, E. M. and Lundin, L. G.**, Genetic variation in the number of pituitary PAS-positive purple cells in the house mouse, *J. Hered.*, 66, 144, 1975.
46. **Leclerc, R. and Pelletier, G.**, Electron microscope immunohistochemical localization of vasopressin in the hypothalamus and neurohypophysis of the normal and Brattleboro rat, *Am. J. Anat.*, 140, 583, 1974.

47. **Gregorová, S., Ivanyi, P., Mickova, M., and Simonová, D.**, The influence of H-2 haplotypes on vesicular gland weight, *Folia Biol.*, (Prague), 22, 44, 1976.
48. **Bailey, D. W.**, Recombinant-inbred strains, *Transplantation*, 11, 325, 1971.
49. **Ruddle, F. H. and Creagan, R. P.**, Parasexual approaches to the genetics of man, *Annu. Rev. Genet.*, 9, 407, 1975.
50. **Papaioannou, V. E., McBurney, M. W., Gardner, R. L., and Evans, M. J.**, Fate of teratocarcinoma cells injected into early mouse embryos, *Nature (London)*, 258, 70, 1975.
51. **Mintz, B. and Illmensee, K.**, Normal genetically mosaic mice produced from malignant teratocarcinoma cells, *Proc. Natl. Acad. Sci., U.S.A.*, 72, 3585, 1975.
52. **Illmensee, K.**, Nuclear and cytoplasmic transplantation in *Drosophila*, in *Insect Development*, Lawrence, P. A., Ed., Blackwell Scientific, Oxford, 1976, 76.
53. **Hall, J. C., Gelbart, W. M., and Kankel, D. R.**, Mosaic systems, in *The Genetics and Biology of Drosophila*, Vol. 1A, Ashburner, M. and Novitski, E., Eds., Academic Press, London, 1976, 265.
54. **Gartler, S. M. and Andina, R. J.**, Mammalian X-chromosome inactivation, *Adv. Hum. Genet.*, 7, 99, 1976.
55. **Coleman, D. L. and Hummel, K. P.**, The influence of genetic background on the expression of the obese (ob) gene in the mouse, *Diabetologia*, 9, 287, 1973.
56. **Webb, S. B., Loria, R. M., Madge, G. E., and Kibrick, S.**, Susceptibility of mice to group B Coxsackie virus is influenced by the diabetic gene, *J. Exp. Med.*, 143, 1239, 1976.
57. **Yoon, J. W., Lesniak, M. A., Fussganger, R., and Notkins, A. L.**, Genetic differences in susceptibility of pancreatic β cells to virus-induced diabetes mellitus, *Nature (London)*, 264, 178, 1976.
58. **Stauffacher, W., Orci, L., Cameron, D. P., Burr, I. M., and Renold, A. E.**, Spontaneous hyperglycemia and/or obesity in laboratory rodents: an example of the possible usefulness of animal disease models with both genetic and environmental components, *Recent Prog. Horm. Res.*, 27, 41, 1971.
59. **Bigger, J. F., Palmberg, P. F., and Zink, H. A.**, In vitro corticosteroids: correlation of response with primary open-angle glaucoma and ocular corticosteroid sensitivity, *Am. J. Ophthalmol.*, 79, 92, 1975.
60. **Wang, D. Y., Bulbrook, R. D., and Hayward, J. L.**, Urinary and plasma androgens and their relation to familial risk of breast cancer, *Eur. J. Cancer*, 11, 873, 1975.
61. **Dobzhansky, T.**, *Genetics and the Origin of Species*, 3rd ed., Columbia University Press, New York, 1951, 1.
62. **Wallis, M.**, The molecular evolution of pituitary hormones, *Biol. Rev.*, 50, 35, 1975.
63. **Lundin, L. G.**, Evolutionary conservation of chromosomal segments, *Clin. Genet.*, in press.
64. **Ohno, S.**, *Sex Chromosomes and Sex-Linked Genes*, Springer, Berlin, 1967, 1.
65. **Sinha, Y. N., Salocks, C. B., Vanderlaan, W. P., and Vlahakis, G.**, Evidence for an influence of mammary tumour virus on prolactin secretion in the mouse, *J. Endocrinol.*, 74, 383, 1977.
66. **Galil, J.**, Fig biology, *Endeavour*, 1, 52, 1977.

Chapter 2

NORMAL AND ABNORMAL ADRENAL STEROIDOGENESIS IN MAN

H. J. Degenhart

TABLE OF CONTENTS

I. INTRODUCTION

The anatomy and histology of the adrenal glands were studied in detail a long time before their function and biochemistry could be described. At present, our knowledge concerning the biochemistry of steroid formation and metabolism is fairly complete. Regulation mechanisms and the modes of action are under study in many laboratories and it is possible to prepare a scheme fitting most experimental data.

A review of the genetically determined variations in the functioning of the adrenal cortex will be presented in this chapter. These can vary from congenital absence of the adrenals to clinically undetectable conditions. Some of the variations mentioned in this review have not yet been described, but the possible clinical consequences seem to warrant their inclusion here. To put them in the right framework, normal adrenal functioning will be described first, starting with some remarks about adrenal anatomy and finishing with the excretion of the steroid metabolites.

II. NORMAL FUNCTION

In man, the two adrenal glands have a combined weight of about 10 g. In the adult 80% of the gland is cortex. A forerunner of this structure, the fetal zone, appears early in fetal life (4 to 6 weeks gestation) followed by the definitive cortex at about 6 to 7 weeks of gestation. The fetal zone develops rapidly and reaches its relative maximal size at about the 15th week of gestation. Its anatomy and histology are well known, but its biochemistry, function, and regulation remain largely obscure at the present time. Shortly before or after birth it involutes suddenly and apart from isolated residues, it has disappeared after 6 months.[1,2] The definitive cortex keeps on growing and becomes one of the most important endocrine glands in man from the time of birth until death.

Mesodermal cells play an important role in the embryological development of the adrenal cortex, the testes, and the ovaries. Their common origin is reflected by the presence of adrenal cortex-like tissues in both testes and ovaries, as found in a significant percentage of all autopsy cases.[3,4]

The adult human adrenal cortex possesses three histologically different, concentric zones.[5] The outer zone is called the zona glomerulosa, the middle zone, the zona fasciculata, and the inner zone, the zona reticularis. Steroid production occurs in all three of them, but each probably has its own "speciality". This is well-proven for the glomerulosa, which is the aldosterone producing zone.

A. Biosynthesis of Cholesterol

Cholesterol is by far the most important precursor for the steroid hormones, although it is probable that sterols like desmosterol and 25-hydroxycholesterol have a function in minor pathways.

De novo cholesterol synthesis by the adrenal cortex is quantitatively less important than cholesterol uptake from the blood,[6,7] a process that will be described below. The biosynthesis of cholesterol in the liver occurs as follows.[8-10]

1. Two acetyl-CoA → acetoacetyl-CoA
2. Acetoacetyl-CoA + acetyl-CoA → 3-hydroxy-3-methylglutaryl-CoA
3. 3-Hydroxy-3-methylglutaryl-CoA → 3R-mevalonic acid
   Reaction 3 is catalyzed by the enzyme HMG-CoA reductase (3-hydroxy-3-methylglutaryl-CoA reductase). Two molecules of NADPH are necessary to supply reducing equivalents for the removal of the CoA and the reduction of the CoA linked

   $$\mathrm{H{-}\underset{\underset{O}{\|}}{C}{-}group.}$$

   A major feedback-inhibition point is located here: cholesterol reduces the rate of mevalonic acid formation, probably by inhibiting the synthesis of the HMG-CoA reductase.[11]
4. Mevalonate → → → squalene
   This is a multistep process, not considered in detail here.
5. Squalene → lanosterol
   In this highly complicated reaction, the linear squalene molecule is folded into the characteristic 4-ring sterol structure.
6. Lanosterol → → → cholesterol
   This is again a multistep process. Lanosterol is a C_{30}-compound, and three methyl-groups must be removed by oxidative processes. In addition one double bond ($C_{24} = C_{25}$) must be saturated and another one shifted ($C_8 = C_9 \rightarrow C_5 = C_6$). The intermediates are known, but several pathways seem to be possible.

B. Cholesterol Uptake

The uptake of circulating cholesterol by the adrenal cortex has not been studied in detail. If this process is analogous to the well-studied case of the cultured human fibroblasts,[11] the cholesterol must be offered in a bound form.

In the fibroblast, a cholesterylester—low-density lipoprotein* complex binds to a specific receptor (which is probably under the control of a single genetic locus). The LDL-cholesterylester enters the cell by endocytosis, where it is hydrolyzed by proteases and one or more acid lipases. The free cholesterol can be stored as such, or is first reesterified. Storage occurs, among other places, in the so-called lipid droplets.[12]

C. Biosynthesis of Adrenal Steroids

The conversion of cholesterol into cortisol or aldosterone asks for the consecutive action of several enzymes (Figure 1). These enzymes belong to three classes: lyases, hydroxylases, and dehydrogenases.

1. Lyases

The most important lyase is pregnenolone synthetase, also called the cholesterol side chain cleaving enzyme system. It is located in the mitochondria. A cytochrome P-450 functions as the terminal oxidase in association with a flavoprotein and a nonheme iron protein called adrenodoxin, adrenal ferredoxin, or cytochrome P-450 reductase.[13] The side chain cleaving enzyme system requires three molecules each of oxygen and NADPH.[14] This suggests the existence of intermediate products. Several authors have

* Cholesterol uptake in the rat adrenal occurs via receptors specific for high-density lipoprotein.[84]

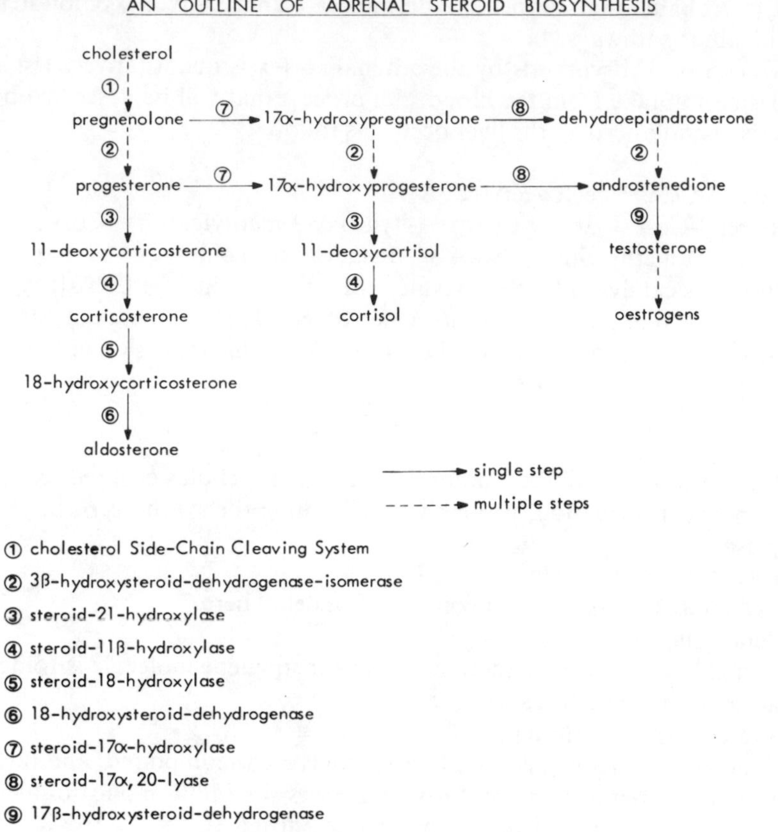

FIGURE 1. An outline of adrenal steroid biosynthesis.

proposed mechanisms involving hydroxylation of cholesterol at positions 20 and 22, followed by a cleavage of the 20—22 bond.[14,15] Early kinetic studies by Burstein and Gut[16] criticized the so-called classical model in which cholesterol is first hydroxylated at C-22 and then at C-20 (Figure 2). They found that the route via 20S-hydroxycholesterol is a very minor pathway and that most of the pregnenolone seemed to be generated via a route not including one of the two hydroxylated sterols.

Recent results obtained by Kraaipoel et al.[17-19] led to the proposal of another model for the side chain cleavage of cholesterol (Figure 3). In this model a Δ^{20-22} unsaturated cholesterol and a 20,22 cholesterol epoxide were introduced as intermediates. The results of Kraaipoel et al.[19] combined with those of Takemoto et al.[20] and Burstein et al.[21] definitely exclude any essential role of 20S-hydroxycholesterol. Whether 22R-hydroxycholesterol is an essential intermediate or a by-product in this process remains to be established. At present, 20R,22R-dihydroxycholesterol is the only intermediate that is generally accepted.

The pathway between 22R-hydroxycholesterol and 20R,22R-dihydroxycholesterol is not entirely clear. As water seems to be involved in this part of the pathway, a conventional hydroxylation step is unlikely.

The formation of adrenal androgens also asks for the cleavage of a C—C — the C_{17}—C_{20} bond. Most, if not all, natural C_{21} steroids with a 20-keto and a 17α-hydroxyl group can undergo C_{17}—C_{20} cleavage. 17α-Hydroxypregnenolone is probably quantitatively the most important substrate in the human adrenal. The C_{17}—C_{20} lyase is located in the microsomal fraction. A cytochrome P-450 is associated with its action, but the detailed mechanism is not known.

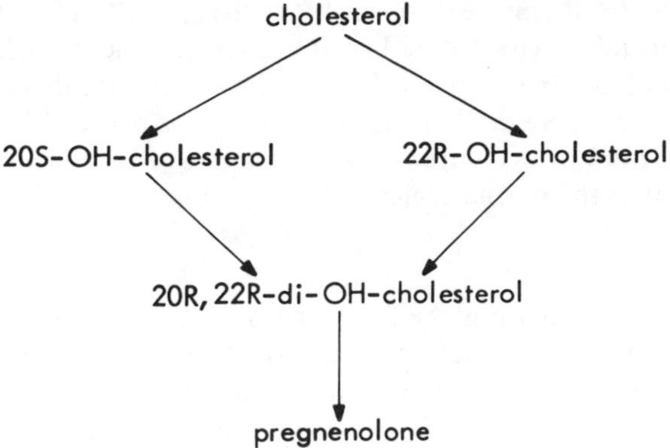

FIGURE 2. Cholesterol side chain cleavage according to the "classical model".

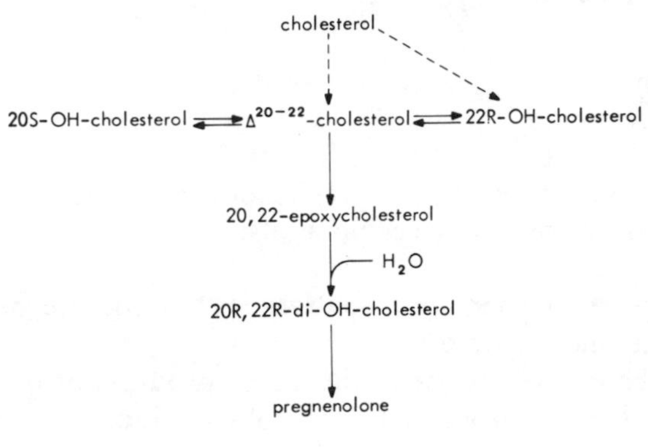

FIGURE 3. Cholesterol side chain cleavage according to the model proposed by Kraaipoel et al.[17-19]

2. *Hydroxylases*

The hydroxylases are partly microsomal (17α- and 21-hydroxylase) and partly mitochondrial (11β- and 18-hydroxylase) The overall reaction equation is

$$\text{steroid-H} + \text{NADPH} + H^+ + O_2 \rightarrow \text{steroid-OH} + \text{NADP}^+ + H_2O.$$

The mitochondrial 11β-hydroxylation reaction is understood relatively well. The NADPH serves to reduce a flavoprotein, which in its turn reduces a nonheme Fe-containing enzyme, also called adrenodoxin, ferredoxin, or (more correctly) cytochrome P-450 reductase. The latter enzyme reduces the cytochrome P-450 responsible for the hydroxylation proper.

The microsomal hydroxylases have a slightly different electron supply chain. They have been studied less thoroughly, but it seems that the electron flow is as follows: NADPH → cytochrome c reductase → cytochrome b_5 → cytochrome P-450. It is not impossible that more proteins will have to be inserted in this chain as more data become available.

It has been proposed that in vivo each of the adrenal hydroxylases has its own supply chain for reducing equivalents. In vitro experiments have demonstrated, however, that these supply chains are not completely specific for a single hydroxylase.

Especially in the older literature, the word "hydroxylase" meant the whole complex of enzymes (flavoprotein, cytochrome P-450 reductase, and cytochrome P-450). The pattern that emerges from the more recent work indicates that there are as many kinds of cytochrome P-450 as there are hydroxylases. It seems preferable to define a steroid hydroxylase as that kind of cytochrome-P-450 that introduces a hydroxyl group on a specific carbon atom of the steroid skeleton.[22]

3. Dehydrogenases

An important dehydrogenase is the 3β-hydroxysteroid dehydrogenase. Its action is virtually always followed by the action of an isomerase, which shifts the double bond from $C_5 = C_6$ to $C_4{=}C_5$. Another important and unusual,[23] dehydrogenase activity is displayed by the enzyme catalyzing the reaction 18-OH-corticosterone → aldosterone. This enzyme is specific for aldosterone formation and occurs only in the zona glomerulosa. Probably less important is the 11β-dehydrogenase. Although essential for the formation of testosterones 17β-hydroxysteroid-dehydrogenase is one of the minor enzymatic activities in the adrenal.

4. The Sulfate Pathway

Parallel with the sequence:

Cholesterol → pregnenolone → 17α-OH-pregnenolone → dehydro-epiandrosterone runs a metabolic pathway of sulfated compounds:

Cholesterol-3-sulfate → pregnenolone-3-sulfate → 17α-OH-pregnenolone-3-sulfate → dehydro-epiandrosterone-3-sulfate.[24]

The latter steroid conjugate is one of the major products of the adrenal cortex, the amount secreted daily often surpasses the cortisol secretion.

D. Regulation

1. The Mechanism of Action of ACTH

The synthesis of glucocorticoids and C_{19} steroids by the adrenal cortex is regulated almost exclusively by ACTH. The mechanism of action of ACTH is very complex and in this section an outline only of the stimulation of steroid production by ACTH will be presented. Comprehensive reviews of the literature can be found elsewhere.[15,25]

ACTH has several effects on the adrenal. Its main short term effects are the stimulation of corticosteroid production (Figure 4) and an increase of adrenal blood flow. In addition to these short term effects, ACTH also influences the growth of the adrenal cortex.

ACTH is bound to receptor sites on the outer surface of the cellular membrane. At least two different receptor systems for ACTH have been found: one with an apparent dissociation constant of approximately 10^{-11} to 10^{-12} M, and another with an apparent K′d of about 10^{-8} M. The latter receptors are present in much larger numbers than the former,[26,27] but the exact function of each of these receptors is unknown. Inside the cell the rate-limiting step in ACTH-stimulated steroid production is situated somewhere between cholesterol and pregnenolone. It may be the transport of cholesterol from extramitochondrial storage sites to the cholesterol side chain cleaving system.[28,29]

A number of steps lie between the binding of ACTH to the cell membrane and the stimulation of pregnenolone synthesis. The first intracellular effect of ACTH is an increased formation of cyclic adenosyl 3′,5′-monophosphate (c-AMP) as a so-called second messenger.[30,31] In the case of ACTH the role of c-AMP as a second messenger seems well established, but the existence of other second messengers cannot be excluded.[32]

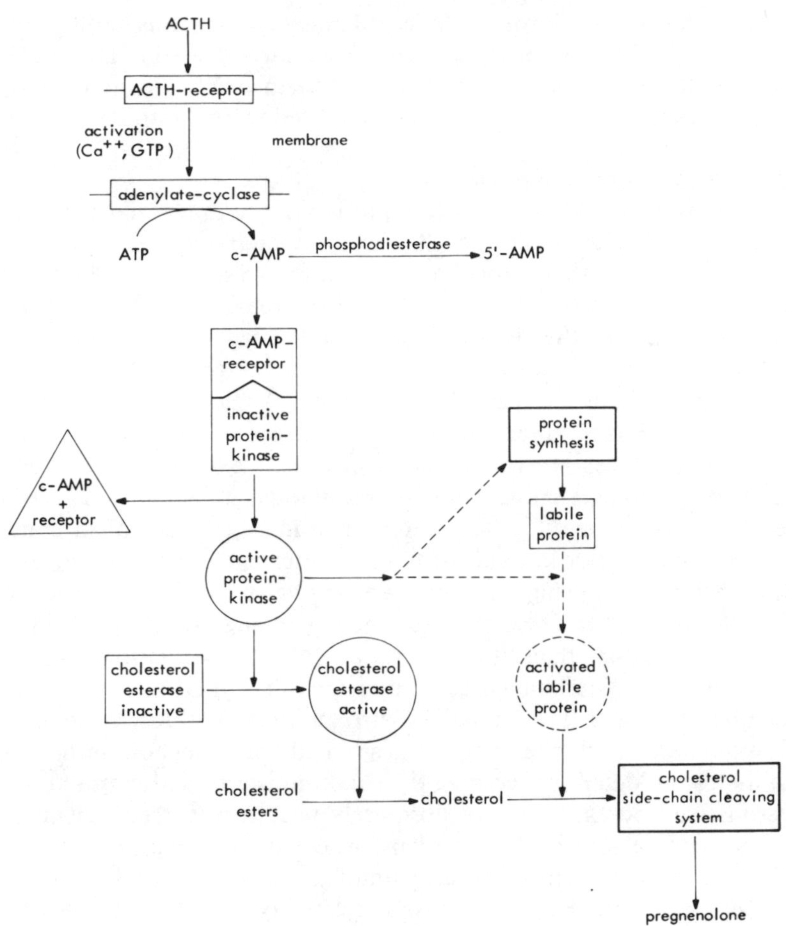

FIGURE 4. A model of the mechanism of action of ACTH.

The activation of adenylate cyclase requires Ca^{++} and seems to be modulated in a still unknown way by several prostaglandins.[33,34] The c-AMP formed can be inactivated by a phosphodiesterase, resulting in the formation of 5′-AMP. Activation of steroid production by c-AMP starts with binding to a c-AMP receptor-inactive protein kinase complex. This process and the next steps have been thoroughly studied by Garren and co-workers.[35] After binding of cyclic AMP, the complex dissociates into a (c-AMP receptor)—c-AMP complex and an active protein kinase, which may form dimers. The active protein kinase can incorporate phosphate from ATP into several proteins, including histones. So far, the only substrate for the protein kinase identified as part of the regulatory mechanism of ACTH is cholesterol esterase,[35,36] which stimulates hydrolysis of cholesterol esters after treatment of adrenal tissue with ACTH. The free cholesterol formed has to be transported from the "lipid droplets" to the cholesterol side chain cleaving system residing in the mitochondria. As cholesterol itself is very hydrophobic, it seems likely that some transport factor, probably a protein (the "labile protein") is needed. At present it is generally accepted that protein synthesis is an essential part of the mechanism of action of ACTH.[15,25]

Several other factors may play a part in the acute stimulation of steroidogenesis by ACTH. Calcium (in addition to its role in the activation of adenylate cyclase), is involved in many other processes in the cell and ACTH is known to influence the uptake of calcium by the adrenal cell and may also influence its intracellular distribution.[15]

There is also evidence for a role of microfilaments in the mechanism of action of ACTH.[37] Finally, ACTH probably does not have an acute stimulating effect on the activity of the cholesterol side chain cleaving system itself, all the cholesterol made available to this enzyme system can be immediately converted into steroids.

2. Regulation of Aldosterone Secretion

The regulation of the aldosterone secretion is very complex and is not understood completely. A complete discussion of all relevant data and opinions could easily fill a 1000 page book and more than a rough outline cannot be given here.[38,39,204]

The main regulatory factor for aldosterone is the renin-angiotensin system.[40] Renin is a protease, produced by the kidney in the juxtaglomerular cells of the afferent arterioles. Renin acts on angiotensinogen, has a molecular weight of about 4×10^4, behaves as an α_2-globulin, and has a remarkable specificity. Angiotensinogen has a molecular weight of 110,000 and is produced in the liver. This protein has the following primary structure: (N-terminal) **asp-arg-val-tyr-ile**-his-pro-phe-his-leu-leu-val-tyr-ser-etc. Renin cleaves off a decapeptide, angiotensin I or proangiotensin: **asp-arg-val-tyr-ile-his-pro-phe-his-leu.** A Cl^--activated, Zn^{++}-containing peptidase, the so-called converting enzyme, removes the dipeptide his-leu, forming angiotensin II or short: angiotensin. This octa‡peptide has the following structure: **asp-arg-val-tyr-ile-his-pro-phe.** An enzyme ("tonin") catalyzing the reaction angiotensinogen → angiotensin II also seems to exist.[194] Angiotensin can be attacked by several angiotensinases. One of these, angiotensinase As, removes the N-terminal asp, yielding angiotensin III.

Both angiotensin II and III stimulate in vitro and in vivo aldosterone production by the glomerulosa cells. Their site of action is situated between cholesterol and pregnenolone, but almost no details concerning their mechanism of action are known. ACTH has a "permissive" action; it is not absolutely necessary for sufficient aldosterone secretion. This can be seen in those patients where the hypophysis is destroyed. The zona fasciculata and zona reticularis have almost disappeared and the cortisol production is virtually nil, while the glomerulosa is relatively less affected, resulting in low-normal aldosterone levels.[41] Long-term administration of additional ACTH results in an increase of aldosterone secretion lasting several days, but after about one week the aldosterone secretion has returned to its basal level.

Serotonin, potassium, prostaglandins, and probably other chemical factors also exert a stimulatory action somewhere between cholesterol and pregnenolone. In addition, Na^+-depletion and K^+-surplus increase aldosterone production (by stimulating hydroxylase activity?) at sites between deoxycorticosterone and aldosterone.[42]

E. Secretion

The secretion of several adrenal steroids is subject to at least two rhythms. One is a mainly ACTH-controlled circadian rhythm, with a frequency of 1c/24 hr.[43] Cortisol levels in blood are highest at about 6:00 a.m. and lowest shortly before midnight. The aldosterone levels show a maximum at about 4:00 a.m. Superimposed is a so-called ultradian rhythm, a more random, pulse-like pattern of secretion with a higher frequency. For cortisol, the distance between two of these maxima is several hours, while ACTH is probably not the only controlling factor.[44,45] In addition, there seem to be very slow variations in adrenal activity with cycles of sometimes more than 2 weeks duration.[46,47]

F. Transport

A large proportion of the circulating steroids is bound to one or more proteins, sometimes dubbed "plasmareceptors". Less then 5% of the circulating cortisol is free, while the α_1-globulin transcortin (a 51,700 dalton molecule) binds the major part. In addition albumin binds some cortisol, but with a low association constant.[48]

The free, unbound, fraction represents the biologically active steroid hormone. In the target tissues the steroid cannot enter the cells before it has dissociated from the carrier. The clearance by the liver of the protein-bound form is much slower than that of the free steroid.

Aldosterone occurs in an albumin-bound, a transcortin-bound, and a free form. Furthermore, one or more specific aldosterone-binding proteins have recently been reported.[195] The free fraction is relatively larger than for most other corticosteroids.

G. Mechanism of Action of Corticosteroids

Much is already known about how steroid hormones exert their effects. As cortisol and aldosterone are the two most important adrenal hormones, these steroids will be used to illustrate the general mechanisms.

1. Glucocorticoids

The biological activities of the glucocorticoids are extremely diverse. Most, if not all, living tissue of the human body reacts with metabolic changes upon contact with, e.g., cortisol. The biochemistry of glucocorticoid action is highly complicated. It has so many aspects, often only superficially studied and poorly understood, that it is impossible to give at present a balanced review.[9,49-51,196]

Some of the most important effects of glucocorticoid hormones are

1. Control of carbohydrate-fat-protein metabolism
2. Antiinflammatory action
3. Suppression of immunoglobulin synthesis
4. Inhibition of bone formation
5. Actions on the CNS

Even this short list suggests that the different target cells have different mechanisms for processing the information offered by the hormone.

A unified picture of what happens when, e.g., cortisol enters the cell has been developed during the last decade by the combined work of many investigators. The rate of entry of a steroid hormone in the cell is determined mainly by diffusion processes: active transport seems to play a minor role. After the entrance, the hormone combines with specific oligomeric proteins, the so-called cytoplasmic receptors (molecular weights 1×10^5 to 3×10^5). The receptors bind glucocorticoids with a remarkable tightness; the dissociation constants are in the order of 10^{-10} M. The receptors are rod-shaped, probably with a binding site for the steroid and a binding site for DNA, not unlike many immunoglobulins, which have an F_{ab} an antigen-combining site, and an F_c site, mediating effector functions.

After a still ill-defined "activation" process the receptor steroid complex moves to the nucleus is translocated and is bound to nuclear receptors. There is at present no consensus as to the exact nature of these, but they are as essential as the cytoplasmic receptors. The two kinds of receptors are probably the main determinants of steroid action. Differences in receptor concentrations and receptor properties are responsible for the manifold reactions seen in the tissues of the body.

After the binding, specific parts of the DNA are activated and changes can occur at three levels:

1. Replication (DNA-synthesis)
2. Transcription (RNA-synthesis)
3. Translation (protein synthesis)

This results in changes in concentrations and activities of enzymes and structural proteins. The "integrated" response, for example an increased gluconeogenesis, can then be observed.

Apart from this main mechanism of action, glucocorticoids have direct, stabilizing, effects on membranes. In addition, they influence cellular metabolism by other, not well-understood means.[52]

2. Aldosterone

Aldosterone's mechanism of action is analogous to that of the glucocorticoids. Because of its low serum concentrations (about 10^3 times less than cortisol), the glucocorticoid activity of aldosterone is unimportant. This hormone is supposed to stimulate the synthesis of enzymes involved in Na^+ and K^+ transport. Much experimental work has been done with the toad bladder but a generally accepted theory valid for the human kidney is still lacking. An indirect action on the Na^+- K^+-dependent ATP'ase in the distal convoluted tubule seems to be an important aspect of aldosterone action.[53-55,205]

H. Metabolism and Excretion

As soon as the steroid hormone has performed its task, it must be removed and/or inactivated. Almost no data are available on steroid release from the receptor. However, it is certain that the steroid does leave the target cell and enters the general circulation.

Many tissues have enzymes that are able to metabolize adrenal steroids. In contrast with the androgens, where, e.g., dihydrotestosterone is a hormone in its own right, metabolic changes in the glucocorticoid or aldosterone molecule drastically reduce the activity.

The major metabolic processes are

1. Reduction of the A-ring
2. Cleavage of the $C_{17}-C_{20}$ bond.
3. Oxidation of the 11β-group
4. Reduction of the 20-keto group
5. Hydroxylations at several positions: 2β, 6β, etc.
6. Reduction of the 17-keto group
7. Conjugation of the free steroids with sulfate or glucuronate

A discussion of all the enzymes involved is far beyond the scope of this chapter. Clinical endocrinologists usually pay little attention to the activity of these enzymes. It does not seem impossible, however, that, analogous to bilirubin metabolism (the Crigler-Najjar syndrome!), deficiencies of inactivating enzymes can play an important role.[56]

III. ABNORMAL FUNCTION

The endocrine system in the human consists of many endocrine "units", each composed of five parts: (1) endocrine tissue(s), (2) a stimulus generator, (3) a hormone transport system, (4) target organs, and (5) a hormone inactivation/removal system. For the adrenal cortex these parts are (1) the three zonae of the adrenal cortex; (2) the pituitary for ACTH and the kidney for renin; (3) blood, with its circulating transport proteins; (4) virtually all tissues of the body; (5) several tissues, but especially the liver. Aberrations have been found in parts 1, 2, 3, 4, and, depending upon definitions, part 5. The letters A, B, C, etc. indicate a group of related disorders. A1, A2, etc. indicate the individual syndromes within such a group.

A. Adrenal Hypoplasia

Anatomical absence of adrenal cortex tissue (A1) is one of the most severe defects in adrenal function. Probably all children with this abnormality die within a few days of birth if not properly treated with steroids. This disorder clearly has an X-linked recessive mode of inheritance.[57,58] No adrenal tissue at all was found at an autopsy.

A recent publication[59] reviews some of the literature on adrenal hypoplasia. Depending upon the capacity of the adrenal, the affected children either die within the first week after birth or survive for only several months. However, a few cases have been described where clinical symptoms developed after the fourth year of life. The longest surviving patients reported are now in the third decade of life. In at least some patients a hypogonadotropic hypogonadism is associated with the adrenal hypoplasia. This suggests that abnormal pituitary function is a factor in the development of adrenal hypoplasia.[60-62] Post-mortem microscopical examination of the pituitary, however, gives evidence that ACTH has been present in many patients with adrenal hypoplasia.[63]

Histologically, there are two main types. The most frequent form is the so-called ''miniature-adult'' adrenal hypoplasia (A2). The fetal cortex is virtually absent (as in anencephaly), the adrenal is reduced in size, but a histologically ''normal'' adult cortex is present. The other form has been called cytomegalic or ''fetal-cortex-only'' adrenal hypoplasia (A3). Here the adult zone is virtually absent and the cells in the remaining tissue have a certain resemblance with normal fetal cortex cells.

The two main types also show genetical differences. It is clear that at least two forms, an autosomal recessive (the ''miniature-adult'' type), and an X-linked recessive form (the cytomegalic type), exist, but it is likely that each of these is genetically heterogeneous.[64-67]

Some authors mention a third type (A4), with a normal fetal/adult ratio, but a subnormal overall size of the adrenals. The mode of inheritance might be X-linked.[68]

B. Idiopathic Addison's Disease

''Idiopathic Addison's disease'' (B1) is a term used rather frequently in current literature. It should be used only for those cases of hypoadrenocorticism, where congenital hypoplasia, infectious or metabolic disease, etc. have been excluded. The diagnosis of *Idiopathic* Addison's disease is therefore reached per *exclusionem*. This is a difficult procedure and it is quite possible that some cases diagnosed as idiopathic are in fact, e.g., tuberculous in origin.

Characteristic of idiopathic Addison's disease is the selective destruction of the adrenal cortex, while the adrenal medulla is reasonably preserved. The hypoadrenalism is often associated with insufficiencies of other endocrine glands (thyroid, parathyroids, gonads). Occurrence of diabetes mellitus, pernicious anemia, and moniliasis also has been described in combination with the idiopathic Addison's disease. The sequence in which these deficiencies become manifest varies considerably. This fact makes it questionable whether all the variants described are really different diseases.

This complex syndrome most probably has an autoimmune basis.[69] About 65% of the patients with idiopathic Addison's disease have detectable antibodies directed against adrenal cortex tissue. It is not clear whether the remaining 35% have undetected antibodies or no adrenal antibodies at all. The possiblity that in some of these patients the hypoadrenocorticism is in fact not idiopathic, must also be considered. Antibodies against other steroid-producing cell types, against the tyroid, etc., are frequently found when these organs are affected.[70]

Many family histories showing clustering of idiopathic Addison's disease in siblings have been published. According to Dunlop,[71] all known cases of proven familial Addison's disease were of the idiopathic type (the reverse statement is not necessarily true!).[72]

Further evidence for one or more genetic factors in the etiology comes from a Danish study, correlating HLA antigens and the occurrence of hypoadrenocorticism. The authors found that HLA-8 positive individuals ran a much higher risk of developing idiopathic Addison's disease than HLA-B8 negative persons.[73] The primary defect(s) is (are) probably not situated in the individual organs, but in the immune system. Eisenbarth et al.[74] speculate that production of one or more factors, under control of gene(s) on chromosome 6 in linkage disequilibrium with HLA-B8, is the genetic basis of idiopathic Addison's disease (and related autoimmune disorders). Interaction with unknown (environmental?) factors then results in development of disease.

The mode of inheritance seems to be autosomal recessive.[75] This holds for the different types: idiopathic Addison's disease, idiopathic Addison's disease with idiopathic hypoparathyroidism, idiopathic Addison's disease with hypothyroidism (Schmidt syndrome), and idiopathic Addison's disease with hypothyroidism and diabetes mellitus (also called Schmidt syndrome).

C. Multiple and Isolated Endocrine Tumors

Besides the group of pluriglandular autoimmune disorders (resulting in adrenal hypofunction), described above, another type of multiple endocrine disfunction (but in this case usually *hyperfunction*) exists: the group of familial endocrine adenomas and, less frequcntly, carcinomas.

Multiple endocrine neoplasia type 1 (MEN—1, Wermer's disease: C1) interferes with the pancreatic islets, the parathyroid glands, the pituitary, and the adrenal cortex. Not all of these endocrine glands need to be affected, while the tumors may or may not be functional. A functional adrenal cortex lesion can result in Cushing's syndrome.[76,77]

In type 2 MEN (Sipple's syndrome: C2) and type 3 MEN (mucosal neuroma syndrome: C3) the adrenal cortex is rarely, if ever, directly involved. Ectopic ACTH production seems to be sometimes responsible for secondary hypersecretion of adrenocortical hormones.[78] Several authors have tried to explain the phenomenon of familial endocrine neoplasia but none of the theories proposed is backed by sufficient evidence to be completely satisfactory. Nevertheless, studies of these remarkable tumors could be of great help in our understanding of the basic mechanisms of carcinogenesis.[79] The mode of inheritance is autosomal dominant, with considerable phenotypic variability (although within a given family the picture is more uniform).[80,81] Even while reading the titles of the many publications on multiple endocrine neoplasia, one is struck by the multitude of symptoms; symptoms which seem to occur in every possible combination.

Familial adrenal neoplasia of a non-MEN type also exists. Adenomas are seen in macrosomia adiposa congenita (C4), carcinomas in the so-called Gardner syndrome (C5), in familial adrenocortical carcinoma (C6), and sometimes in the Beckwith-Wiedemann syndrome (C7).[82]

D. Inborn Errors of Steroid Biosynthesis

Most of the cholesterol necessary for steroid biosynthesis in the adrenal cortex, is derived from the blood. Impaired cholesterol synthesis, limited to the adrenal, will therefore be hard to detect, if such a condition exists at all. No serious clinical problems are to be expected in those cases.

Impaired cholesterol uptake from the circulation caused by defects in the LDL-cholesterol receptors is also still an hypothetical condition. It will probably present as several adrenal hypofunction with ACTH and angiotensin unresponsiveness. It is quite possible that some patients with adrenal hypoplasia, in fact, are lacking the proper mechanism for cholesterol uptake. However, at present this is speculation, although mutations affecting LDL-cholesteryl ester uptake in human fibroblasts have been described.[83]

Much more is known about the deficiencies in the enzymes involved in cortisol, aldosterone, and adrenal C_{19}-steroid biosynthesis. Those described in the literature are summarized in Table 1.

There are six different enzyme-systems (1, 2, 3, 4, 5, and 6) necessary for the transformation of cholesterol into aldosterone and five enzymes (1, 2, 3, 4, and 7), probably in part the same biochemical entities, are necessary for cortisol biosynhhesis. If one of these latter enzymes is deficient, cortisol production will be inappropriate. This is sensed by the feedback mechanism controlling cortisol levels. In response, ACTH production by the pituitary is adjusted, i.e., blood ACTH levels increase. The correction maneuver often, but certainly not always, succeeds, resulting in normal or low-normal cortisol secretion, but at the cost of adrenal hyperplasia and increased production of cortisol precursors.

In the case of deficiencies 3, 4, and (to a lesser degree) 2, part of these precursors can be converted into the potent androgen testosterone or, like dehydroepiandrosterone, have a (weak) intrinsic androgenic activity. Intrauterine exposure to these high levels of testosterone or other androgens, leads to marked virilization of the external genitalia in the female. The internal genitalia are normal. The genital abnormalities in male neonates are much less expressed, but both boys and girls manifest progressive virilization when they grow older.[85-87]

Enzymes 9, 10, and 11 are borderline cases. In the first place, their activities in the adrenal are low and their relative importance in adrenal steroidogenesis is not well known. In the second place, they can also be classified as inactivating enzymes. On the other side, one can argue that in principle they belong to the group of enzymes, necessary for adrenal C_{19}-steroid formation or activity.

The literature on the inborn errors of steroidogenesis is very extensive.[88-92] Table 2 gives the main characteristics of the several syndromes.

1. Congenital Lipoid Adrenal Hyperplasia

This (D1) is the biochemical counterpart of severe adrenal hypoplasia.[93] Virtually no adrenal (and testicular) steroids are produced, because the very first step of steroidogenesis, pregnenolone formation, is blocked.[94,95] The patients suffer from salt wasting and the mortality is high.

TABLE 1

Enzyme Defects Known to Affect Steroid Biosynthesis with the EC-Numbers of the Enzymes

	Deficiency	EC-number of the enzyme involved
1.	Cholesterol side chain cleaving system deficiency (identical with pregnenolone synthetase deficiency and congenital lipoid adrenal hyperplasia; "Prader's disease".)	1.14.15.X.
2.	3β-Hydroxysteroid-dehydrogenase-isomerase deficiency	1.1.1.145 and 5.3.3.1.
3.	Steroid-21-hydroxylase deficiency	1.14.99.10.
4.	Steroid 11β-hydroxylase deficiency	1.14.15.4.
5.	Steroid-18-hydroxylase deficiency (= corticosterone methyloxidase I deficiency)	1.14.15.5.
6.	18-Hydroxysteroid-dehydrogenase deficiency (= corticosterone methyloxidase II deficiency)	1.1.3.X.
7.	Steroid-17α-hydroxylase deficiency	1.14.99.9.
8.	Steroid-17α,20-lyase deficiency	4.1.2.30.
9.	17β-Hydroxysteroid-dehydrogenase deficiency (= 17-ketosteroid reductase deficiency)	1.1.1.63/1.1.1.64.
10.	5α-Steroid-reductase deficiency	1.3.1.22.
11.	3β-Steroid-sulfatase deficiency	3.1.6.2.

TABLE 2

Some Important Characteristics of the Enzyme Defects Described

Deficiency	Adrenal cortex hyperplasia	Cortisol production	Aldosterone production	Testosterone production	Signs of androgen excess or deficiency: Females	Signs of androgen excess or deficiency: Males	Mode of inheritance
1. Pregnenolone synthetase	Yes	Depressed	Depressed; salt wasting	Depressed	No[a]	Def.	Autosomal recessive
2. 3β-HSD	Yes	Depressed	Depressed; salt wasting	Depressed	Exc. (usually slight)	Def.	Autosomal recessive
3. 21-hydroxylase	Yes	Depressed	Variable[b]	Increased	Exc.	Exc. (usually slight)	Autosomal recessive
4. 11β-hydroxylase	Yes	Depressed	Depressed: salt wasting rare	Increased	Exc.	Exc. (usually slight)	Autosomal recessive
5. 18-hydroxylase	No[c]	Normal	Depressed; salt wasting	Normal	No[a]	No[a]	Autosomal recessive
6. 18-dehydrogenase	No[d]	Normal	Depressed; salt wasting	Normal	No[a]	No[a]	Autosomal recessive
7. 17α-hydroxylase	Yes	Depressed	Depressed;[b] no salt wasting	Depressed	Estrogen deficiency	Def.	Autosomal recessive
8. 17α,20-lyase	No[d]	Normal[d]	Normal;[d] no salt wasting	Depressed	?	Def.	X-linked recessive
9. 17β-HSD	No[d]	Normal[d]	Normal[d] no salt wasting	Depressed	?	Def.	Male limited autosomal recessive
10. 5α-reductase	No[d]	Normal[d]	Normal;[d] no salt wasting	Normal	?	Def.	Male limited autosomal recessive
11. 3β-sulfatase	No[d]	Normal[d]	Normal;[d] no salt wasting	Normal[d]	?	No[a]	X-linked recessive

[a] Normal biological activity of the sex hormones.
[b] See text.
[c] Normal adrenal weight, but remarkable histological changes.
[d] Probably normal, but not known with absolute certainty.

In male children, the syndrome is characterized by various degrees of incomplete masculine differentiation. In girls the external genitalia are normal or very slightly virilized. It seems possible that in these patients direct cleavage of cholesterol by a 17α,20 lyase (normally a nonexistent or very minor pathway), leads to formation of small amounts of androgenic C_{19}-steroids.

There are some indications that the clinical picture is further aggravated by the secondary formation of toxic sterols.[96]

This disorder is certainly not a homogenous one, as several different enzyme-activities are present in preparations of the side chain cleaving enzyme system. In his thesis, Kraaipoel[97] speculates upon the biochemistry of the possible variants.

2. 3β-Hydroxysteroid-Dehydrogenase Deficiency

Male patients with this syndrome (D2) usually have hypospadias, while the girls are normal or slightly virilized, i.e., have enlargement of the clitoris.[98,99] The intrinsic androgenic activity of dehydroepiandro‡sterone is believed to be responsible for the latter phenomenon. Salt loss also occurs here. Long term survival has been reported for several patients, but mortality is high.

The 3β-hydroxysteroid-dehydrogenase of the adrenal differs from the testis enzyme. Several authors[100,101] have described boys in which the enzyme defect was complete in the adrenal, but partial in the testis, while peripheral enzyme activity was close to normal. A reasonable explanation is, that the enzyme consists of two (or more) polypeptide chains (A and L, from adrenal and liver). If this molecule resembles lactate dehydrogenase, five different forms are possible: A_4, A_3L, A_2L_2, AL_3, and L_4. Mutations in A would not affect L_4, the liver form. The testicular enzyme could have intermediate activity, if its structure were A_3L, A_2L_2 or AL_3.[102] The isomerase shifting the double bond ($\Delta^5 \rightarrow \Delta^4$) is closely associated with the 3β-dehydrogenase, but apart from some studies in patients with adrenal tumors, no congenital isomerase deficiency has been reported.

3. 21-Hydroxylase Deficiency

This is by far the most common enzyme-defect (D3) in steroid biosynthesis. Table 3 lists the incidences found by different authors. The highest frequency is found among Alaskan Eskimos, an unexplained phenomenon.[103] Salt wasting occurs in about 30% of all patients. This has been (and still is) the subject of much discussion. It seems, however, that at present a majority of investigators holds the view that three main factors are responsible.[104]

TABLE 3

Observed Incidences of Congenital Adrenal Hyperplasia (steroid-21-hydroxylase deficiencies)

Author	Homozygotes	Heterozygotes (calculated)
Prader (Switzerland)	1/5000 [a]	1/35
Childs (Maryland)	1/67000[a]	1/129
Hubble (Birmingham)	1/7300 [a]	1/43
Rosenbloom (Wisconsin)	1/15000[a]	1/61
Qazi (Toronto)	1/27000[b]	1/82
Hirschfeld (Alaska)	1/1480 [b]	1/19
Hirschfeld (Yupik Eskimos)	1/490 [b]	1/11

[a] Salt losers and non-salt-losers
[b] Salt losers only

1. The mutation in the steroid-21-hydroxylase of salt losers is more severe than the one occurring in nonsalt losers. K_M and/or V_{max} for progesterone 21-hydroxylase, one of the first steps in aldosterone formation, and for 17α-hydroxyprogesterone 21-hydroxylase, a decisive step in cortisol formation, are highly abnormal. In non-salt-losers only the K_M and/or V_{max} for 17α-hydroxyprogesterone are changed by the mutation. Untreated non-salt-losers in fact often show *elevated* aldosterone production.[105] Whether or not multiple forms of the steroid-21-hydroxylase exist, is one problem. This makes, however, no essential difference: mutations in one enzyme with two binding sites — one for progesterone (site I) and one for 17α-hydroxyprogesterone (site II) — are on the basis of the available data hard to distinguish from mutations in two enzymes (enzyme I for progesterone and enzyme II for 17α-OH-progesterone) having one polypeptide chain in common.
2. In consequence the aldosterone production in the salt-loser is insufficient, even under normal, unstressed conditions. As it reflects the maximal capacity of the adrenal, no further increase is possible, not even during salt restriction.
3. Circulating weak aldosterone-antagonists such as progesterone, 16α-OH-progesterone, 17α-OH-progesterone, inhibit aldosterone action in the kidney. When the aldosterone levels are already low, this inhibition leads to salt loss in the urine. At normal aldosterone concentrations, the inhibition by these steroids is insignificant and there is no salt loss.[106,107]

Whether or not salt-excreting factors are produced by the adrenal cortex is still an unsettled question. In the first few days of life, salt-losing crises are very rare. This is probably due to the low rate of metabolic inactivation of aldosterone.

The definitive diagnosis is rather difficult to establish in the early postnatal period, especially when only urinary steroid excretion data are available. Plasma 17α-hydroxyprogesterone determinations are to be preferred.[108] Interpretation of buccal smear chromatin, still used in some clinics for sex assignment, is not always easy.[109] It should be replaced by uaryotype analysis.

The 21-hydroxylase deficiency is in fact the only inborn error in group D, for which an autosomal-recessive mode of inheritance is well established. Precise genetic studies for the other defects are difficult, because the incidences are low or long-term studies have not yet been made. It is likely that several different mutations in the steroid-21-hydroxylase gene exist. So many different clinical and biochemical pictures are found in the literature that the occurrence of one and the same mutation in all these cases is highly improbable.[197,198]

The present techniques do not permit unequivocal heterozygote detection and prenatal diagnosis. Successes have been reported, but 100% has not yet been reached.[110] The recent finding that a very close genetic linkage exists between the HLA-complex and the steroid-21-hydroxylase opens up new ways for both genetic counseling of parents, and for basic studies. Assuming that a structural gene is involved, it can already be stated that the gene for the steroid 21-hydroxylase is located on chromosome 6.[111,206]

4. 11β-Hydroxylase Deficiency

This deficiency (D4) has much in common with the 21-hydroxylase deficiency. Females have masculinized external genitalia, but the internal genitalia are virtually normal. In male children signs of virilization are present at birth or develop later. The excessive androgen production results in early closure of the epiphyses, leading to short adult stature.[112,113] Salt wasting in *untreated* patients is very rare, if it occurs at all.[104] A prominent feature is the hypertension seen in the majority (but not all!) of the cases described.[114]

As can be seen in Figure 1, both the pathways to aldosterone and cortisol are affected. The prominent precursors produced in spurious amounts are 11-deoxycortisol, C_{19}-steroids, and deoxycorticosterone (DOC). Of these, 11-deoxycortisol and its main metabolite, tetrahydrodeoxycortisol, have only a feeble biological activity but the C_{19}-compounds are responsible for the signs of androgen excess while the DOC induces the hypertension. In normal individuals, plasma DOC is less than 20 ng/100 mℓ, but in patients with 11β-hydroxylase deficiencies values up to 2000 ng/100 mℓ have been reported. It is, however, still a matter of doubt whether DOC is solely responsible. Other steroids, for example 18-hydroxylated ones, could be involved.[115,116]

Gregory and Gardner[199] wrote in 1976 that approximately 50 cases are known in the literature, an incidence less than reported for the 21-hydroxylase deficiency. Several biochemical variants have been described.[117] New and Levine[89] even state: "This enzyme deficiency has the most pleomorphic presentation." Long-term administration of the drug metyrapone, a blocker of the 11β-hydroxylase, induce s a symptom-complex mimicking the genetic disease. Although real proof is lacking, the mode of inheritance seems to be autosomal recessive. The discussion about the mutations involved is analogous to the one given for the 21-hydroxylase deficiency.

5. Aldosterone Biosynthesis Defects

The two enzymic defects affecting only the biosynthesis of aldosterone have much in common. Varying degrees of sodium loss, hyperkalemia, dehydration, and failure to thrive are seen in the patients with an 18-hydroxylase deficiency (corticosterone methyl oxidase deficiency I: (D5) and in those with an 18-dehydrogenase deficiency (corticosterone methyl oxidase deficiency II: (D6). The production of cortisol and adrenal C_{19}-steroids is normal, as expected. No genital abnormalities are found.[118]

The aldosterone production is very low, while the plasma renin activity, if determined is found elevated. Not all authors report exact data about the production of corticosterone and deoxycorticosterone, but in general it can be said that (again, as expected) both steroids are present in elevated amounts. Obviously this is not enough to compensate for the aldosterone deficit. It is remarkable that treatment with deoxycorticosterone acetate could often be stopped when the children grew older. A positive Na^+ balance seems to be maintained by an elevated salt intake in unstressed conditions. This fact suggests, that the so-called transient hypoaldosteronism could be a very mild deficiency in the 18-oxidation process.[200]

The main difference between the two defects is in the production of 18-hydroxycorticosterone. The cases of 18-hydroxylase deficiencies reported by Visser and Cost,[119] investigated further by Degenhart et al.,[201] the patient of Jean et al.[121] and the twins described by Ravussin et al.,[122] all had a subnormal 18-hydroxycorticosterone secretion. The patients with an 18-dehydrogenase deficiency, in contrast, had moderate to grossly elevated secretion rates.[123-127] The pedigree of the family described by Visser and Cost[119] could be traced back for six generations. The six parents of the three affected children had the same great-grandparents four generations ago!

An autosomal-recessive mode of inheritance for both defects is compatible with the literature data. Considerable clinical and biochemical heterogeneity exists, however, even in the small groups of patients known at present.

6. 17α-Hydroxylase Deficiency

The patients with this very rare deficiency present with hypertension and hypokalemia. Additional symptoms in females are primary amenorrhea, absent pubic hair, and other signs of sexual infantilism. In males the differentiation of the (androgen-dependent) external genitalia is markedly incomplete, but testes, though small, are present. There is no testosterone unresponsiveness.

This deficiency blocks the formation of cortisol at an early level: the conversion of progesterone and pregnenolone into their 17α-hydroxylated derivatives. As a consequence, the formation of both androgens and estrogens is impaired, leading to a deficiency of all sex hormones.

In the pathway to aldosterone, no block is present and the elevated plasma ACTH levels stimulate the production of deoxycorticosterone and corticosterone which is therefore sometimes 100 times higher than normal. The high levels of these mineralocorticoids induce hypertension while, as a secondary effect, the renin activity is suppressed. Consequently, aldosterone production is very low. It is possible that deoxycorticosterone and corticosterone reduce the production of aldosterone even further by substrate inhibition or a feed-forward inhibition of the 18-dehydrogenase system.[128-131] As corticosterone is also a glucocorticoid, the patients show no evidence of cortisol deficiency, although the plasma levels of the latter steroid are usually very low.

Detailed studies are necessary to establish whether or not this syndrome is genetically homogeneous. This author expects that the steroid 17α-hydroxylase deficiency is, at least biochemically, as heterogeneous as, for example, the 21- and 11β-deficiencies. According to McKusick,[120] autosomal-recessive inheritance is possible.

7. 17α,20-Desmolase Deficiency

This defect (D8) is even rarer than D5, D6, or D7. It was proven to exist in three related XY individuals with ambiguous external genitalia and inguinal testes. These cases reported by Zachmann et al.[132] were carefully studied. Clinical data, urinary and blood steroid analyses, and the results of an incubation experiment with testicular tissue implicated a defect in both testes and adrenals. Strikingly, the urinary 17-ketosteroid excretion was normal, with the notable exception of dehydroepiandrosterone, which was absent. An explanation for this curious fact might be that the step: 17α-OH-pregnenolone → dehydroepiandrosterone is more affected than the alternative one: 17α-OH-progesterone → androstenedione. The mode of inheritance might be X-linked recessive.

8. 17β-Hydroxysteroid Dehydrogenase Deficiency

About ten cases are known at present, all of them XY individuals[133] with defective testicular-steroidogenesis (D9). The majority of the patients are phenotypically female, but at puberty they develop hirsutism and clitoromegaly. Plasma testosterone is subnormal, while plasma androstenedione is elevated severalfold. The estrone production is also elevated. The latter hormone is probably responsible for the breast development which occurs in 50% of these children.

It is not known with certainty if this deficiency is expressed in the adrenal, but the 17β-hydroxysteroid dehydrogenase of the liver and other, nonendocrine, tissues is not severely affected, suggesting that this enzyme is under different genetic control. The 17β-hydroxysteroid dehydrogenase deficiency is, on clinical grounds, difficult to distinguish from several other forms of hereditary incomplete male pseudohermaphroditism, like the syndromes of Lubs, Gilbert-Dreyfus, Reifenstein, and Rosewater. However, these latter four syndromes probably represent variable phenotypic manifestations of partial androgen *insensitivity* without hereditary defects in testicular or adrenal androgen *synthesis*.[134,135]

9. 5α-Reductase Deficiency

This defect (D10) causes another form of familial incomplete male pseudohermaphroditism. A number of patients were found in a Dominican village.[136,137] The description by Imperato-McGinley et al.[136] is very impressive:

"The affected males (46 XY) are born with marked ambiguity of the external genitalia, and before the disorder became obvious to the community were raised as girls. . . . At puberty, their voice deepens and they develop a typical male phenotype with a substantial increase in muscle mass; there is no breast enlargment. The phallus enlarges to become a functional penis, and the change is so striking that these individuals are referred to by the townspeople as "guevedoces" — penis at 12 (years of age)."

Plasma testosterone is within the normal male range, but plasma dihydrotestosterone is subnormal. In the urine the ratio of $5\alpha/5\beta$ steroids is much lower than normal. The abnormality is due to a defect in the Δ^4-steroid-5α-reductase, leading to insufficient conversion of testosterone into dihydrotestosterone. As adrenal steroids can also undergo reduction of the C_4=C_5 double bond, this enzyme defect is described here. Since both testosterone and dihydrotestosterone are involved in male sexual differentiation and development, the male reproductive track shows remarkable anatomical aberrations. No symptoms are described in affected females, although they may have clinical consequences not yet appreciated. Several 5β-steroids (remember the $5\alpha/5\beta$ ratio is subnormal!), are known to cause exacerbations in porphyria, for example.[207]

The pedigree,[136] illustrating the transmission of the defect through seven generations, merits close attention. The mode of inheritance is autosomal recessive with male-limited expression.

10. 3β-Hydroxysteroid Sulfate-Sulfatase Deficiency

This was first described as a placental disorder (D11), marked by pre- and perinatal manifestations. It is usually discovered when after 40 weeks of pregnancy spontaneous labor does not develop. Urinary estrogen excretion is found to be very low, without signs of fetal distress.

Later the 3β-sulfatase deficiency (which always occurred in male fetuses) was also demonstrated in other tissues and found to persist an indefinite time after birth without significant changes in plasma steroid levels.[138-141] More recently[142,143] it was found that the sulfatase deficiency occurred together with X-linked ichthyosis, a noninflammatory skin disease and it seems that both syndromes are causally related.

This deficiency probably affects the sulfated steroid pathway at several stages, since the conversion of cholesterolsulfate and the other conjugated steroids into the free compounds is impaired. The lysosomal aryl sulfatases A and B are generally not affected, although a few patients have been reported with generalized sulfatase deficiencies. Studies on placental aryl sulfatase C activity demonstrate that *this* enzyme is severely affected. The skin manifestations might therefore indicate that other compounds (mucopolysaccharides?) too, are substrates for the deficient enzyme(s). In the syndrome reported by Cret et al.[203] adrenal insufficiency is present together with abnormalities of the connective tissues. X-linked ichthyosis is not uncommon (about 1 in 6000 males). This suggests that steroid sulfatase deficiency, once considered to be very rare, is in fact not so rare at all.

E. Nonspecific Metabolic Defects

1. Wolman's Disease

Wolman's disease is a lipid storage disease, characterized by the presence of large amounts of triglycerides and cholesterol esters in the lysosomes of many organs. The clinical symptoms are hepatosplenomegaly, persistent steatorrhea, vomiting, and adrenal insufficiency. The adrenals are enlarged and calcified. The most severe form of this lipidosis has its onset in early infancy and despite treatment with steroids is virtually always fatal within the first 6 months of life.[144,145] This results from the congenital deficiency of a lysosomal acid lipase.[146] The effect on the adrenal is probably an inhibition of the very first steps in steroid biosynthesis. The LDL-cholesteryl ester complex is taken up by the cells, but cannot be hydrolyzed and therefore the supply of free cholesterol for side chain cleavage will be too small. Secondary damage is done by the calcification and the swollen lysosomes, presenting as vacuoles.[147] The mode of inheritance is autosomal recessive. The abnormal enzyme seems to be present in many tissues. This provides the possibility of prenatal diagnosis by investigating amniotic fluid cells.[148]

2. Cholesterol Ester Storage Disease

Cholesterol ester storage disease (CESD) is, when compared to Wolman's disease, relatively benign. Here too one finds hepatosplenomegaly, enlarged adrenals, and storage of cholesterol esters and triglycerides. Adrenal calcification is uncommon and adrenal steroid production is not severely depressed.[149] McKusick[120] therefore lists CESD as "cholesterol ester storage disease of *liver*".

CESD is also caused by a deficiency in a lysosomal acid lipase, but this is clearly a different mutation, possibly at the same locus. Cortner and co-workers[150] describe how electrophoresis of the acid lipases demonstrates that in normal cells at least two enzymes are present, called A and B by them. A is absent in Wolman's disease and CESD. At present the discussion is still in qualitative terms, such as "the acute infantile form of Wolman's disease", "less severe clinical variants of Wolman's disease", and "cholesterol ester storage disease". Biochemical data are still largely lacking. The mode of inheritance is again autosomal recessive.

3. Adrenoleukodystrophy

Adrenoleukodystrophy is a term introduced by Blaw[151] in 1971. This disorder is characterized by progressive cerebral demyelination and adrenal atrophy. It has been described under various other names: Schilder's disease, Addison-Schilder's disease, diffuse cerebral sclerosis, sudanophilic leukodystrophy, Siemerling-Creutzfeldt disease, etc. The time of onset is in general between 4 and 9 years of age, but in one case the patient was already 50 years old at the time the symptoms occurred.

Livet et al.[156] studied plasma cortisol and ACTH and urinary aldosterone in five diseased children. Plasma cortisol was low-normal to low, but the ACTH levels were always elevated. Exogenous ACTH had almost no effect on the plasma cortisol. The basal aldosterone excretion was normal, although one child showed abnormal urinary salt loss. Sodium deprivation stimulated the aldosterone excretion.[156] In another series, normal or even elevated plasma cortisol levels were found, but here too most patients did not respond to ACTH.[157]

It is noteworthy that histological changes occur mainly in the zona fasciculata and reticularis, while the glomerulosa, the aldosterone producer, is only slightly affected. Several biochemical aberrations have been described: storage of abnormal cholesterol esters, abnormal kinetics of cholesterol metabolism, and presence of abnormal fatty acids. At present there is, however, no general agreement as to the primary metabolic error. Findings reported by some authors can not be reproduced by others, indicating the existence of considerable heterogeneity.[154,208] In the endocrinological textbooks this disorder is usually treated less thoroughly than in the neurological literature,[152] probably because the endocrine aspects are less striking than the dramatic neurological deterioration seen in these patients. Several authors have pointed out that the adrenal cortex function varies from virtually normal to clear-cut insufficiency. Schaumburg even states: ". . . it is evident that the majority of patients do not have clinical signs of adrenal insufficiency."[157] It seems likely that adrenoleukodystrophy is not one single syndrome, but a group of related X-linked diseases, caused by different mutations at the same locus.* It would be of importance to see whether in these patients basal and ACTH-stimulated cholesterol uptake by the adrenal is normal.

* Familial Addison's disease with spastic paraplegia, a poorly defined disorder, is probably not identical with adrenoleukodystrophy.[155]

F. Defects in Regulation

1. ACTH Deficiencies

ACTH deficiencies are caused by insufficient pituitary action. Plasma ACTH levels are low, leading to partial adrenal atrophy and poor cortisol production. They can have a genetic origin,[120] e.g., either autosomal panhypopituitarism (F1) or X-linked panhypopituitarism (F2), but will not be further described here.

2. Angiotensin and Renin Deficiencies

As far as the author knows, there has been no report of proven familial hyporeninemic hypoaldosteronism.* The cases with hyporeninemic hypoaldosteronism described, were mainly adults. Their hyporeninemia usually resulted from nonspecific renal damage. A high percentage also had diabetes mellitus.[159] There is, however, no reason why this syndrome could not exist as a separate entity. Several heritable forms can be expected to exist: congenital absence or inactivity of the renin producing cells, production of a renin with abnormal structure and low or absent activity, familial absence of angiotensinogen, familial absence of the converting enzyme, etc.

If "big renin" (a 63,000 dalton renin precursor) is really *the* precursor of renin in man, defective conversion of "big" into "normal" renin also could occur. Some (but not all) anephric patients seem to be able to maintain significant blood aldosterone levels in the absence of kidney-produced renin. Other stimuli like calcium,[209] ectopically produced renin or a high "tonin" activity, for example, must be responsible for the zona glomerulosa action. People with, e.g., kidneys lacking the juxtaglomerular apparatus, but possessing these compensating mechanisms could be lacking renin, but still go clinically undetected. Is this an extreme end of normal variation?

2. ACTH Unresponsiveness

Hereditary unresponsiveness to ACTH, also named "familial glucocorticoid deficiency", has been described several times.[160-163,202] One of the early reports[164] has the following title: "Familial Addison's disease. Case reports of two sisters with corticoid deficiency unassociated with hypoaldosteronism". This indicates at once the main characteristics: ACTH blood levels are high, while cortisol production is low and does not change significantly after ACTH administration. As expected, hypoglycemia, convulsions, muscular weakness, and skin pigmentation have been recorded. Several of the affected patients were tall. Mild swelling of the face and hands is sometimes seen during hypoglycemia.

When investigated, the zona fasciculata and zona reticularis were found to be degenerated. The zona glomerulosa, however, often functioned in a normal way. In, e.g., the case described by Kershnar et al.[165] deoxycorticosterone, corticosterone, and aldosterone secretion were normal.

It is not clear if the ACTH unresponsiveness is really always due to absent ACTH receptors or another part of the information-processing system proper (primary, or "real" ACTH unresponsiveness; see Figure 4).

Moshang stated:[166] "It is our contention that familial glucocorticoid insufficiency is often an inherited progressive degenerative disorder of the adrenal cortex . . . It may be that there is an inherited disorder of ACTH receptors, but this possibility has not yet been documented."

A non-ACTH-related, genetically determined degeneration of the adrenal cortex with poor responses towards endogenous and exogenous ACTH is also present in adrenoleukodystrophy and in idiopathic Addison's disease (secondary, or "pseudo" ACTH unresponsiveness)! Only by detailed in vitro studies of ACTH effects (of

* Liddle[158] described a family disorder characterized by hypoaldosteronism, hyporeninemia, and low angiotensin. These patients present, however, as cases of hyperaldosteronism, due to a renal tubular defect.

course, often impossible) will it in a given case be feasible to decide which of the several possible defects is actually present.

In view of the above mentioned facts, it comes as no surprise that genetically the patients with adrenal unresponsiveness to ACTH form a heterogeneous group. McKusick[120] suggests that there may be both autosomal recessive (F3) and X-linked (F4) forms.

4. Angiotensin Unresponsiveness

A very able endocrinologist[168] while discussing an article[167] reporting two cases of angiotensin unresponsiveness wrote: "Despite the authors best efforts, I'm not sure what has gone awry in these two patients. Particularly obscure is the pathogenesis of the hypertension in the face of hypoaldosteronism." There is also no entry of such a syndrome in McKusick's catalog.[120] As the list of known inherited disorders caused by hormone unresponsiveness is already long (HGH, ACTH, ADH, PTH, insulin, aldosterone, testosterone, 1α,25-di-OH-cholecalciferol, etc.), I see no reason why angiotensin unresponsiveness (F5) should not exist. Convincing reports, however are scarce.

An absent or degenerated zona glomerulosa (in the presence of normal zonae fasciculata and reticularis) also could mimic primary angiotensin unresponsiveness, analogous to the situation described for ACTH.

G. Glucocorticoid-Suppressible Hyperaldosteronism

Glucocorticoid-suppressible hyperaldosteronism is an entity in which hyperplasia of the adrenal cortex occurs in the absence of any known enzyme deficiency.[169-172] The patients present with varying degrees of hypertension, hypokalemia, metabolic alkalosis, and suppressed renin activity. There is oversecretion of aldosterone without clear-cut abnormalities in the production of cortisol and C_{19}-steroids. The ACTH levels are not far off the normal range.[173] Dexamethasone, in doses of 1 to 2 mg/day is able to correct the hyperaldosteronism, although some patients may require several weeks of treatment before a satisfactory response is obtained. The defect responsible for the hyperaldosteronism in these patients could be situated in abnormal ACTH sensitivity of the glomerulosa cells, or the presence of aldosterone-producing fasciculata cells. The hypertension might be caused by an as yet unknown factor also produced by the adrenal cortex. An autosomal dominant model of inheritance is compatible with the family histories described.[174]

H. Malfunction of the Transport Proteins

The transport of adrenal steroids to the target tissues is partly dependent upon the carrier proteins. It is, therefore, remarkable that neither congenital deficiency of transcortin (H1: X-linked dominant?), nor hereditary analbuminemia (H2: autosomal recessive) have detectable clinical consequences. Funder[175] and Burke[176] give interesting short reviews of this matter. Lohrenz et al.[177] described an increase in transcortin (H3) levels in two siblings, brother and sister, discovered: " . . . during a screening procedure of healthy employees of the company". They did not have any offspring and the genetic status of this abnormality is therefore uncertain.

I. Rhythms and Their Disorders

The rhythms in the plasma steroid concentrations (ultradian, circadian, and infradian) probably have a physiological meaning, although it is still largely obscure. Besides the plasma hormone concentration, $\{H\}$, the first derivative of the concentration, $d\{H\}/dt$, could play a role in the information transfer in the endocrine system. Hereditary disturbances of the rhythms and their possible consequences are not known. It is, however, certain that in Cushing's disease (which is as a matter of fact rarely a genetic disease) the rhythms can be drastically altered.[46,47,178]

J. Bartter's Syndrome

This syndrome is although not quite correct, often described under the heading "genetic disorders of the adrenal". The clinical and biochemical picture of this puzzling disorder varies considerably from patient to patient. Constant features are hypokalemia, metabolic alkalosis, and hyperaldosteronism (secondary to hyperplasia of the juxtaglomerular apparatus) without hypertension. Dwarfism is often present.[179-182] The primary defect is not to be found in the adrenal cortex, for even total adrenalectomy does not stop the potassium wasting.[183] Evidence is accumulating that abnormalities in prostaglandin synthesis play an important role in the pathogenesis of this autosomal-recessive disease.[184,185]

K. Congenital Unresponsiveness to Corticosteroids

Cortisol resistance (K1) was described in 1976 by Vingerhoeds et al.[186] They found high plasma ACTH and cortisol levels and a high cortisol production rate (up to 140 mg/24 hr) in a hypertensive, hypokalemic male. The transcortin levels were normal and there were no signs of Cushing's syndrome. During a follow-up of several years no changes were noted. Unfortunately, the patient "has been less than cooperative with regard to extensive investigation of his family", but probably the syndrome is hereditary.

Aldosterone resistance or pseudohypoaldosteronism, (K2) is a condition known for about 20 years. Roy[187] has collected most of the reports and added five new cases. The disease occurs in infancy and is characterized by severe salt-wasting, hyperkalemia and high aldosterone and renin plasma levels. There is no evidence of hypocortisolism or androgen excess. The salt loss in the urine is probably due to a defect in the renal tubular cells. Whether this defect is in the intracellular cytosol receptors or in another part of the complex system is completely unknown. The several forms described in the literature might represent defects at different levels of intracellular reception. A very interesting variant is described by Anand et al.[188] where sodium loss did not occur via the urine, but was due to sweat gland disfunction. The few data available point to an autosomal dominant mode of inheritance.

Contrary to the situation in vivo, studies in vitro with *tumor cells* have demonstrated defects in most stages of steroid hormone action.[189] The "genetic approach" has been invaluable for the elucidation of the mechanisms.[190]

It can be expected that in vitro work with cells obtained from the patients with steroid hormone resistance will be most helpful in confirming and extending the results obtained with animal and tumor tissues.

L. Secondary Steroid Metabolism

A large number of enzymes are involved in steroid inactivation and degradation. It is, therefore, surprising that almost nothing is known about genetic variation in these mechanisms. The 5α-reductase deficiency and the 17α,20-desmolase deficiency, are in fact the only enzyme defects that could be classified as specific disorders of steroid inactivation/degradation.

There is some evidence that in the Crigler-Najjar syndrome,[191] in addition to the impaired conjugation of bilirubin with glucuronide, a defect occurs in steroid glucuronide formation.[192] However, compared with the severe jaundice and disturbance of the central nervous system seen in this disease, the effect on steroid metabolism is insignificant. Several other conditions (liver disease, thyroid disorders, etiocholanolone fever, etc.) exist, where steroid metabolism is altered.[193] The effects of these conditions on the inactivation enzymes are often secondary, or not known at all. They have at present no place in a review of hereditary variation of adrenal cortex functioning.

TABLE 4

The Inherited Disorders Mentioned in this Article with the Corresponding Numbers of McKusick's Catalogue[120]

		Number in McKusick's catalogue
Adrenal Cortex		
Adrenal cortex hypoplasia	A.1.	30020
	A.2.	
	A.3.	
	A.4.	
Idiopathic Addison's disease		24030
Endocrine neoplasia		
MEN-1	C.1.	13110
MEN-2	C.2.	17140
MEN-3	C.3.	16230
Macrosomia adiposa congenita	C.4.	24810
Gardner syndrome	C.5.	17530
Familial adrenocortical carcinoma	C.6.	20230
Beckwith-Wiedemann syndrome	C.7.	22560
Enzyme defects		
Congenital lipoid adrenal hyperplasia	D.1.	20171
3β-HSD-deficiency	D.2.	20181
21-hydroxylase deficiency	D.3.	20191
11β-hydroxylase deficiency	D.4.	20201
18-hydroxylase deficiency	D.5.	20340
18-dehydrogenase deficiency	D.6.	20340
17α-hydroxylase deficiency	D.7.	20211
17α,20-desmolase deficiency	D.8.	30915
17β-HSD- deficiency (status in adrenal uncertain)	D.9.	26430
5α-reductase deficiency (status in adrenal uncertain)	D.10.	26460
3β-sulfatase deficiency (status in adrenal uncertain)	D.11.	26275, 30810
Cret's syndrome (defect completely unknown)		—
Nonspecific metabolic defects		
Wolman's disease	E.1.	27800
Cholesterol ester storage disease	E.2.	21500
Adrenoleukodystrophy	E.3.	30010
Addison's disease with spastic paraplegia	E.4. (?)	20150
Stimuli		
ACTH-deficiency	F.1.	20140
	F.2.	31200
ACTH-unresponsiveness	F.3., F.4.	20220, 30025, 24020
Angiotensin-unresponsiveness	F.5. (?)	—
Glucocorticoid-suppressible hyperaldosteronism	G.1.	10390
Transport		
Transcortin deficiency	H.1.	12250
Albumin deficiency	H.2.	20530
Transcortin excess	H.3.	12250

TABLE 4 (continued)

		Number in McKusick's catalogue
Target Organs		
5α-reductase deficiency	D.10.	26460
Bartter's syndrome	J.1.	24120
Cortisol resistance	K.1.	—
Aldosterone resistance	K.2.	—
Hypersensitivity for aldosterone (Liddle's syndrome)	K.3.	17720
Secondary Metabolism		
17α,20-desmolase deficiency (status in periferal tissues uncertain)	D.8.	30915
5α-reductase deficiency	D.10.	26460
Crigler-Najjar syndrome		21880

REFERENCES

1. **Seely, J. Rodman,** The fetal and neonatal adrenal cortex, in *Metabolic, Endocrine and Genetic Disorders of Children,* Kelley, V. C., Ed., Harper and Row, Hagerstown, 1974, 225.
2. **Jost, A.,** The fetal adrenal cortex, in *Handbook of Physiology, Section 7: Endocrinology,* Vol. 6, Blaschko, H., Sayers, G., and Smith, A. D., Eds., American Physiological Society, Washington DC., 1975, 107.
3. **Dahl, E. V. and Bahn, R. C.,** Aberrant adrenal cortical tissue near the testis in human infants, *Am. J. Pathol.,* 40, 587, 1962.
4. **Siebenmann, R. E., Steiner, H., and Uehlinger, E.,** Die pathologische Morphologie der endokrinen Regulationsstörungen, in *Handbuch der Allgemeinen Pathologie* Vol. 8 (Part 1), Seifert, G., Ed., Springer, Berlin, 1971, 290.
5. **Long, J. A.,** Zonation of the mammalian adrenal cortex, in *Handbook of physiology. Section 7: Endocrinology,* Vol. 6, Blaschko, H., Sayers, G., and Smith, A. D., Eds., American Physiological Society, Washington, D.C., 1975, 13.
6. **Borkowski, A., Delcroix, C., and Levin, S.,** Metabolism of adrenal cholesterol in man: I. In vivo studies, *J. Clin. Invest.,* 51, 1664, 1972.
7. **Borkowski, A., Delcroix, C., and Levin, S.,** Metabolism of adrenal cholesterol in man: II. In vitro studies, *J. Clin. Invest.,* 51, 1679, 1972.
8. **Nes, W. R. and McKean, M. L.,** *Biochemistry of Steroids and Other Isopentenoids,* University Park Press, Baltimore, 1977.
9. **Träger, L.,** *Steroidhormone,* Springer, Berlin, 1977, chap. 4.
10. **Olson, J. A.,** The biosynthesis of cholesterol, *Rev. Physiol.,* 56, 173, 1965.
11. **Goldstein, J. L. and Brown, M. S.,** The low-density lipo-protein pathway and its relation to atherosclerosis, *Annu. Rev. Biochem.,* 46, 897, 1977.
12. **Moses, H. L., Davis, W. W., Rosenthal, A. S., and Garren, L. D.,** Adrenal cholesterol: localization by electron-microscope autoradiography, *Science,* 163, 1203, 1969.
13. **De Alvare, L. R., Kimura, T., Singhakowinta, A., Honn, K. V., and Chavin, W.,** Mitochondrial redox components of human adrenocortical steroid hydroxylases under physiological conditions and in focal hyperplasia of the zona fasciculata, *Acta Endocrinol. (Copenhagen).,* 84, 780, 1977.
14. **Shikita, M. and Hall, P. F.,** The stoichiometry of the conversion of cholesterol and hydroxycholesterols to pregnenolone (3β-hydroxypregn-5-en-20-one) catalysed by adrenal cytochrome P-450, *Proc. Natl. Acad. Sci., U.S.A.,* 71, 1441, 1974.

15. **Schulster, D., Burstein, S., and Cooke, B. A.,** *Molecular Endocrinology of the Steroid Hormones,* John Wiley & Sons, New York, 1976.
16. **Burstein, S. and Gut, M.,** Biosynthesis of pregnenolone, *Recent Prog. Horm. Res.,* 27, 303, 1971.
17. **Kraaipoel, R. J., Degenhart, H. J., Leferink, J. G., van Beek, V., De Leeuw-Boon, H., and Visser, H. K. A.,** Pregnenolone formation from cholesterol in bovine adrenal cortex mitochondria: proposal of a new mechanism, *FEBS Lett.,* 50, 204, 1975.
18. **Kraaipoel, R. J., Degenhart, H. J., Van Beek, V., De Leeuw-Boon, H., Abeln, G., Visser H. K. A., and Leferink, J. G.,** Evidence for 20,22-epoxycholesterol as an intermediate in side-chain cleavage of 22R-OH-cholesterol by adrenal cortex mitochondria, *FEBS Lett.,* 54, 172, 1975.
19. **Kraaipoel, R. J., Degenhart, H. J., and Leferink, J. G.,** Incorporation of $H_2{}^{18}O$ into 20α,22R-di-OH-cholesterol: evidence for an epoxide-diol pathway in the adrenocortical cholesterol side-chain cleavage mechanism, *FEBS Lett.,* 57, 294, 1975.
20. **Takemoto, C., Nakano, H., Sato, H., and Tamaoki, D.,** Fate of molecular oxygen required by endocrine enzymes for the side-chain cleavage of cholesterol, *Biochim. Biophys. Acta,* 152, 749, 1968.
21. **Burstein, S., Middleditch, B. S., and Gut, M.,** Enzymatic formation of (20R, 22R)-20,22-dihydroxycholesterol from cholesterol and a mixture of $^{16}O_2$ and $^{18}O_2$: random incorporation of oxygen atoms, *Biochem. Biophys. Res. Commun.,* 61, 692, 1974.
22. **Hayaishi, O.,** *Molecular Mechanisms of Oxygen Activation,* Academic Press, New York, 1974.
23. **Ulick, S.,** Diagnosis and nomenclature of the disorders of the terminal portion of the aldosterone biosynthetic pathway, *J. Clin. Endocrinol. Metab.,* 43, 92, 1976.
24. **Domínguez, O. V., Valencia, S. A., and Loza, A. C.,** On the role of steroid sulfates in hormone biosynthesis, *J. Steroid Biochem.,* 6, 301, 1975.
25. **Tell, G. P. E., Morera, A. M., and Saez, J. M.,** Mechanism of action of adrenocorticotropic hormone, in *Congenital Adrenal Hyperplasia,* Lee, P. A., Plotnick, L. P., Kowarski, A. A., and Migeon, C. J., Eds., University Park Press, Baltimore, 1977, 33.
26. **Lefkowitz, R. J., Roth, J., and Pastan, I.,** ACTH-receptor interaction in the adrenal: a model for the initial step in the action of hormones that stimulate adenyl cyclase, *Ann. N.Y. Acad. Sci.,* 185, 195, 1971.
27. **McIlhinney, R. A. J. and Schulster, D.,** Studies on the binding of ^{125}I labelled corticotropin to isolated rat adrenocortical cells, *J. Endocrinol.,* 64, 175, 1975.
28. **Garren, L. D., Gill, G. N., Masui, H., and Walton, G. M.,** On the mechanism of action of ACTH, *Recent Prog. Horm. Res.,* 27, 433, 1971.
29. **Mahaffee, D., Reitz, R. C., and Ney, R. L.,** The mechanism of action of adrenocorticotropic hormone, *J. Biol. Chem.,* 249, 227, 1974.
30. **Grahame-Smith, D. G., Butcher, R. W., Ney, R. L. and Sutherland, E. W.,** Adenosine 3′,5′-monophosphate as the intracellular mediator of the action of adrenocorticotropic hormone on the adrenal cortex, *J. Biol. Chem.,* 242, 5535, 1967.
31. **Robinson, G. A., Butcher, R. W., and Sutherland, E. W.,** *Cyclic AMP,* Academic Press, New York, 1971.
32. **Sharma, R. K., Ahmed, N. K., Sutliff, L. S., and Brush, J. S.,** Metabolic regulation of steroidogenesis in isolated adrenal cells of the rat: ACTH regulation of cGMP and cAMP levels and steroidogenesis, *FEBS Lett.,* 45, 107, 1974.
33. **Lefkowitz, R. J., Roth, J., and Pastan, I.,** Effects of calcium on ACTH stimulation of the adrenal: separation of hormone binding from adenyl cyclase activation, *Nature (London),* 228, 864, 1970.
34. **Honn, K. V. and Chavin, W.,** Prostaglandin modulation of the mechanism of ACTH action in the human adrenal, *Biochem. Biophys. Res. Commun.,* 73, 164, 1976.
35. **Garren, L. D., Gill, G. N., Masui, H., and Walton, G. M.,** On the mechanism of action of ACTH, *Recent Prog. Horm. Res.,* 27, 443, 1971.
36. **Trzeciak, W. H. and Boyd, G. S.,** Activation of cholesteryl esterase in bovine adrenal cortex, *Eur. J. Biochem.,* 46, 201, 1974.
37. **Mrotek, J. J. and Hall, P. F.,**The influence of cytochalasin B on the response of adrenal tumor cells to ACTH and cyclic AMP, *Biochem. Biophys. Res. Commun.,* 64, 891, 1975.
38. **Stockigt, J. R.,** Mineralocorticoid hormones, *Adv. Steroid Biochem. Pharmacol.,* 5, 161, 1976.
39. **Ross, R. J.,** *Aldosterone and Aldosteronism,* Year Book Medical Publishers, Chicago, 1975.
40. Advances in Our Knowledge of the Renin-Angiotensin System (Symposium; April 1976), *Fed. Proc.,* 36, 1753, 1977.
41. **Ganong, W. F. and Van Brunt, E. E.,** Control of aldosterone secretion, in *Handbook of Experimental Pharmacology, The Adrenocortical Hormones,* Vol. 14/3, Deane, H. W. and Rubin, B. L., Eds., Springer, Berlin, 1968, chap. 9.
42. **Williams, G. H. and Braley, L. M.,** Effects of dietary sodium and potassium intake and acute stimulation on aldosterone output by isolated human adrenal cells, *J. Clin. Endocrinol. Metab.,* 45, 55, 1977.

43. **Rastogi, G. K., Dash, R. J., Sharma, B. R., Sawhney, R. C., and Sialy, R.**, Circadian responsiveness of the hypothalamic-pituitary axis, *J. Clin. Endocrinol. Metab.*, 42, 798, 1976.
44. **Krieger, D. T., Allen, W., Rizzo, F., and Krieger, H. P.**, Characterization of the normal temporal pattern of plasma corticosteroid levels, *J. Clin. Endocrinol. Metab.*, 32, 266, 1971.
45. **Holaday, J. W., Martinez, H. M., and Natelson, B. H.**, Synchronized ultradian cortisol rhythms in monkeys: persistence during corticotropin infusion, *Science*, 198, 56, 1977.
46. **Brown, R. D., van Loon, G. R., Orth, D. N., and Liddle, G. W.**, Cushing's disease with periodic hormonogenesis: one explanation for paradoxical response to dexamethasone, *J. Clin. Endocrinol. Metab.*, 36, 445, 1973.
47. **Liberman, B., Wajchenberg, B. L. Tambascia, M. A. and Mesquita, C. H.**, Periodic remission in Cushing's disease with paradoxical dexamethasone response: an expression of periodic hormonogenesis, *J. Clin. Endocrinol. Metab.*, 43, 913, 1976.
48. **Westphal, U.**, Binding of corticosteroids by plasma proteins, in *Handbook of Physiology. Section 7: Endocrinology*, Vol. 6, Blaschko, H., Sayers, G., and Smith, A. D., Eds., American Physiological Society, Washington D.C., 1975, chap. 9.
49. **Cake, M. H. and Litwack, G.**, The glucocorticoid receptor, in *Biochemical Actions of Hormones*, Vol. 3, Litwack, G., Ed. Academic Press, New York, 1975, chap. 10.
50. **King, R. J. B.**, Intracellular reception of steroid hormones, *Essays in Biochemistry*, 12, 41, 1976.
51. **Malkinson, A. M.**, *Hormone Action*, Chapman and Hall, London, 1975.
52. **Janoski, A. H., Shaver, J. C., Christy, N. P., and Rosner, W.**, On the pharmacologic actions of 21-carbon hormonal steroids ("glucocorticoids") of the adrenal cortex in mammals, in *Handbook of Experimental Pharmacology, The Adrenocortical Hormones*, Vol. 14/3, Deane, H. W. and Rubin, B. L., Eds., Springer, Berlin, 1968, chap. 12.
53. **Schmidt, U., Schmid, J., Schmid, H., and Dubach, U.C.**, Sodium and potassium activated ATP-ase. A possible target of aldosterone, *J. Clin. Invest.*, 55, 655, 1975.
54. **Porter, G. H.**, Action of aldosterone on transepithelial sodium transport, in *Basic Life Sciences, (Enzyme Induction)*, Vol. 6, Parke, D. V., Ed., Plenum Press, New York, 1975, 105.
55. **Stewart, J.**, Genetic studies on the mechanism of action of aldosterone in mice, *Endocrinology*, 96, 711, 1975.
56. **Träger, L.**, *Steroidhormone*, Springer, Berlin, 1977, chap. 9.
57. **Sperling, M. A., Wolfsen, A. R., and Fisher, D. A.**, Congenital adrenal hypoplasia: an isolated defect of organogenesis, *J. Pediatr.*, 82, 444, 1973.
58. **Pakravan, P., Kenny, F. M., Depp, R., and Allen, A. C.**, Familial congenital absence of adrenal glands; evaluation of glucocorticoid, mineralocorticoid, and estrogen metabolism in the perinatal period, *J. Pediatr.*, 84, 74, 1974.
59. **Petersen, K. E., Tygstrup, I., and Thamdrup, E.**, Familial adrenocortical hypoplasia with early clinical and biochemical signs of mineralocorticoid deficiency (Hypoaldosteronism), *Acta endocrinol. (Copenhagen)*, 84, 605, 1977.
60. **Prader, A., Zachmann, M., and Illig, R.**, Luteinizing hormone deficiency in hereditary congenital adrenal hypoplasia, *J. Pediatr.*, 86, 421, 1975.
61. **Golden, M. P., Lippe, B. M., and Kaplan, S. A.**, Congenital adrenal hypoplasia and hypogonadotropic hypogonadism, *Am. J. Dis. Child.*, 131, 1117, 1977.
62. **Kelly, W. F., Joplin, G. F., and Pearson, G. W.**, Gonadotrophin deficiency and adrenocortical insufficiency in children: a new syndrome, *Br. Med. J.*, 2, 98, 1977.
63. **Utley, W. S.**, Familial congenital adrenal hypoplasia, *Arch. Dis. Child.*, 43, 724, 1968.
64. **Kerenyi, N.**, Congenital adrenal hypoplasia, *Arch. Pathol.*, 71, 336, 1961.
65. **O'Donohoe, N. V. and Holland, P. D. J.**, Familial congenital adrenal hypoplasia, *Arch. Dis. Child.*, 43, 717, 1968.
66. **Weiss, L. and Mellinger, R. C.**, Congenital adrenal hypoplasia — an X-linked disease, *J. Med. Genet.*, 7, 27, 1970.
67. **Martin, M. M.**, Familial Addison's disease, in: *The Clinical Delineation of Birth Defects X*, Williams & Wilkins, Baltimore, 1971, 98.
68. **Laverty, C. R. A., Fortune, D. W., and Beischer, N. A.**, Congenital idiopathic adrenal hypoplasia, *Obstet. Gynecol.*, 41, 655, 1973.
69. **Irvine, W. J. and Barnes, E. W.**, Addison's disease, ovarian failure and hypoparathyroidism, *Clin. Endocrinol. Metab.*, 4, 379, 1975.
70. **Blizzard, R. M., Chee, D., and Davis, W.**, The incidence of adrenal and other antibodies in the sera of patients with idiopathic adrenal insufficiency (Addison's disease), *Clin. Exp. Immunol.*, 2, 19, 1967.
71. **Dunlop, D. M.**, Eighty-six cases of Addison's disease, *Br. Med. J.*, 2, 887, 1963.
72. **Frey, M. M., Vogt, J. H., and Nerup, J.**, Familial poly-endocrinopathy, *Acta endocrinol. (Copenhagen)*, 72, 401, 1974.

73. **Platz, P., Ryder, L., Nielsen, L. S., Svejgaard, A., Thomsen, M., Nerup, J., and Christy, M,.** HL-A and idiopathic Addison's disease, *Lancet,* 2, 289, 1974.
74. **Eisenbarth, G., Wilson, P., Ward, F., and Lebovitz, H. E.,** HLA type and occurrence of disease in familial polyglandular failure, *N. Engl. J. Med.,* 298, 92, 1978.
75. **Spinner, M. W., Blizzard, R. M., and Childs, B.,** Clinical and genetic heterogeneity in idiopathic Addison's disease and hypoparathyroidism, *J. Clin. Endocrinol.,* 28, 795, 1968.
76. **Schimke, R. N.,** Multiple endocrine adenomatosis syndromes, *Adv. Intern. Med.,* 21, 249, 1976.
77. **Wermer, P.,** Genetic aspects of adenomatosis of endocrine glands, *Am. J. Med.,* 16, 363, 1954.
78. **Pearse, A. G. E. and Polak, J. M.,** Endocrine tumors of neural crest origin, *Med. Biol.,* 52, 3, 1974.
79. **Mulvihill, J. J., Miller, R. W., and Fraumeni, J. F.,** *Genetics of Human Cancer,* Raven Press, New York, 1977.
80. **Johnson, G. J., Summerskil, W. H. J., Anderson, V. E., and Keating, F. R.,** Clinical and genetic investigation of a large kindred with multiple endocrine adenomatosis, *N. Engl. J. Med.,* 277, 1379, 1967.
81. **Vance, J. E., Stoll, R. W., Kitabchi, A. E., Buchanan, K. D., Hollander, D., and Williams, R. H.,** Familial nesidioblastosis as the predominant manifestation of multiple endocrine adenomatosis, *Am. J. Med.,* 52, 211, 1972.
82. **Fraumeni, J. F. and Miller, R. W.,** Adrenocortical neoplasms with hemihypertrophy, brain tumors, and other disorders, *J. Pediatr.,* 70, 129, 1967.
83. **Anderson, R. G. W., Goldstein, J. L., and Brown, M. S.,** A mutation that impairs the ability of lipoprotein receptors to localize in coated pits on the cell surface of human fibroblasts, *Nature (London),* 270, 695, 1977.
84. **Gwynne, J. T., Mahaffee, D., Brewer, H. B., and Ney, R. L.,** Adrenal cholesterol uptake from plasma lipoproteins: regulation by corticotropin, *Proc. Natl. Acad. Sci., U.S.A.,* 73, 4329, 1976.
85. **Wilkins, L.,** *The Diagnosis and Treatment of Endocrine Disorders in Childhood and Adolescence,* Charles C Thomas, Springfield, Ill., 1965, chap. 17.
86. **Prader, A.,** Der Genitalbefund beim Pseudohermaphroditismus feminus des kongenitalen adrenogenitalen Syndroms, *Helv. Paediatr. Acta,* 9, 231, 1954.
87. **Huffstadt, A. and Visser, H. K. A.,** Surgical correction of the external genitalia in girls with congenital adrenal hyperplasia, *Maandschr. Kindergeneeskd.,* 34, 385, 1966.
88. **Lee, P. A., Plotnick, L. P., Kowarski, A. A., and Migeon, C. J.,** *Congenital Adrenal Hyperplasia,* University Park Press, Baltimore, 1977.
89. **New, M. I. and Levine, L. S.,** Congenital adrenal hyperplasia, *Adv. Hum. Genet.,* 4, 251, 1973.
90. **Zurbrügg, R. P.,** Congenital adrenal hyperplasia, in *Endocrine and Genetic Diseases of Childhood and Adolescence,* 2nd ed., Gardner, L. I., Ed., W. B. Saunders, Philadelphia, 1975, 372.
91. **Bongiovanni, A. M.,** Congenital adrenal hyperplasia and related disorders, in *The Metabolic Basis of Inherited Disease,* 4th ed., Stanbury, J. B., Wyngaarden, J. B., and Fredrickson, D. S., Eds., McGraw-Hill, New York, 1978, chap. 41.
92. **Visser, H. K. A.,** The adrenal cortex in childhood. Part 2: Pathological aspects, *Arch. Dis. Child.,* 41, 113, 1966.
93. **Prader, A. and Siebenmann, R. E.,** Nebenniereninsuffizienz bei kongenitaler lipoid Hyperplasie der Nebennieren, *Helv. Paediatr. Acta,* 12, 569, 1957.
94. **Degenhart, H. J., Visser, H. K. A., Boon, H., and O'Doherty,** N. J. O., Evidence for deficient 20α-cholesterol-hydroxylase activity in adrenal tissue of a patient with lipoid adrenal hyperplasia, *Acta Endocrinol. (Copenhagen),* 71, 512, 1972.
95. **Koizumi, S., et al.,** Cholesterol side-chain cleavage enzyme activity and cytochrome P-450 content in adrenal mitochondria of a patient with congenital lipoid adrenal hyperplasia (Prader disease), *Clin. Chim. Acta,* 77, 301, 1977.
96. **Falke, H. E., Degenhart, H. J., Abeln, G. J. A., and Visser, H. K. A.,** Effects of 25-hydroxycholesterol and aminoglutethimide in isolated rat adrenal cells. A model for congenital lipoid adrenal hyperplasia? *Mol. Cell. Endocrinol.,* 4, 107, 1976.
97. **Kraaipoel, R. J.,** Studies on Cholesterol Side-chain Cleavage, thesis, Rotterdam, 1978.
98. **Bongiovanni, A. M.,** The adrenogenital syndrome with deficiency of 3β-hydroxysteroid dehydrogenase, *J. Clin. Invest.,* 41, 2086, 1962.
99. **Kenny, F. M., Reynolds, J. W. and Green, O. C.,** Partial 3β-hydroxysteroid dehydrogenase (3β-HSD) deficiency in a family with congenital adrenal hyperplasia: evidence for increasing 3β-HSD activity with age, *Pediatrics,* 48, 756, 1971.
100. **Schneider, G., Genel, M., Bongiovanni, A. M., Goldman, A. S., and Rosenfield, R. L.,** Persistent testicular Δ^5-isomerase-3β-hydroxysteroid dehydrogenase (Δ^5-3β-HSD) deficiency in the Δ^5-3β-HSD form of congenital adrenal hyperplasia, *J. Clin. Invest.,* 55, 681, 1975.
101. **Jänne, O., Perheentupa, J., Viinikka, L., and Vihko, R.,** Testicular endocrine function in a pubertal boy with 3β-hydroxysteroid dehydrogenase deficiency, *J. Clin. Endocrinol. Metab.,* 39, 206, 1974.

102. **Degenhart, H. J., Visser, H. K. A., and Boon, H.,** Aspects of the enzymology of perinatal steroid metabolism, *Excerpta Med. Int. Congr. Ser.,* 219, 522, 1971.
103. **Hirschfeld, H. J. and Fleshman, J. K.,** An unusually high incidence of salt-losing congenital adrenal hyperplasia in the Alaskan Eskimo, *J. Pediatr.,* 75, 492, 1969.
104. **Kowarski, A. A.,** Mechanism of salt loss in congenital virilizing adrenal hyperplasia, in *Congenital Adrenal Hyperplasia,* Lee, P. A., Ed., University Park Press, Baltimore, 1977, 113.
105. **Loras, B., Haour, F., and Bertrand, J.,** Exchangeable sodium and aldosterone secretion in children with congenital adrenal hyperplasia due to 21-hydroxylase deficiency, *Pediatr. Res.,* 4, 145, 1970.
106. **Janoski, A. H.,** Naturally occurring adrenal steroids with salt-losing properties. Relationship to congenital adrenal hyperplasia, in *Congenital Adrenal Hyperplasia,* Lee, P. A. Ed., University Park Press, Baltimore, 1977, 99.
107. **Degenhart, H. J., Visser, H. K. A., Wilmink, R., and Croughs, W.,** Aldosterone and cortisol secretion rates in infants and children with congenital adrenal hyperplasia suggesting different 21-hydroxylation defects in salt-losers and non-salt-losers, *Acta Endocrinol. (Copenhagen),* 48, 587, 1965.
108. **Hughes, I. A. and Winter, J. S. D.,** The application of a serum 17OH-progesterone radioimmunoassay to the diagnosis and management of congenital adrenal hyperplasia, *J. Pediatr.,* 88, 766, 1976.
109. **Gareis, F. J., Asper, A. C., and Smith, D. W.,** Low X-chromatin frequency in untreated congenital adrenal hyperplasia, *Lancet,* 2, 373, 1971.
110. **New, M. I.,** Present status of prenatal diagnosis of congenital adrenal hyperplasia, in *Congenital Adrenal Hyperplasia,* Lee, P. A., Ed., University Park Press, Baltimore, 1977, 511.
111. **Dupont, B., Oberfield, S. E., Smithwick, E. M., Lee, T. D., and Levine, L. S.,** Close genetic linkage between HLA and congenital adrenal hyperplasia (21-hydroxylase deficiency), *Lancet,* 2, 1309, 1977.
112. **Frasier, S. D., Horton, R., and Ulstrom, R. A.,** Androgen metabolism in congenital adrenal hyperplasia due to 11β-hydroxylase deficiency, *Pediatrics,* 44, 201, 1969.
113. **Shepard, T. H. and Clausen, S. W.,** Case of adrenogenital syndrome with hypertension treated with cortisone, *Pediatrics,* 8, 805, 1951.
114. **Gandy, H. M., Keutmann, E. H., and Izzo, A. J.,** Characterization of urinary steroids in adrenal hyperplasia: isolation of metabolites of cortisol, compound-S and deoxycorticosterone from a normotensive patient with adrenogenital syndrome, *J. Clin. Invest.,* 39, 364, 1960.
115. **Genest, J., Nowaczynski, W., Kuchel, O., Boucher, R., Rojo-Ortega, J. M., Constantopoulos, G., Ganten, D., and Messerli, F.,** The adrenal cortex and essential hypertension, *Recent Progr. Horm. Res.,* 32, 377, 1976.
116. **Biglieri, E. G.,** Plasma deoxycorticosterone concentrations in the adrenal enzymatic deficiencies causing hypertension, in *Juvenile Hypertension,* New, M. I. and Levine, L. S., Eds., Raven Press, New York, 1977.
117. **Maschler, I., Weidenfeld, J., Muller, A., Slavin, S., Shaefer, J., Chowers, I., and Finkelstein, M.,** A case of adrenogenital syndrome with aberrant 11β-hydroxylation, *Acta Endocrinol (Copenhagen),* 85, 832, 1977.
118. **Visser, H. K. A.,** Hypoadrenocorticism, in *Endocrine and Genetic Diseases of Childhood and Adolescence,* 2nd ed., Gardner, L. I., Ed., W. B. Saunders, Philadelphia, 1975, 513.
119. **Visser, H. K. A. and Cost, W. S.,** A new hereditary defect in the biosynthesis of aldosterone: urinary C_{21}-corticosteroid pattern in three related patients with a salt-losing syndrome, suggesting an 18-oxidation defect, *Acta Endocrinol. (Copenhagen),* 47, 589, 1964.
120. **McKusick, V. A.,** *Mendelian Inheritance in Man,* Johns Hopkins University Press, Baltimore, 1975.
121. **Jean, R., Legrand, J. C., Meylan, F., Rieu, D., and Astruc, J.,** Hypoaldostéronisme primaire par anomalie probable de la 18-hydroxylation, *Arch. Fr. Pédiatr.,* 26, 769, 1969.
122. **Ravussin, J.-J., De Martinville, B., Lauras, B., Chatelain, Ph., and Freycon, F.,** Hypoaldostéronisme chez les jumeaux. Déficit en 18-hydroxylase probable, *Pédiatrie,* 32, 781, 1977.
123. **Milla, P. J., Trompeter, R., Dillon, M. J., Robins, D., and Shackleton, C.,** Salt-losing syndrome in 2 infants with defective 18-dehydrogenation in aldosterone biosynthesis, *Arch. Dis. Child.,* 52, 580, 1977.
124. **Rösler, A., Rabinowitz, D., Theodor, R., Ramirez, L. C., and Ulick, S.,** The nature of the defect in a salt-wasting disorder in Jews of Iran, *J. Clin. Endocrinol. Metab.,* 44, 279, 1977.
125. **Ulick, S., Gautier, E., Vetter, K. K., Markello, J. R., Yaffe, S., and Lowe, C. U.,** An aldosterone biosynthetic defect in a salt-losing disorder, *J. Clin. Endocrinol. Metab.,* 24, 669, 1964.
126. **Hamilton, W., McCandless, A. E., Ireland, J. T., and Gray, C. E.,** Hypoaldosteronism in three sibs due to 18-dehydrogenase deficiency, *Arch. Dis. Child.,* 51, 576, 1976.
127. **David, R. Golan, S., and Drucker, W.,** Familial aldosterone deficiency: enzyme defect, diagnosis and clinical course, *Pediatrics,* 41, 403, 1968.
128. **Tourniaire, J., Audi-Parera, L., Loras, B., Blum, J., Castelnovo, P., and Forest, M. G.,** Male pseudohermaphroditism with hypertension due to a 17α-hydroxylation deficiency, *Clin. Endocrinol.,* 5, 53, 1976.

129. **Kershnar, A. K., Borut, D., Kogut, M. D., Biglieri, E. G., and Schambelan, M.**, Studies in a phenotypic female with 17-α-hydroxylase deficiency, *J. Pediatr.*, 89, 395, 1976.
130. **Biglieri, E. G., Herron, M. A., and Brust, N.**, 17-Hydroxylation deficiency in man, *J. Clin. Invest.*, 45, 1946, 1966.
131. **Alvarez, M. N., Cloutier, M. D., and Hayles, A. B.**, Male pseudohermaphroditism due to 17-α-hydroxylase deficiency in two siblings, *Pediatr. Res.*, 7, 325, 1973.
132. **Zachmann, M., Völlmin, J. A., Hamilton, W., and Prader, A.**, Steroid 17,20-desmolase deficiency, *Clin. Endocrinol.*, 1, 369, 1972.
133. **Virdis, R., Saenger, P., Senior, B., and New, M. I.**, Endocrine studies in a pubertal male pseudohermaphrodite with 17-keto-steroid reductase deficiency, *Acta Endocrinol. (Copenhagen)*, 87, 212, 1978.
134. **Wilson, J. D., Harrod, M. J., Goldstein, J. L., Hemsell, D. L., and MacDonald, P. C.**, Familial incomplete male pseudohermaphroditism, Type 1, *N. Engl. J. Med.*, 290, 1097, 1974.
135. **Amrhein, J. A., Jones Klingensmith, G., Walsh, P. C., McKusick, V. A., and Migeon, C. J.**, Partial androgen insensitivity. The Reifenstein syndrome revisited, *N. Engl. J. Med.*, 297, 350, 1977.
136. **Imperato-McGinley, J., Guerrero, L., Gautier, T., and Peterson, R. E.**, Steroid 5α-reductase deficiency in man: an inherited form of male pseudohermaphroditism, *Science*, 186, 1213, 1974.
137. **Walsh, P. C., Madden, J. D., Harrod, M. J., Goldstein, J. L., MacDonald, P. C., and Wilson, J. D.**, Familial incomplete male pseudohermaphroditism, type 2, *N. Engl. J. Med.*, 291, 944, 1974.
138. **Osathanondh, R., Canick, J., Ryan, K. J., and Tulchinsky, D.**, Placental sulfatase deficiency: a case study, *J. Clin. Endocrinol. Metab.*, 43, 208, 1976.
139. **Shapiro, L. J., Cousins, L., Fluharty, A. L., Stevens, R. L., and Kihara, H.**, Steroid sulfatase deficiency, *Pediatr. Res.*, 11, 894, 1977.
140. **France, J. T. and Liggins, G. C.**, Placental sulfatase deficiency, *J. Clin. Endocrinol. Metab.*, 29, 138, 1969.
141. **Tabei, T. and Heinrichs, W. L.**, Diagnosis of placental sulfatase deficiency, *Am. J. Obstet. Gynecol.*, 124, 409, 1976.
142. **Jöbsis, A. C., Van Duuren, C. Y., De Vries, G. P., Koppe, J. G., Rijken, Y., Van Kempen, G. M. J., and De Groot, W. P.**, Trophoblast sulphatase deficiency associated with X-chromosomal ichthyosis, *Ned. Tijdschr. Geneesk.*, 120, 1980, 1976.
143. **Shapiro, L. J., Weiss, R., Webster, D., and France, J. T.**, X-linked ichthyosis due to steroid-sulphatase deficiency, *Lancet*, 1, 70, 1978.
144. **Wolman, M., Sterk, V. V., Gatt, S., and Frenkel, M.**, Primary familial xanthomatosis with involvement and calcification of the adrenals, *Pediatrics*, 28, 742, 1961.
145. **Patrick, A. D. and Lake, B. D.**, Wolman's disease, in *Lysosomes and Storage Diseases*, Hers, H. G. and Van Hoof, F., Eds., Academic Press, New York, 1973, 217.
146. **Patrick, A. D. and Lake, B. D.**, Deficiency of an acid lipase in Wolman's disease, *Nature (London)*, 222, 1067, 1969.
147. **Lake, B. D. and Patrick, A. D.**, Wolman's disease: deficiency of E 600-resistant acid esterase activity with storage of lipids in lysosomes, *J. Pediatr.*, 76, 262, 1970.
148. **Patrick, A. D., Willcox, P., Stephens, R., and Kenyon, V. G.**, Prenatal diagnosis of Wolman's disease, *J. Med. Genet.*, 13, 49, 1976.
149. **Beaudet, A. L., Ferry, G. D., Nichols, B. L., and Rosenberg, H. S.**, Cholesterol ester storage disease: clinical, biochemical, and pathological studies, *J. Pediatr.*, 90, 910, 1977.
150. **Cortner, J. A., Coates, P. M., Swoboda, E., and Schnatz, J. D.**, Genetic variation of lysosomal acid lipase, *Pediatr. Res.*, 10, 927, 1976.
151. **Blaw, M. E.**, Melanodermic type leucodystrophy (adreno-leucodystrophy) in *Handbook of Clinical Neurology*, Vol. 10, Vinken, P. G. and Bruyn, G. W., Eds., American Elsevier, New York, 1970, 128.
152. **Sanchez, J. E. and Lopez, V. F.**, Sex-linked sudanophilic leukodystrophy with adrenocortical atrophy (so-called Schilder's disease), *Neurology*, 26, 261, 1976.
153. **Ohno, F. Harada, H., Komatsu, K., Saijo, K., and Miyoshki, K.**, Two cases of pseudoaldosteronism (Liddle's syndrome) in siblings, *Endocrinol. Jpn.*, 22, 163, 1975.
154. **Yavin, E., Milunsky, A., DeLong, G. R., Nash, A. H., and Kolodny, E. H.**, Cholesterol metabolism in cultured fibroblasts in adrenoleukodystrophy, *Pediatr. Res.*, 10, 540, 1976.
155. **Gumbinas, M., Mei Liu, H., Dawson, G., Larsen, M., and Green, O.**, Progressive spastic paraparesis and adrenal insufficiency, *Arch. Neurol.*, 33, 678, 1976.
156. **Livet, M. O., Chaussain, J. L., Lyon, G.**, La maladie de Schilder avec insuffisance surrenale (Adreno-leucodystrophy), *Arch. Fr. Pédiatr.*, 34, 232, 1977.
157. **Schaumburg, H. H., Powers, J. M., Raine, C. S., Suzuki, K., and Richardson, E. P.**, Adrenoleucodystrophy, *Arch. Neurol.*, 32, 577, 1975.
158. **Liddle, G. W., Bledsoe, T., and Coppage, W. S.**, A familial renal disorder simulating primary aldosteronism but with negligible aldosterone secretion, *Trans. Assoc. Am. Physicians.*, 76, 199, 1963.

159. **De Leiva, A., Christlieb, A. R., Melby, J. C., Graham, C. A., Day, R. P., Luetscher, J. A., Zager, P. G.**, Big renin and biosynthetic defect of aldosterone in diabetes mellitus, *N. Engl. J. Med.*, 295, 639, 1976.
160. **Williams, H. E. and Freeman, M.**, Primary familial Addison's disease, *Aust. Paediatr. J.*, 1, 93, 1965.
161. **Migeon, C. J., Kenny, F. M., Kowarski, A., Snipes, C. A., Spaulding, J. S., Finkelstein, J. W., and Blizzard, R. M.**, The syndrome of congenital adrenocortical unresponsiveness to ACTH. Report of six cases, *Pediatr. Res.*, 2, 501, 1968.
162. **Kelch, R. P., Kaplan, S. L., Biglieri, E. G., Daniels, G. H., Epstein, C. J., and Grumbach, M. M.**, Hereditary adrenocortical unresponsiveness to adrenocorticotropic hormone, *J. Pediatr.*, 81, 726, 1972.
163. **Thistlethwaite, D., Darling, J. A. B., Fraser, R., Mason, P. A., Rees, L. H., and Harkness, R. A.**, Familial glucocorticoid deficiency, *Arch. Dis. Child.*, 50, 291, 1975.
164. **Shepard, T. H., Landing, B. H., and Mason, D. G.**, Familial Addison's disease. Case report of two sisters with corticoid deficiency unassociated with hypoaldosteronism, *Am. J. Dis. Child.*, 97, 154, 1959.
165. **Kershnar, A. K., Roe, T. F., and Kogut, M. D.**, Adrenocorticotropic hormone unresponsiveness: report of a girl with excessive growth and review of 16 reported cases, *J. Pediatr.*, 80, 610, 1972.
166. **Moshang, T.**, Familial glucocorticoid deficiency, *N. Engl. J. Med.*, 298, 282, 1978.
167. **Christlieb, A. R., Hickler, R. B., Lauler, D. P., and Williams, G. H.**, Hypertension with inappropriate aldosterone stimulation, *N. Engl. J. Med.*, 281, 128, 1969.
168. **Schwartz, Th. B., Ed.**, *The Yearbook of Endocrinology 1970,* Yearbook Medical Publishing, Chicago, 1970, 277.
169. **Sutherland, D. J. A., Ruse, J. L., and Laidlaw, J. C.**, Hypertension, increased aldosterone secretion and low plasma renin relieved by dexamethasone, *Can. Med. Assoc. J.*, 95, 1109, 1966.
170. **Miura, K., Yoshinaga, K., Goto, K., Katsushima, I., Maebashi, M., Demura, H., Iino, M., Demura, R., and Torikai, T.**, A case of glucocorticoid-responsive hyperaldosteronism, *J. Clin. Endocrinol. Metab.*, 28, 1807, 1968.
171. **Giebink, G. S., Gotlin, R. W., Biglieri, E. G., and Katz, F. A.**, A kindred with familial glucocorticoid-suppressible aldosteronism, *J. Clin. Endocrinol. Metab.*, 36, 715, 1973.
172. **New, M. I. and Peterson, R. E.**, A new form of congenital adrenal hyperplasia, *J. Clin. Endocrinol. Metab.*, 27, 300, 1967.
173. **New, M. I., Siegal, E. J., and Peterson, R. E.**, Dexamethasone-suppressible hyperaldosteronism, *J. Clin. Endocrinol. Metab.*, 37, 93, 1973.
174. **Grim, C. E., Weinberger, M. H., and Anand, S. K.**, Familial dexamethasone-suppressible, normokalemic hyperaldosteronism, in *Juvenile Hypertension,* New, M. I. and Levine, L. S., Eds., Raven Press, New York, 1977, 109.
175. **Funder, J. W.**, Physiological significance of steroid binding proteins, *Excerpta Med. Int. Congr. Ser.*, No. 403, 459, 1977.
176. **Burke, C. W.**, Clinical significance of steroid-binding proteins in plasma, in *Excerpta Med. Int. Congr. Ser.*, No. 403, 463, 1977.
177. **Lohrenz, F., Doe, R. P., Seal, U. S.**, Idiopathic or genetic elevation of corticosteroid-binding globulin? *J. Clin. Endocrinol. Metab.*, 28, 1073, 1968.
178. **Krieger, D. T., Ed.**, *Endocrine Rhythms,* Raven Press, New York, 1978.
179. **Bartter, F. C., Pronove, P., Gell, J. R., and MacCardle, R. C.**, Hyperplasia of the juxtaglomerular complex with hyperaldosteronism and hypokalemic alkalosis. A new syndrome, *Am. J. Med.*, 33, 811, 1962.
180. **Cannon, P. J., Leeming, J. M., Sommers, S. C., Winters, R. W., and Laragh, J. H.**, Juxtaglomerular cell hyperplasia and secondary hyperaldosteronism (Bartter's syndrome): a reevaluation of the pathophysiology, *Medicine,* 47, 107, 1968.
181. **Gardner, J. D., Simopoulos, A. P., Lapey, A., and Shibolet, S.**, Altered membrane sodium transport in Bartter's syndrome, *J. Clin. Invest.*, 51, 1565, 1972.
182. **Visser, H. K. A., Degenhart, H. J., Desmit, E., and Cost, W. S.**, Mineralocorticoid excess in two brothers with dwarfism, hypokalaemic alkalosis and normal blood pressure, *Acta endocrinol. (Copenhagen),* 55, 661, 1967.
183. **Trygstad, C. W., Mangos, J. A., Bloodworth, J. M. B., and Lobeck,** C. C., A sibship with Bartter's syndrome: failure of total adrenalectomy to correct the potassium wasting, *Pediatrics,* 44, 234, 1969.
184. **Gill, J. R., Fröhlich, J. C., Bowden, R. E., Taylor, A. A., Keiser, H. R., Seyberth, H. W., Oates, J. A., and Bartter, F. C.**, Bartter's syndrome: a disorder characterized by high urinary prostaglandins and a dependence of hyperreninemia on prostaglandin synthesis, *Am. J. Med.*, 61, 43, 1976.
185. **Bowden, R. E., Gill, J. R., Radfar, N., Taylor, A. A., and Keiser,** H. R., Prostaglandin synthetase inhibitors in Bartter's syndrome, *J. Am. Med. Assoc.*, 239, 117, 1978.

186. **Vingerhoeds, A. C. M., Thijssen, J. H. H., and Schwartz, F.**, Spontaneous hypercortisolism without Cushing's syndrome, *J. Clin. Endocrinol. Metab.*, 43, 1128, 1976.
187. **Roy, C.**, Pseudohypoaldosteronisme familial, *Arch. Fr. Pediatr.*, 34, 37, 1977.
188. **Anand, S. K., Froberg, L., Northway, J. D., Weinberger, M., and Wright, J. C.**, Pseudohypoaldosteronism due to sweat gland dysfunction, *Pediatr. Res.*, 10, 677, 1976.
189. **Thompson, E. B., Norman, M. R., and Lippman, M. E.**, Steroid hormone actions in tissue culture cells and cell hybrids. Their relation to human malignancies, *Recent Progr. Horm. Res.*, 33, 571, 1977.
190. **Yamamoto, K. R., Gehring, U., Stampfer, M. R., and Sibley, C. H.**, Genetic approaches to steroid hormone action, *Recent Progr. Horm. Res.*, 32, 3, 1976.
191. **Crigler, J. F. and Najjar, V. A.**, Congenital familial nonhemolytic jaundice with Kernicterus, *Pediatrics*, 10, 169, 1952.
192. **Peterson, R. E. and Schmid, R.**, A clinical syndrome associated with a defect in steroid glucuronide formation, *J. Clin. Endocrinol. Metab.*, 17, 1485, 1957.
193. **Bondy, P. K.**, The adrenal cortex, in *Duncan's Diseases of Metabolism*, 7th ed., Bondy, P. K. and Rosenberg, L. E., Eds., W. B. Saunders, Philadelphia, 1974, chap. 18.
194. **Boucher, R., Asselin, J., and Genest, J.**, A new enzyme leading to the direct formation of angiotensin II, *Circ. Res., Suppl. I*, 34—35, I-203, 1974.
195. **Richardson, K. S. C., Nowaczynski, W., and Genest, J.**, Aldosterone-binding proteins in human plasma, *N. Engl. J. Med.*, 295, 114, 1976.
196. **King, R. J. B. and Mainwaring, W. I. P.**, *Steroid-Cell Interactions*, University Park Press, Baltimore, 1974.
197. **Riddick, D. H. and Hammond, C. B.**, Adrenal virilism due to 21-hydroxylase deficiency in the postmenarchial female, *Obstet. Gynecol.*, 45, 21, 1975.
198. **Qazi, Q. H. and Thompson, M. W.**, Incidence of salt-losing form of congenital virilizing adrenal hyperplasia, *Arch. Dis. Child.*, 47, 302, 1972.
199. **Gregory, T. and Gardner, L. I.**, Hypertensive virilizing adrenal hyperplasia with minimal impairment of synthetic route to cortisol, *J. Clin. Endocrinol. Metab.*, 43, 769, 1976.
200. **Russell, A., Levin, B., Sinclair, L., and Oberholzer, V. G.**, A reversible salt-wasting syndrome of the newborn and infant, *Arch. Dis. Child.*, 38, 313, 1963.
201. **Degenhart, H. J., Frankena, L., Visser, H. K. A., Cost, W. S., and Van Seters, A. P.**, Further investigation of a new hereditary defect in the biosynthesis of aldosterone: evidence for a defect in 18-hydroxylation of corticosterone, *Acta Physiol. Pharmacol. Neerl.*, 14, 88, 1966.
202. **Spark, R. F. and Etzkorn, J. R.**, Absent aldosterone response to ACTH in familial glucocorticoid deficiency, *N. Engl. J. Med.*, 297, 917, 1977.
203. **Cret, L., Bourgeois, J., Souillet, G., Thomas, A., David, M., and Jeune, M.**, Nanisme chondrodysplasique avec insuffisance surrénale congénitale et lymphopénie chronique. Un nouveau syndrome familial? *Pédiatrie*, 31, 616, 1976.
204. **Reid, I. A., Morris, B. J., and Ganong, W. F.**, The reninangiotensin system, *Annu. Rev. Physiol.*, 40, 377, 1978.
205. **Bentley, P. J. and Scott, W. N.**, The actions of aldosterone, in *General, Comparative and Clinical Endocrinology of the Adrenal Cortex*, Vol. 2, Chester-Jones, I. and Henderson, E. W., Eds., Academic Press, London, 1978, chap. 6, p. 497.
206. **Levine, L. S., Zachmann, M., New, M. I., Prader, A., Pollock, M. S., O'Neill, G. J., Yang, S. Y., Oberfield, S. E., and Dupont, B.**, Genetic mapping of the 21-hydroxylase-deficiency gene within the HLA linkage group, *N. Engl. J. Med.*, 299, 911, 1978.
207. **Fisher, L. K., Kogut, M. D., Moore, R. J., Goebelsmann, U., Weitzmann, J. J., Isaacs, H., Griffin, J. E., and Wilson, J. D.**, Clinical, endocrinological, and enzymatic characterization of two patients with 5α-reductase deficiency: evidence that a single enzyme is responsible for the 5α-reduction of cortisol and testosterone, *J. Clin. Endocrinol. Metab.*, 47, 653, 1978.
208. **Schaumberg, H. H., Powers, J. M., Raine, C. S., Spencer, P. S., Griffin, J. W., Prineas, J. W., and Boehme, D. M.**, Adrenomyeloneuropathy: a probable variant of adrenoleukodystrophy, *Neurology*, 27, 114, 1977.
209. **Ølgaard, K., Madsen, S., Hammer, M., and Ladefoged, J.**, Calcium dependent aldosterone secretion in anephric and nonnephrectomized patients on regular hemodialysis, *J. Clin. Endocrinol. Metab.*, 46, 740, 1978.

Chapter 3

CORTICOSTEROIDS AND ADRENOCORTICAL FUNCTION IN ANIMALS

J. G. M. Shire

TABLE OF CONTENTS

I. INTRODUCTION

Studies of genetic variation in the adrenal function of experimental animals complement those on variation in human adrenocortical function. Most investigations in man have been concerned with pathological mutations which interfere with steroid synthesis.[1] In contrast, most work on laboratory and domestic animals has been concerned with variation within the range of normality. The following sections deal with the structure of the adrenal cortex, the factors which regulate blood levels of corticosteroids, and the responses of target tissues to these hormones. Whenever possible, I have tried to discuss how many genes underlie particular phenotypic differences and where their primary sites of action may be. The emphasis given to studies on mice is a consequence of the existence of well-defined inbred strains in a species with a short generation time.

II. CORTICAL MORPHOLOGY

The position of the adrenal glands and the degree of left-right asymmetry differ greatly between strains of mice.[2-4] Genetic variation affecting the weight of the adrenals is also widespread. Threefold differences between strains have been described in mice[4-7] and arctic foxes.[8] Adrenal weight varied more than twofold in rats[4,9,10] and guinea pigs.[11] Wild rats and mice had larger adrenals than animals from laboratory strains, even when reared by foster mothers of the laboratory strain.[4,12,13] Biometric investigations have shown significant heritabilities for adrenal weight in mice[3] and pigs.[14] Lines of mice have been successfully selected for high and low relative adrenal weight.[15,16] Correlated responses in adrenal weight were found when selection experiments were carried out for other characters in mice,[17-20] rats,[4,21-24] and chickens.[25] In the mouse, the dominant mutation Oligosyndactyly *(Os)* is associated with increased adrenal weight, but only in certain genetic backgrounds.[26] Several mutations, which result in adrenal hyperplasia accompanied by elevated plasma levels of corticosteroids, are described in Section III.A.4.

The adrenal cortex is made up of several zones, which are usually considered to have different functions. The ultrastructural appearance of the fascicular and glomerular zones differed between rats of the spontaneously hypertensive (SHR) and Kyoto-Wistar (W/KY) strains and between W/KY and W/CFN Wistars.[27] Several ultrastructural parameters of the zona fasciculata differed between Wistar, Sprague-Dawley, and AGUS rats.[28] The width of the zona glomerulosa varies between strains of mice.[29] Variation at the *Ezg* locus is responsible for the difference in this zone between CBA and Peru mice.[30,31] When on the DI background, the *Os* mutation caused, probably indirectly, hypertrophy of the zona glomerulosa.[26] The zona glomerulosa is intensely sudanophilic in DBA mice, but not in mice of any other strain.[32] The zona fasciculata shows marked quantitative differences between strains.[4] Those between the A and CBA strains were attributed to variation at two loci.[33] The fascicular zones of adult DBA and AKR mice do not stain with lipophilic stains like Sudan.[34-37] This is discussed further in Sections III.A.1 and 2.

The juxtamedullary X-zone, which undergoes marked changes during postnatal development, shows at least a fourfold variation in volume between strains.[4,38] The adrenals of pituitary dwarf mice, both *dw*[39,40] and *df*,[41] have no X-zone. Involution occurs at puberty in male mice, and the body weight at which it occurs differs between strains.[42] In females, involution of the X-zone occurs during first pregnancy, some time after puberty. Strains differ greatly in how long the zone persists before involuting.[4] Degeneration occurs very early, around the age of 5 to 6 weeks, in A strain mice and in mice carrying the dominant *Ex* allele.[43] Genetic variation also affects the form that X-zone degeneration takes. Fatty degeneration of the zone, in which the cells become replaced by large lipid-filled vacuoles, occurs in females of many strains. Collapse of the X-zone, with pycnosis of the nuclei and without the accumulation of lipid, takes place spontaneously in C57BL, SF, and Peru mice.[4] Degeneration of the X-zone takes place later in nude, *nu nu*,[44] and obese, *ob ob*,[45] mice than in their normal sibs, probably as a consequence of their delayed maturation. The control of the X-zone and its degeneration is discussed in Sections IV.B. and C.

Brown degeneration of the inner part of the cortex occurs in the adrenals of female mice of certain strains.[46] The incidence of senescent changes varies from strain to strain.[47] As DE mice grow old, their adrenals enlarge greatly and become filled with acellular material.[5]

III. STEROID PRODUCTION

The secretions of the adrenals can be measured directly by sampling from the veins carrying blood away from the glands. The production rate of individual steroids can also be measured using portions of adrenal tissue incubated or superfused in vitro or by incubating suspensions of dissociated cortical cells. Indirect estimates of steroid production can be made from measurements of their concentration in peripheral plasma. However, differences in steroid degradation will interact with differences in secretion rate, and this may make the situation more difficult to interpret.

One of the functions of the adrenal is to secrete corticosteroids in response to stress. Thus, distinctions must be made between factors affecting the resting level of steroids in plasma and those affecting the size and duration of responses to stress. The following sections deal with some of the genetic variation affecting corticosteroid levels in mice, rats, and domestic animals.

A. Mice

1. C57 Black and DBA

In 1964 Levine and Treiman[48] described marked differences between male mice of four strains in their plasma corticosterone levels following an electric shock. C57BL/10J mice had a large and prolonged rise in corticosteroid levels, while the rise in DBA/2J mice was small and of shorter duration. These observations fitted with earlier reports that C57BR and C57BL/6 males showed a dramatic fall in the numbers of circulating eosinophils after handling.[49,50] Handling did not affect mice of other strains, including DBA/1, in this way. Indications that the explanation of the differences in stress response would be complex were given by the finding that cortisone produced eosinopenia in adrenalectomized C57 mice at much lower doses than in adrenalectomized mice of other strains.[49] The levels of hepatic tyrosine aminotransferase, an enzyme induced by corticosteroids, were increased by fasting in C57BL/6J mice but not in DBA/2J mice.[51]

Later studies have confirmed that the stress-induced rise in corticosterone concentration above resting levels is greater in C57BL/10J than in DBA/2J,[52,53] even when the stressor used was an injection of saline.[32] In a study in which the control values for plasma corticosterone were higher than those usually reported, reciprocal F1 males had responses that were similar to those of their maternal strains.[52] This could be due to sex-linked genes, to positive maternal effects, or to both.

The resting level of corticosterone in C57BL males was similar to[32,48,54] or slightly lower than[53] that in DBA males. Corticosterone breakdown was investigated to see if its rate differed between the strains. Unexpectedly, it was found to be more efficient in C57BL/10J and C57BL/6J mice than in mice of other strains.[55,56] This implies the existence of large differences in steroid output between C57 and DBA males. The adrenal weights of C57 and DBA are very similar,[57-59] although one study[3] found that C57BL/10J had smaller adrenals than DBA/1J. The adrenal weights of reciprocal F1 mice differed.[3] A positive maternal effect would seem to have been present, since both female and male F1 mice resembled the maternal strain. When adrenal slices were incubated in vitro with ACTH, adrenals from C57BL/10J males produced more corticosterone than adrenals from DBA/2J males.[32] Adrenals from reciprocal F1 males produced similar, intermediate, amounts of corticosterone per milligram of tissue.[37] Suspensions of C57BL/Tb adrenal cells which had been enzymically dissociated[60] produced more corticosterone than those of DBA/2J cells.[61] The cells from F1 males showed a tendency to resemble those of their maternal strain.

The microscopic appearance of the adrenals of mice in the two strains differs. The nuclei of the zona fasciculata are larger in DBA/2J than in C57BL/6J.[62] The adrenal cortex of most strains of mice, including C57BL, stains strongly with fat stains like Sudan. The adrenals of DBA do not.[32,34] The phenotype of unstressed F1 mice depends on the way that sudanophilia is scored. They are either intermediate[37,63] or like C57.[64,65] Backcross to DBA mice showed increased variance[37] and apparent bimodality.[65] Unstressed backcross to C57 mice all had strongly sudanophilic adrenals.[64,65] Unstressed F2 mice[64] showed a pattern of results compatible with a single locus controlling lipid depletion. Crosses of DBA/2J with the phenotypically identical AKR/J strain, which carries the adrenal lipid depletion allele, *ald*, showed that DBA must carry an allele at a different locus.[37] This locus should be designated *ald-2*.

The difference in sudanophilia is a reflection of the five- to sevenfold differences in the amount of esterified cholesterol stored in the glands.[32,37,59] All esters of cholesterol are affected, but the most striking difference, a 12-fold one, is in the concentration of cholesteryl adrenate (C22:4).[66] The acute stimulation of adrenals in vivo with large doses of ACTH depleted the cholesterol ester stores of DBA/2J males, but not those of C57BL/10J.[67] Some chronically stressed C57BL/6J and C57 × DBA F1 males had lipid-depleted adrenals.[64]

Corticosterone output by adrenal slices[37] and disaggregated cells[68] from genetically heterogeneous hybrids was more variable than the output of adrenal tissue from either strain. This suggests that genes affecting the specific activity of cortical cells were segregating. The strong correlation found across the strains between cholesterol ester content and corticosterone output was found to be greatly reduced in backcross mice.[37] Thus, there must be at least two differences between C57 and DBA, one affecting the storage of cholesterol esters and the other the output of corticosterone. The possibility that part of the difference in output may lie within the adrenal cells is suggested by the lesser response of DBA/2J cells to ACTH.[61] Despite the similarity in adrenal weight, the differences in adrenal output may be due to acute or long-term differences in stimulation by ACTH. The interpretation of the observation[32] that 100 mU of ACTH produced a larger rise in plasma corticosterone in DBA/2J males than in C57BL/10J males is difficult, given the absence of any dose-response data and the existence of the difference in steroid degradation. Three hours after the injection of a smaller dose of ACTH, plasma corticosterone levels were higher in C57BL/6J mice than in DBA/1J mice.[54]

It is possible that the difference between C57 and DBA mice is at least partly due to differences in the perception of stimuli as stressful. Most investigators have used a fixed period of foot-shock and assumed that this represented a standard stress. However, DBA mice actively avoid foot-shocks by jumping into the air. C57BL/6J mice accumulated 50 μAsec of charge in 1.7 sec while DBA/2J mice took 3.6 sec.[64] The F1 mice took 2.5 sec. Although the shock actually received by the mice may have been equalized, other differences may have been introduced into the stressful situation. DBA mice are intolerant of ethanol while C57BL mice prefer to drink 10% ethanol rather than water.[69] When an injection of alcohol was used as a stressor, the rise in plasma corticosterone was much larger and more prolonged in DBA/2J than in C57BL/6J.[70] Experiments in which plasma ACTH levels were measured would be very helpful in tracking down the sites of action of the genes which differentiate DBA and C57.

The adrenals of DBA mice become depleted of lipid at puberty.[37] Lipid repletion can be brought about by castration and depletion by the injection of testosterone.[37] All esters of cholesterol are affected, most particularly cholesteryl adrenate.[66] The plasma corticosterone rise following stress was significantly greater in castrated DBA/2 males than in sham-operated or intact males.[53] Adrenal sudanophilia,[63,71] cholesterol ester stores,[66] and the stress-induced rise in corticosterone[53] are effectively unaffected in C57BL males either by castration or by testosterone. Even daily injections of 2.5 mg of testosterone produced only a very small decrease in the sudanophilia of castrated C57BL/TbO males.[71] Several other systems in C57 mice are relatively insensitive to testosterone.[72-74]

Relatively little is known about differences in the adrenocortical function of C57 and DBA females. Differences in sudanophilia are less marked,[63] and interpretations are complicated by the presence of estrus cycles and an X-zone whose development differs between the strains (Section II). Treiman et al.[52] found that stress induced a much greater rise in plasma corticosterone level in DBA/2J females than in C57BL/10J females. Control levels of corticosterone were, however, very high. Diez et al.,[75] using litters of mixed sex, found that the rise in plasma corticosterone after stress was higher in DBA/1Bg than in C57BL/10Bg between the ages of 20 and 30 days. Surgical stress greatly increased the resistance of C57BL/6J females, but not DBA/2J females, to 650 rads of radiation.[76] The cholesterol ester stores of C57BL/10J females, but not those of DBA/2J females, can be altered by castration and then normalized by the injection of estrogen.[66]

2. Lipid Depletion in AKR

Adrenal lipid depletion in adult AKR mice is caused by homozygosity for the *ald* allele,[35] at a locus on chromosome 1 close to the dipeptidase, *Dip-1*, locus.[77] AC strain mice, which were derived from a cross of the AKR and WLO strains, are homozygous for *ald*. They do not suffer from the lethal leukemia typical of AKR mice, showing that homozygosity for *ald* is not a sufficient cause of such leukemia.[36] The lipid-depleted cortex of *ald ald* mice has very low levels of esterified cholesterol[37,59] and lacks the vesicles in which it is stored.[36]

Lipid depletion occurs at puberty, at the same time as X-zone involution and changes in the seminiferous tubules in males.[78] It can be prevented or reversed by castration.[35] Injections of 12.5 μg of testosterone were sufficient to cause depletion of the cholesterol esters stored in the adrenals of castrated *ald ald* mice.[71] The corticosterone output of adrenals of *ald ald* mice stimulated with ACTH was the same as that of normal mice before puberty, but less than normal after puberty, both in vivo and in vitro.[79] The corticosterone response to stress of AKR/J mice was slightly less than that of DBA/2J,[48] and resting levels of corticosterone were very low.[54]

Hypophysectomy leads to repletion of the cortex, presumably by stopping the endogenous secretion of testosterone. ACTH treatment of such hypophysectomized *ald ald* mice slightly reduced the sudanophilia of their adrenals.[80] Studies on adrenal weight,[81] cortical nuclear morphology,[82] and corticosterone output[79] did not, however, support the idea of hypersecretion of ACTH in intact *ald ald* mice. No studies of the relation between cholesterol ester stores and corticosterone output have been made in hybrid mice segregating for *ald*, in contrast to those on mice segregating for *ald-2*.[37]

Personal observations on some of the adrenals from the AKR-CBA chimeras studied by Tuffrey et al.[83] suggested that the patch size for the lipid-depletion phenotype was equal to the size of the whole cortex. If the cortex is multiclonal in origin, as suggested by observations using β-glucuronidase as a marker,[84] this implies that the primary site of action of *ald* is not in the cortical cells themselves.

3. Other Inbred Strains

BALB/c males had resting levels of corticosterone about twice those of C57BL/6 males, both in the By[85] and J sublines.[54,70] Plasma levels were higher in BALB/c than in C3H, both when unstressed[86] and after 15 min in an open field situation.[87] Even 3 hr after an injection of ACTH, the plasma corticosterone level was three times its resting value in BALB/cJ mice.[54]

Measurements on backcrosses and recombinant inbred strains produced by crossing the BALB/cBy and C57BL/6By strains suggested that variation at two loci, *Cpl-1* and *Cpl-2*, was most likely.[85] One locus might be involved with corticosterone breakdown, since this appeared to be relatively inefficient in BALB/cJ mice.[56] Several observations suggest that pituitary feedback relations may be altered in BALB/c mice. Corticosterone levels were not completely suppressed by dexamethasone administration.[86] Cold stress reduced the plasma corticosterone levels in BALB/cJ, but elevated them in C57BL/10J.[88] The finding of larger spleens in BALB/cJ mice than in C57BL/10J indicates that there may be differences in the sensitivity of target tissues to corticosteroids.[89] Even after adrenalectomy, significant amounts of corticosterone remained in circulation.[86] This may have been a consequence of the high frequency of accessory adrenal nodules in BALB/c.[2]

Differences within the adrenal cells themselves may also exist between BALB mice and mice of other strains. Metopirone, which blocks steroid biosynthesis, reduced plasma corticosterone levels to zero in C3H but not in BALB/c mice.[86] The difference may lie in the metabolism of the injected metopirone or in the effectiveness of this inhibitor in BALB/c adrenal cells. BALB/c adrenals, ulike C3H adrenals, seem to have the capacity to produce cortisol and 11-dehydrocorticosterone as well as corticosterone.[90]

Differences within the adrenal cells must also underlie variation in the proportions of different corticosteroids synthesized in vitro from progesterone. CBA/FaCam and SF/Cam mice synthesized more of a compound identified as 11-deoxycortisol than corticosterone, while A/Cam mice synthesized less.[91] Relatively high production of corticosterone was inherited as an autosomal dominant. The specific activity of the adrenal cells differed between the three strains.[41] Both compounds were found, in appropriate ratios, in peripheral plasma from mice of the three strains.[92] The situation would closely resemble that found in rats by Rapp and Dahl,[23] if the alternative to corticosterone were 18-hydroxycorticosterone (Section III.B.1).

Strain differences in plasma corticosterone levels whose sites of action are unknown have been reported between SJL/J and C57BL/10J[38] and between nonagouti males of the YS/Wf and VY/Wf strains.[93] The output of corticosterone per milligram of adrenal tissue in response to ACTH was greater for tissue from wild mice and laboratory-fostered wild mice than for tissue from "Swiss Wistar" mice.[13] Genetic variation in the adrenal cortex does not always lead to differences in steroid production. CBA and Peru mice, which differ at the *ezg* locus, had identical plasma levels and synthesis rates of aldosterone.[94,95]

4. Hyperfunctional Mutants

Lethargic, *lh*, is an autosomal recessive whose effects first show around the age of 15 days when homozygotes develop abnormalities of gait and balance.[96] Around this age, hyperplasia of the adrenal develops, the cortex becomes partially depleted of lipid, and the corticosterone levels in plasma rise much above those in normal sibs.[96,97] Many lethargic mice die around this age. After this age, survivors have lower than normal corticosterone levels, even though their adrenals are still enlarged. The marked thymic involution found in homozygotes appears to be a consequence of adrenocortical hyperfunction. Thymic involution is retarded and the chances of survival are increased if lethargic mice are hemiadrenalectomized before they are 15 days old.[97] Both the adrenal and the behavioral alterations could be pleiotropic effects of a primary action within the hypothalamic region.

Obese, *ob*, and diabetic, *db*, mice show signs of hyperfunction of the adrenal cortex. In obese mice the adrenal glands are enlarged.[45,98,99] Plasma levels of corticosterone were elevated[100] even though the pool size for tritiated corticosterone was enlarged.[101] Similarly, older diabetic mice had larger adrenals, and higher corticosterone levels, than their normal sibs.[102] While the adrenals play some role in the development of the full syndrome, as shown by the reduced insulin resistance of adrenalectomized *db* mice,[103] most of the adrenocortical changes are probably secondary. The in vitro responses of adrenal tissue are the same on a per milligram basis in obese and normal mice.[104] The 14-fold elevation in pituitary ACTH in fat *ob ob* mice can be normalized, along with body weight, by restricting food intake.[99] It is possible that the radioimmunoassays used measured different mixtures of hormone, prohormone,[105] and fragments.[106,107]

The yellow mutations A^y and A^{vy} cause mice to become fat, but have only secondary[108] or marginal[93] effects on adrenocrotical function.

B. Rats

1. Hypertensive Strains

Rat strains differ in their susceptibility to hypertension. Hypertension can easily be induced in many lines of Sprague-Dawley rats by treatment with 11-deoxycorticosterone (DOC), a high sodium diet, or by unilateral nephrectomy.[109-115] One line of CD Sprague-Dawleys was resistant to the combined effects of a high salt diet and nephrectomy.[110] Long-Evans rats are resistant to all three procedures, unless their regulation of sodium intake is overcome by adding sucrose to saline drinking water.[110,113,116] Long-Evans rats, as well as Sprague-Dawleys and some Wistars, develop hypertension during the adrenal regeneration which follows adrenal nucleation.[113,117] Adrenal hyperplasia after unilateral adrenalectomy was less in W/Fu Wistars than in Holtzman Sprague-Dawleys and was not accompanied by hypertension.[112,118] Genetic variation in susceptibility to adrenal regeneration hypertension is also suggested by the finding that some, but not all, of a genetically undefined colony of "Wistars" developed it after a standard surgical procedure.[119] Adrenal regeneration may involve neural signals, as well as hormonal ones, to and from the hypothalamus.[120] F344 rats are effectively resistant to DOC, saline, and nephrectomy, separately or in combination.[110,114-116] Their control over sodium intake does not break down when the saline is sweetened.[116] They are, however, susceptible to hypertension induced by renal disease[116] and to that induced by a tumor secreting ACTH, prolactin, and growth hormone.[111]

Dahl et al.[23,109] selected lines that were resistant to, and susceptible to, hypertension induced by a high salt diet from a single colony of Sprague-Dawleys. Biometric analysis suggested that four to six genes distinguished the lines. Variation at one locus accounted for about 16% of the difference in blood pressure between the lines. This locus controlled the relative amounts of 18-hydroxydeoxycorticosterone (18OH-DOC), an effective mineralocorticoid[119] whose production is not suppressed by a high sodium diet, and corticosterone synthesized from DOC.[23,122] In susceptible rats, homozygous for the high allele, almost 40% of DOC was 18-hydroxylated. The difference in the proportions of 18- and 11-hydroxylation between the homozygotes seems to be the result of structural differences in the cytochrome P450 common to both reactions.[123] Stress induced by experimental reward-punishment conflict induced hypertension much more rapidly in the susceptible line, presumably because it led to excessive secretion of 18OH-DOC.[124] The original Sprague-Dawley colony must have been polymorphic at the cytochrome locus, as were at least one colony of CD Sprague-Dawleys.[23] All the CFN Wistars and SHR rats tested were homozygous for the allele producing relatively high levels of 18OH-DOC.[23]

SHR rats are spontaneously hypertensive and have larger adrenals than Wistars,[24,125] but produce less aldosterone, corticosterone, DOC, and 18OH-DOC per milligram of adrenal tissue,[125] which contains less cytochrome P450.[126] Since SHR rats also have disturbances of thyroid function[125] and prostaglandin metabolism,[128] the relationship between the adrenal changes and hypertension is unclear.

2. Other Rat Strains

As well as the differences between strains in the production of 18OH-DOC described above, there are differences between the Wistar and Long-Evans strains in 17-hydroxylation during adrenal regeneration.[117,129] Testosterone production by adrenal tissue in vitro varied over a fivefold range when Wistars, Listers, and Sprague-Dawleys were compared.[130] These strains also differed in the rate of production of corticosterone in vitro. Wistars produced the least amounts of both steroids. Adrenals from Sprague-Dawleys had the highest rate of corticosterone production, while those from Listers produced the most testosterone.[130] In vivo Sprague-Dawleys that were probably a different stock showed the least response to ether stress. Lister rats had the heaviest adrenals, the large response to exogenous ACTH, and the greatest response to ether stress.[131] Comparison of the in vivo and in vitro findings suggests that there may be differences in corticosteroid degradation between these strains. Wistar rats had small adrenals and a proportionately lesser response to ACTH.[131] Wild rats were much less responsive to exogenous ACTH than were a different stock of Wistars.[132] Rats selected for emotional reactivity had larger adrenals and greater stores of esterified cholesterol, but lower plasma corticosterone levels and greater numbers of eosinophils, than rats selected for unreactivity.[133]

C. Domestic Animals

Even though very marked differences have been found between breeds of dogs in pituitary and thyroid morphology,[134] there appears to be only one report on breed differences in adrenal function. Boston terriers appear to be unusually susceptible to a canine equivalent of Cushing's syndrome.[135] Four inbred strains of rabbit were found to have differences in levels of corticosterone at rest, after ACTH injections, and after pituitary suppression with dexamethasone.[54]

The adrenals of Africander cattle contain twice as much esterified cholesterol as those of Brahman cattle.[136] Significant sire effects were found in a study of the effects of transport stress on plasma corticosteroids in Holstein cattle.[137] A heritability of 82% has been found in longhorn cattle for the rise in plasma corticosteroids 2 hr after the injection of ACTH.[138]

The porcine stress syndrome (PSS) is characterized by malignant hyperthermia, electrolyte disturbances, dyspnea, and muscle tremor after exercise or stress.[139] It is often fatal. Pig breeds differ in their susceptibility to PSS. Dense lipid-staining masses were found in the adrenals of Poland-China swine, which are susceptible to PSS.[140] Breed differences in corticosteroid levels exist, but are not related to susceptibility.[141,142] High plasma clearance rates for corticosteroids were found in susceptible pigs.[139] The rise in plasma corticosteroids after an injection of ACTH was less in susceptible pigs than in resistant ones,[143] even though plasma levels of ACTH were very high in susceptible pigs.[141] These measurements were made by radioimmunoassay, and so different proportions of the different sizes of ACTH may be present in the two phenotypes.[105] Evidence for the basic disturbance in PSS being within the hypothalamus comes from the finding that dexamethasone will suppress plasma ACTH levels in resistant pigs, but not in susceptible ones.[143] Further support for a central cause of PSS is given by the finding that susceptibility can be predicted by rapid, adverse reactions to halothane anesthesia. Halothane susceptibility is inherited as an autosomal recessive.[144] The allele frequency varies from 1.0 in Dutch and 0.8 in French Pietrains to 0.0 in Durocs and French Large Whites.[144] The correlation of PSS with H blood group alleles may be due to linkage or to pleiotropy.[145] A possible homologue may exist in human populations.[146]

Turkeys have been successfully selected for high and low corticosterone responses to cold stress.[147] Correlated responses were found in the steroid responses to heat stress and to exogenous ACTH. The low line showed favorable correlated responses in a number of economic characteristics. These included weight gain, egg production, docility, and resistance to *Mycoplasma meleagridis.* Chickens have been selected for high and low responses to injected ACTH.[148] The line relatively unresponsive to ACTH also showed a lesser response to heat stress. No analyses have yet been made on segregating stocks produced by crossing the high and low lines of either chickens or turkeys.

IV. DEGRADATION AND TRANSPORT

A. Steroid Catabolism

The metabolic clearance of corticosteroids is increased in pigs with PSS, but the enzymes affected are not yet known (Section III.C). Strain differences in the breakdown of corticosteroids by the liver are known in guinea pigs, rats, and mice. The difference between Hartley strain guinea pigs and those of strains 2 and 13 was mainly in the 2α-hydroxylation of cortisol. The rate of 2α-hydroxylation was seven times higher in the strain 2 and 13 guinea pigs.[149] The elevated levels of cortisol found by Whipp et al.[150] in their strain of guinea pigs could have been due to an alteration of hepatic hydroxylation. The livers of FW49 rats have much more Δ^4-5α-reductase activity, and much less steroid hydroxylase activity, than the livers of SpD/UL rats.[151] As well as alterations in the metabolic clearance rates of steroids, these differences will lead to differences in the proportions of the various metabolites. Threefold differences in steroid sulfatases have been demonstrated between a pair of rat strains.[152]

The degradative reduction of corticosterone is much less dependent on an exogenous supply of NADPH in C57BL mice than it is in mice of other strains, including DBA/2, BALB/c, and AC.[55,56] Differences in the apparent affinity of the enzymes for NADP, and in the hepatic levels of NADPH generating dehydrogenases, may, together or separately, underlie the differences in steroid reduction.[63] The extent of the difference between C57BL/10ScSn and DBA/2J mice depends on their diet. The difference is most marked after the mice have been on a fat-free diet for 3 days.[153] This procedure increased the levels of NADPH-generating dehydrogenases in the C57 mice as expected,[154] but produced a slight, but unexpected, fall in their levels in DBA. The F1 hybrids resembled their C57 parents in their response to the fat-free diet. Segregating backcross mice have not been used to analyze the situation.

The differences in reductive capacity could be consequences of the differences between C57 and DBA mice in thyroid function.[127] Alternatively they could be due to differences in the strains' responses to estrogen[66] or androgen (see Section III.B.1), since sex steroids are known to affect the pattern of steroid degradation in rats.[155]

Breakdown of corticosteroids also takes place within the adrenal cortex. 2α- and 6β-hydroxylation were found to be nine and seven times more active in strain 13 guinea pigs than in Hartley guinea pigs. Two apparent Kms for 2α-hydroxylation were found in guinea pigs with active intra-adrenal degradation, suggesting that there may be two different hydroxylase enzymes.[156] Plasma corticosterone levels are higher in *Tfm* rats than in normal male sibs.[157] The levels of adrenal 5α-reductase and 3β-hydroxysteroid dehydrogenase remain at the high levels found before puberty in normal sibs. Prolactin injections normalized these levels in *Tfm* rats and lowered the levels found in normal males and females.[158]

Differences in the pattern of ring A reduction of androgens have been found between the adrenal tissue of NH and LACA mice.[159] Reductive degradation of corticosterone was more active in homogenates of adrenals from C57BL/10ScSn mice than from DBA/2J mice.[63]

B. Binding Proteins

Differences in the plasma levels of corticosteroid-binding globulin (CBG) have been shown between strains of rats[131] and breeds of pigs.[142] In man the locus controlling variation in levels of CBG is on the X chromosome.[160] It would be interesting to see if it were also X-linked, by comparing reciprocal F1 males, in other species of mammals, given the strong evidence for the conservation of sex-linked genes in evolution.[161]

V. TROPHIC INFLUENCES

A. ACTH

Some genetic variation affecting the degree of stimulation by, and responsiveness to, ACTH has already been described in earlier sections. Guernsey[162] and Holstein-Friesian[163] cattle with inherited pituitary hypoplasia completely lack ACTH. The resultant adrenocortical aplasia leads to prolonged gestation of homozygous fetuses, since corticosteroids are important in the initiation of parturition. No deficiencies of corticotropin releasing factor or monotropic deficiencies of ACTH are known. Similarly, there is no evidence yet for differences in the amino acid sequence of ACTH within a species, although there are differences between species.

ACTH, MSH, the endorphins, and the enkephalins all seem to be derived from a common precursor protein.[164] Endorphins are produced in equimolar proportions to ACTH, and production of both molecules is suppressed by dexamethasone.[165] Some of the genetic differences in the suppressibility of ACTH levels by dexamethasone (see Sections III.A.1 and 3 and III.C) might be consequences of differences in the systems controlling endorphin production. This might also be true for the differences in the effect of dexamethasone on the acquisition of passive avoidance responses in A/J and DBA/2J mice.[166]

Some of the complexities of studying the control of ACTH release are shown by the way that the size of the stress response depends greatly on the circumstances of the test. A/J mice showed stress responses as large as those of C57BL mice when kept in a novel environment,[48] but not when returned to their home cage after a short exposure to stress.[167] Ketamine stimulates ACTH release by influencing aminergic transmission.[168] The interpretation of strain differences in the plasma corticosterone response to ketamine in mice (twofold) and rabbits (threefold)[54] is complicated by the possibility of differences in adrenal responsiveness to ACTH and in the metabolic clearance of corticosterone.

Evidence for strain differences in the average levels of effectiveness of ACTH comes from two kinds of observations on mice. Homozygosity for *ezg* causes Peru mice to have an indistinct zona glomerulosa. A similar histological appearance can be produced in the adrenals of CBA mice by treatment with ACTH.[31] There was a wide zona glomerulosa in the adrenals of Peru mice treated with sufficient dexamethasone to cause a marked reduction of the zona fasciculata.[31] Peru mice have relatively large adrenals, but the correlation between zona glomerulosa width and adrenal weight disappeared when mice of the backcrosses to CBA and Peru were measured.[169] This implies that these two parameters are affected by different functions of plasma ACTH level. ACTH produces premature collapse of the X-zone in female mice.[31] The X-zone of Peru females, though large, normally collapses[41] as does that of C57BL females.[57,170] Other evidence suggesting that C57 mice may have higher average levels of ACTH is described in Section III.A.1.

B. Prolactin

The adrenal X-zone in mice is controlled by the pituitary and involutes after hypophysectomy.[171] Pituitary dwarf mice have no X-zone (see Section II), but do have a zona fasciculata of normal size.[172] This suggests that ACTH is not the trophic hormone for the X-zone, substantiated by the following observations. The X-zone remained intact when ACTH production was suppressed by dexamethasone in Peru and CBA mice.[31] Administration of ACTH to females of these strains induced involution of their X-zones,[31] as did increased population density.[173] Variation in the volume of the zona fasciculata, dependent on ACTH, and in the volume of the X-zone were not correlated when mice of three strains were compared.[174] The percentage of the adrenal cortex occupied by the X-zone varied from 15 to 55% between strains.[174,175] Chester-Jones[171] maintained the X-zones of hypophysectomized mice with injections of a pituitary extract rich in gonadotropins. If a gonadotropin were the trophic hormone for the X-zone, then the zone should be present in the adrenals of dwarf mice since these do not lack gonadotropins,[176,177] only prolactin and growth hormone. Furthermore, the X-zones are intact in male and female hypogonadic, *hyp*, mice which lack gonadotropin-releasing factor,[178] but not prolactin or growth hormone. SJL females have a large X-zone which involutes late in life. They also have many prolactin cells in their pituitaries.[38] In rats, both *Tfm*[158] and normal males and females,[179] prolactin affects the reduction of steroids within the adrenal cortex. 20α-Hydroxysteroid dehydrogenase is restricted to the X-zone of adult female adrenals in mice of several strains[63,180,181] and is absent after testosterone treatment.[180] Prolactin levels are less in males than in females, and the X-zone involutes earlier in males. Prolactin levels are reduced in female rodents during the first part of pregnancy, which would coincide with the involution of the zone at this time. Secondary X-zones appear in males after castration and after estrogen treatment in some strains,[182] as does 20α-hydroxysteroid dehydrogenase activity.[180] A reappearance of the X-zone during lactation has been reported in one colony of mice.[183] It is also intriguing that Peru mice, which have very large X-zones, show very marked maternal behavior,[63] which may also be dependent on prolactin.[184] Nest building ability was correlated with X-zone size over three strains,[185,186] but the correlation was not tested on segregating generations.

Studies on the X-zones of pygmy (*pg*) mice (which seem to be insensitive to growth hormone),[187] little (*lit*) mice (which are deficient in prolactin),[188] and torpid (*td*) mice (which may be)[189] would be interesting.

C. Sex Steroids

In C57BL/10J mice, but not in DBA/2J mice, the presence of ovaries or the administration of estrogens causes cholesterol esters to accumulate in the adrenal cortex.[66] Chronic estrogen treatment increased the adrenal weights of males of four strains. The responses of females differed. Hypertrophy occurred in C57BL and BALB/c. There was a fall in the relative weight of the adrenals of A/He mice and no change in the weight of those of C3H/He mice.[182] Estrogen treatment enhanced the onset of ceroid deposition ("brown degeneration") in all except the C3H mice.

Castration affects the adrenocortical function of males. It resulted in a greater rise in plasma corticosterone in YS/Wf males than in VY/Wf males.[93] Alterations in testosterone levels, whether upwards or downwards, have very marked effects on the adrenals of mice like AKR and DBA which are homozygous for the *ald* or *ald-2* genes (see Sections III.A.1 and 2).

X-zone involution occurs rapidly at puberty in males and can be induced in intact mice by relatively large doses of testosterone.[190] It is not yet established whether the steroid acts directly on the cells of the X-zone or indirectly. Mice with testicular feminization (*Tfm*/Y) had X-zones which underwent fatty degeneration,[191] showing that conventional sensitivity to testosterone is not essential for this process. However, involution occurred later than in sibling *Tfm*/+ and +/+ females. Perhaps in females testosterone influences the withdrawal of trophic support for the X-zone.

D. Renin and Angiotensin

Angiotensin, which plays a part in the regulation of aldosterone, is cleaved from its precursor by renin. Mice selected for high juxtaglomerular granularity (JGI) had higher renin concentrations in their kidneys than mice from the low JGI line.[18] CD rats selectively bred for high JGI had higher renal and plasma renin activity (PRA), but lower blood pressure, than the rats of the corresponding low JGI line.[192] The low JGI rats secreted less aldosterone[193] and carried the allele for high 18OH-DOC production.[194] It is not clear whether the renin differences are secondary to the mineralocorticoid differences or are caused by separable genes. Sprague-Dawley rats selectively bred for spontaneous hypertension had higher PRA than those from the line with normal blood pressure.[195] PRA is higher in F344 rats than in Sprague-Dawleys[115] and is higher in DBA/2J mice than in BALB/c.[196]

Renin is also found in the submaxillary glands of mice. The largest amounts were found in males of the NZB strain and SSI colony. DBA mice had intermediate amounts while CBA and BALB mice had very little.[196] The concentration of renin in the submaxillary glands of SWR/J mice was 100 times that in the glands of C57BL/10J mice. This was true for untreated males and for males injected with 5-dihydrotestosterone. The difference between these two strains is controlled by variation at a single autosomal locus. Heterozygotes are intermediate.[197]

The strength of the angiotensin signal to adrenal tissue depends not only on the concentration of renin but also on the level of the angiotensinogen substrate. This differed between strains.[196] The rise in angiotensinogen concentration which took place after nephrectomy was much greater in DBA/2J mice than in NZB mice.[196]

The vasculature of NZ genetically hypertensive rats is more responsive to exogenous angiotensin than are the blood vessels of normotensive controls.[198] It is not known whether there is also a difference in the responsiveness of adrenal tissue.

E. Abnormal Function

Pituitary and adrenal hyperplasia follow neonatal castration in the BALB/c, CBA, CE, C3H, DBA, H, NH, and Z strains.[46,199] A, C57BL, C57BR, F, and ICRC mice do not develop hyperplasia of either the pituitary or adrenal.[199,200] Hyperplastic adrenals from BALB/c mice produce androgens, while those from DBA and CE mice produce estrogens. Those from CBA and C3H synthesize both estrogens and androgens.[46] The hyperplastic adrenals become neoplastic in CE and NH mice.[199] Adrenocortical carcinoma occurs at a high freqency in intact Osborne-Mendel rats.[201]

VI. TARGET ORGANS

A. Whole Tissues

There is evidence for genetic variation affecting the corticosteroid receptor systems of rats and mice. Fewer receptors specific for DOC were found in the hypothalamus of Long-Evans rats than in the same region of the brain in Sprague-Dawleys.[202] Measurements on appropriate hybrids could test whether this difference was causally related to the resistance of Long-Evans rats to salt-induced hypertension (Section III.B.1). Measurements of the binding of DOC in the hypothalamus of W/Fu rats would be interesting since these rats had high plasma levels of DOC during adrenal regeneration, but did not become hypertensive.[118]

Injections of aldosterone caused sodium retention in CBA/FaCam mice but not in Peru mice. Aldosterone did, however, stimulate potassium excretion in mice of both strains, but to a much lesser extent in CBA.[203] Peru mice, unlike mice of CBA and other strains, were resistant to spironolactone, an antagonist of type I, aldosterone-specific, corticosteroid binding.[204] The nuclear binding of tritiated aldosterone was twice as great in kidney tissue from CBA mice as in tissue from Peru mice.[203] The F1 mice resembled their Peru parents in both the physiological effects of aldosterone and in the low level of nuclear binding. The correlation between total aldosterone binding and urinary electrolyte output did not hold for backcross to CBA mice. The correlation between the type of nuclear binding, defined by its relative resistance to KC1 extraction, and the type of electrolyte response did, however, hold.[203] This implies that aldosterone may have two separable actions; one on sodium retention mediated by type I receptors and another one on potassium excretion.

Variation in the response to exogenous hormone is not necessarily caused by differences in the target organs being studied.[169] The sites of action of the genetic differences in the hormonal and behavioral responses to dexamethasone, described in Sections III and V, are unknown and could be either peripheral or central. Differences between strains[205] and selected lines[206] of rats in the frequency of stomach ulceration may well have been secondary to differences in the output of corticosteroids. Corticosteroids increase the levels of duodenal alkaline phosphatase activity. Differences between AKR and DBA mice in the activity of this enzyme[207] could have been due to differences in its inducibility since both strains produce relatively low amounts of corticosterone (Section III.A.1 and 2).

The relatively strong eosinopenic effect of cortisone in C57BL mice[49] cannot have been due to reduced degradation of exogenous steroid. Studies on congenic pairs of strains have suggested that increased sensitivity of a subpopulation of thymocytes, in vivo and in culture, was associated with the *H-2a* histocompatibility haplotype.[208] Low doses of dexamethasone caused a paradoxical[209] increase in the incorporation of thymidine by cells from the mesenteric lymph node of CBA/FaCam mice, but not by those from C57BL/Tb or DBA/2J mice.[65]

B. Cells in Culture

Stable variants of established cell-culture lines can be isolated by selective procedures, which may involve exposure to mutagens. S49 mouse lymphoma cells are usually killed by corticosteroids, but several lines have been selected which were resistant to dexamethasone.[210] Most of these lines had lost the ability to bind dexamethasone specifically and with high affinity. Similar r^- variants have been obtained from W7 thymoma cells[211] and L929 fibroblasts.[212] Normal amounts of dexamethasone were bound by the cytoplasm of some resistant lines of S49. These variants could be divided into those in which the nuclear transfer of steroid was absent (nt^-) or increased (nt^i) and those in which it was normal but the cells remained alive (deathless, d^-).[213] Complementation tests, carried out by fusing cells of two different resistant lines, showed that r^-, nt^-, and nt^i variants did not complement. They may, thus, all have had altered receptor molecules. Indeed, the receptors from nt^i lines had a molecular weight half that of wild-type receptors and an axial ratio of 4:1 instead of the usual 8:1. The binding characteristics of *nt⁻* and *ntⁱ* receptors to DNA-cellulose columns also differed and may have accounted for their different concentrations within the nucleus.[213] Resistant *d⁻* lines had wild-type receptor molecules. Complementation tests on several *d⁻* lines might reveal several classes, corresponding to variants with defects in locus-specific recognition or lesions in the individual steps of the suicide pathway. W7 cells contained twice the concentration of receptor molecules found in S49 cells, and resistant clones arose at 1000th of the rate found for S49 cells.[211] These observations, together with the recessiveness of the *r⁻* phenotype in hybrid cells, suggest that the S49 cells may be functionally haploid at the receptor locus. This raises the question of whether the second copy of the structural locus for the receptor protein has been lost or deleted or whether it has been permanently inactivated. In normal lymphoid cells, allelic exclusion limits the expression of immunoglobin loci to those coded for one haploid set of DNA.[214]

Tyrosine aminotransferase (TAT) can be induced with dexamethasone in HTC rat hepatoma cells. Variant clones have been isolated in which TAT was not inducible. Some were *r⁻*,[215] while others had normal amounts of receptor and must have been blocked in later stages of enzyme induction.[216] Mouse 3T3 cells in which arylhydrocarbon hydroxylase (AHH) but not TAT was inducible were fused with *r⁻* HTC cells. TAT inducibility was recessive while AHH inducibility was dominant.[217] TAT inducibility reappeared in a hybrid clone after it had lost more than one third of its chromosomes,[218] suggesting that the genes concerned could be mapped by chromosome-loss methods.[219]

Pituitary cell lines[220-223] in which the synthesis of growth hormone can be induced by glucocorticoids may provide another promising system for analyzing the mechanism of action of corticosteroids.

C. Multiorganism Situations

1. Fetal Systems

The frequency with which fetal abnormality or death follows the administration of a standard dose of corticosteroids to the mother varies between strains. The most reliable information comes from studies in which the responses to a range of doses have been observed. There are several sites at which differences in response to exogenous hormone could arise. There are likely to be differences in maternal metabolism, producing differences in the level of hormone to which the feto-placental unit is exposed. There may be differences in the metabolism of the hormone by the placenta and by the fetus. There may also be differences between fetuses in the responsiveness of individual target tissues. The gene loci involved may be different in the mother and in the fetus, even when the fetus has exactly the same genotype as its mother. The situation becomes even more complex in hybrid pregnancies, in which fetal and maternal genotypes differ. Attempts to partition the variation in susceptibility between mother and offspring have been of two kinds. In the first, the susceptibility of fetuses with the same genotype, but from uterine mothers of different genotype, have been compared. In the second, the susceptibility of genetically different fetuses raised in the same maternal environment have been compared.

Cleft palate can be induced in A/J mice with a low dose of corticosteroids, while the median effective dose is much higher in CBA/J and C57BL mice. Studies on the susceptibility of reciprocal F1 female fetuses, which have the identical genotypes but different maternal environments, have shown that there were maternal effects in both the A × CBA[224] and A × C57BL/6 crosses.[225] The A maternal environment increased the susceptibility of the F1 fetuses. Unsexed fetuses of the reciprocal F1 crosses between the congenic strains C57BL/10ScSn and B10.A showed that the B10.A maternal environment increased the frequency of cleft palate.[226] In all cases there was also evidence for a contribution of fetal genotype to susceptibility. However, when blastocysts were transferred between A and CBA mice, the susceptibility of the transferred embryos was unaffected,[224] implying that the maternal effect occurred before implantation, perhaps through the cytoplasm of the egg.

In two studies, observations have been made on backcross fetuses, compared within standard maternal environments. Francis[227] found evidence for sex-linked, as well as autosomal, factors influencing differences in fetal susceptibility. Biddle and Fraser,[225,228] who also compared A/J with C57BL/6J but used a different treatment protocol, could find no evidence from the comparison of male and female reciprocal F1 hybrids for sex-linked genes affecting fetal susceptibility. They did, however, show that at least two autosomal loci controlled the responsiveness of the fetus. A factor increasing the frequency of cleft palate appeared to be linked to the *H-2a* histocompatibility allele. This would fit with the observations of higher frequencies of cleft palate in B10.A mice, which have the *H-2a* allele like A/J mice, compared with their congenic strain C57BL/10ScSn. The possible association of the *H-2a* haplotype with the responsiveness of thymocytes to corticosteroids has already been described (Section VI.A).

There have been several studies that have attempted to sort out the physiological bases of the maternal and fetal differences. Increasing the amount of fat in the diet of C57BL/6J mice greatly increased their susceptibility to cleft palate induced by cortisone,[229] presumably by decreasing the maternal breakdown of corticosteroids (see Section IV.A). An interesting approach to partitioning susceptibility compared the effectiveness of steroids administered intramuscularly to the mother and intra-amniotically to the fetus.[230] Unfortunately, single different doses of different corticosteroids were administered by the two routes. More of a standard dose of cortisol given to the mother on day 11 of pregnancy was retained by A/J fetuses than by CBA/J fetuses.[231] On day 14[232] and on day 18,[233] the A fetuses retained more of a maternal injection of corticosterone than CBA fetuses. However, there was no difference in retention between A fetuses which had been transferred as blastocysts and CBA fetuses within the same CBA mother.[232] Thus, there was not only a maternal difference in the metabolism of corticosterone but also an embryonic difference that must lie within the target tissue rather than in the general metabolism of the fetus. Facial mesenchyme from A/J embryos bound about twice as much dexamethasone[234] and cortisone,[235] as did the same tissue from C57BL/6J mice. Three strains (A/J, DBA/1J and B.10A) with high levels of binding were all susceptible to cleft palate, while three strains (C57BL/6J, C57BL/10ScSn, and CBA/J) with low binding capacity were all relatively resistant. C3H/HeJ, with intermediate susceptibility to cleft palate, had intermediate amounts of binding protein.[235] There was some evidence for a difference in affinity between the A and C57BL receptors.[234] These findings also suggest an association of *H-2a* with fetal susceptibility, but non*H-2* loci must also be involved for both C3H and CBA are *H-2k*. The chromosomal region around *H-2* would also seem to be involved in the maternal differences between B10 and B10.A.[226]

The inbred strains which are susceptible to embryonic mortality induced by corticosteroids differ from those susceptible to cleft palate.[225,227] Strain differences in the incorporation into the fetus of maternal glucose in response to dexamethasone might be involved.[236] Corticosteroid-induced mortality might be the cause of the high preimplantation losses of BALB/cJ mice when stressed during pregnancy,[237] given the high plasma corticosterone levels in this strain (Section IV.A.3). Some mutations at the lid-gap locus, *lg*, can be repaired by injections of cortisone on day 15 of fetal life.[238] Discrepancies between different investigators[233,238,239] may have been caused by the use of different single doses of cortisone and by differences in the genetic backgrounds of the several alleles studied.

Studies on genetic variation affecting the role of corticosteroids in the initiation of labor and the maturation of fetal lung function[240] could be rewarding.

2. Virus Induction

A single injection of dexamethasone greatly increased the number of C-type virus particles in the pancreas of C57BL/6J and C57BL/He mice. Dexamethasone did not induce any such virus in C3H/fDp and BALB/c mice.[241] In crosses with BALB/c mice, inducibility was recessive and showed a 1:1 segregation in the backcross. It was dominant in F1 crosses with C3H mice.

The induction of mammary tumor virus (MTV) in cultured mammary cell lines seems to depend on corticosteroid receptors.[242-244] Differences in the level of cytoplasmic receptors were not the cause of differences in the amount of MTV produced per cell by different sublines of the C3H MT6 cell line.[245] In this system the possibility exists of altering the viral genome as well as modifying that of the host cell.

VII. FUTURE PROSPECTS

The previous sections show how much genetic variation within the range of normality there is that affects the production and metabolism of adrenal steroids. The study of the interaction of such genetic variation with environmental variation will become increasingly important. It will help us to understand the genetic basis of susceptibility to hypertension and other diseases induced by stress. Other environmental factors whose effects may depend on the genotype of the individual include diet and drugs. Knowledge of the genetics of adrenal function is already being applied in agriculture to improve economic traits by minimizing the consequences of stressful stimuli.

The proper study of the ecological consequences[246,247] of genetic variation in the endocrine responses to population density and other stresses has yet to begin. This is partly because of a lack of characters for which an individual's genotype can be determined, irrespective of its age or physiological state. Studies on polymorphisms are easiest when the genetic variants can be identified by differences in protein structure. Studies of the possible pleiotropic effects of alleles at polymorphic coat-color loci in species like the arctic fox,[8] domestic cat[248] and dog, horse, rat,[10] and mouse could be worthwhile.

Many of the strain differences described in this chapter are of a quantitative nature and need to be analyzed using recombinant inbred strains. The relationship between the genes responsible for such quantitative variation and those causing the enzyme defects found in the human population[1] will be of interest. The location of genes in one species may suggest possibilities for their location in other species.[161,249] Thus, the locus for transcortin might be sex linked in rodents as well as in man, and some of the genes concerned with corticosteroid receptors might be associated with the HLA region of the human chromosome.

Studies on variant cells in culture have revealed much about the receptor system for dexamethasone, and appropriate systems should tell us about the other corticosteroid receptors.[250,251] Understanding the control of the receptors and of their pattern of differentiation will, however, require a combination of somatic and meiotic analysis, using both cultured cells and whole organisms.

A recessively inherited homolog of lipoid adrenal hyperphasia, one of the inherited defects of corticosteroid biosynthesis in man, has recently been described in rabbits.[121]

REFERENCES

1. **Degenhart, H. J.,** Normal and abnormal adrenal steroidogenesis in man, in *Genetic Variation in Hormone Systems,* Vol. 1, Shire, J. G. M., Ed., CRC Press, Boca Raton, Fla., 1979, chap. 2.
2. **Hummel, K. P.,** Accessory adrenal cortical nodules in the mouse, *Anat. Rec.,* 132, 281, 1958.
3. **Meckler, R. J. and Collins, R. L.,** Histology and weight of the mouse adrenal: a diallel genetic study, *J. Endocrinol.,* 31, 95, 1965.
4. **Shire, J. G. M.,** Endocrine genetics of the adrenal gland, *J. Endocrinol.,* 62, 173, 1974.
5. **Chai, C. K. and Dickie, M. M.,** Endocrine variations, in *The Biology of the Laboratory Mouse,* 2nd ed., Green, E. L., Ed., McGraw-Hill, New York, 1966, 387.
6. **Crispens, C. G.,** *Handbook on the Laboratory Mouse,* Charles C Thomas, Springfield, Ill., 1975, 82.
7. **Schüler, L., Borodin, P. M., and Belyaev, D. K.,** Problems of stress genetics. II. Genetic analysis of relative weight of endocrine glands in normal and stressful conditions, *Genetika,* 12, 72, 1976.
8. **Keeler, C. E., Ridgway, S., Lipscomb, L., and Fromm, E.,** The genetics of adrenal size and tameness in colorphase foxes, *J. Hered.,* 59, 82, 1968.
9. **Mullen, R. J. and Hoornbeek, F. K.,** Genetic aspects of fertility and endocrine organ size in rats, *Genet. Res.,* 16, 251, 1971.
10. **Keeler, C. E.,** Modification of brain and endocrine glands, as an explanation of altered behavior trends, in coat-character mutant strains of the Norway Rat, *J. Tenn. Acad. Sci.,* 22, 202, 1947.
11. **Eaton, O. N.,** Weights and measurements of the parts and organs of mature inbred and crossbred guinea-pigs, *Am. J. Anat.,* 63, 273, 1938.
12. **Donaldson, J. C.,** Note on the weight of the adrenals in crosses between the albino and the wild Norway rat, *Proc. Soc. Exp. Biol. Med.,* 21, 157, 1924.
13. **Seabloom, R. W. and Seabloom, N. R.,** Response to ACTH by superfused adrenals of wild and domestic house mice, *Life Sci.,* 15, 73, 1975.
14. **Wegner, W.,** Zur biologischen Variation einiger quantitativfunktioneller Merkmale der Nebennieren, *Endokrinologie,* 58, 140, 1971.
15. **Badr, F. M. and Spickett, S. G.,** Genetic variation in adrenal weight relative to bodyweight in mice, *Acta Endocrinol. (Copenhagen) Suppl.,* 100, 92, 1965.
16. **Badr, F. M.,** Selection for high and low adrenal weight, *J. Endocrinol.,* 70, 457, 1976.
17. **Stewart, J. and Spickett, S. G.,** Genetic variation in diuretic responses: further and correlated responses to selection, *Genet. Res.,* 10, 95, 1967.
18. **Rapp, J. P.,** Effects of DCA and Na intake on mice bred for high and low juxtaglomerular indices, *Am. J. Physiol.,* 212, 1135, 1967.
19. **Chai, C. K. and Melloh, A.,** Selective breeding for variations in thyroidal iodine release rate in mice, *J. Endocrinol.,* 55, 233, 1972.
20. **Dawson, N. J.,** A study of some organs and tissues in mice subjected to genetic selection for different body-proportions, *Comp. Biochem. Physiol. A,* 50, 353, 1975.
21. **Cole, V. V. and Harned, B. K.,** Adrenal and pituitary weights in rats with reduced glucose tolerance, *Endocrinology,* 30, 146, 1942.
22. **Geiss, M. A.,** Adrenal volume in male rats with reduced glucose tolerance, *Proc. Soc. Exp. Biol. Med.,* 53, 107, 1943.
23. **Rapp, J. P. and Dahl, L. K.,** Adrenal steroidogenesis in rats bred for susceptibility to the hypertensive effect of salt, *Endocrinology,* 88, 52, 1971.
24. **Kojima, A., Takahashi, Y., Ohno, S., Sato, A., Yamada, T., Kubota, T., Yamori, Y., and Okamoto, K.,** An elevation of plasma TSH concentration in spontaneously hypertensive rats, *Proc. Soc. Exp. Biol. Med.,* 149, 661, 1975.
25. **Farrington, A. J. and Mellen, W. J.,** Thyroid activity and endocrine gland weight in fast- and slow-growing chickens, *Growth,* 31, 43, 1967.
26. **Stewart, A. D. and Stewart, J.,** Studies on the syndrome of diabetes insipidus associated with oligosyndactyly, *Am. J. Physiol.,* 217, 1191, 1969.
27. **Nickerson, P. A.,** The adrenal cortex in spontaneously hypertensive rats: a quantitative ultrastructural study, *Am. J. Pathol.,* 84, 545, 1976.
28. **Shilov, A. G., Khristolyubova, N. B., and Kolesnikova, L. V.,** A comparative study of the ultrastructure of the zona fasciculata cells of the adrenal cortex in rats of different strains, *Tsitologiya,* 19, 122, 1977.
29. **Shire, J. G. M. and Spickett, S. G.,** Genetic variation in adrenal structure: qualitative differences in the zona glomerulosa, *J. Endocrinol.,* 39, 277, 1967.
30. **Shire, J. G. M.,** A strain difference in the adrenal zona glomerulosa determined by one gene-locus, *Endocrinology,* 85, 415, 1969.
31. **Shire, J. G. M. and Stewart, J.,** The zona glomerulosa and corticotrophin: a genetic study in mice, *J. Endocrinol.,* 55, 185, 1972.

32. **Doering, C. H., Shire, J. G. M., Kessler, S., and Clayton, R. B.,** Cholesterol ester concentration and corticosterone production in adrenals of the C57BL/10 and DBA/2 strains in relation to adrenal lipid depletion, *Endocrinology,* 90, 93, 1972.
33. **Shire, J. G. M. and Spickett, S. G.,** Genetic variation in adrenal structure: strain differences in quantitative characters, *J. Endocrinol.,* 40, 215, 1968.
34. **Vicari, E. M.,** The adrenal lipids of mice with high and low mammary gland tumor incidences, *Anat. Rec.,* 86, 523, 1943.
35. **Arnesen, K.,** The adrenothymic constitution and susceptibility to leukemia in mice, *Acta Pathol. Microbiol. Scand. Suppl.,* 109, 1, 1956.
36. **Arnesen, K.,** Adrenocortical lipid depletion and leukemia in mice, *Acta Pathol. Microbiol. Scand. Suppl.,* 248, 15, 1974.
37. **Doering, C. H., Shire, J. G. M., Kessler, S., and Clayton, R. B.,** Genetic and biochemical studies of adrenal lipid depletion in mice, *Biochem. Genet.,* 8, 101, 1973.
38. **Pierpaoli, W., Haraa-Ghera, N., Bianchi, E., Müller, J., Meshorer, A., and Bree, M.,** Endocrine disorders a contributory factor to neoplasia in SJL/J mice, *J. Natl. Cancer Inst.,* 53, 731, 1974.
39. **Deanesly, R.,** Adrenal cortex differences in male and female mice, *Nature (London),* 141, 79, 1938.
40. **Bartels, E. D.,** Studies on hereditary dwarfism. III. Development of the adrenals in dwarf mice, *Acta Pathol. Microbiol. Scand.,* 18, 20, 1941.
41. **Spickett, S. G., Shire, J. G. M., and Stewart, J.,** Genetic variation in adrenal and renal structure and function, *Mem. Soc. Endocrinol.,* 15, 271, 1967.
42. **Badr, F. M., Shire, J. G. M., and Spickett, S. G.,** Genetic variation in adrenal weight: strain differences in the development of the adrenal glands of mice, *Acta Endocrinol. (Copenhagen),* 58, 191, 1968.
43. **Shire, J. G. M. and Spickett, S. G.,** A strain difference in the time and mode of regression of the adrenal X-zone in female mice, *Gen. Comp. Endocrinol.,* 11, 355, 1968.
44. **Shire, J. G. M. and Pantelouris, E. M.,** Comparison of endocrine function in normal and genetically athymic mice, *Comp. Biochem. Physiol. A,* 47, 93, 1974.
45. **Naeser, P.,** Structure of the adrenal glands in mice with the obese hyperglycemic syndrome (gene symbol ob), *Acta Pathol. Microbiol. Scand. Sect. A,* 83, 120, 1975.
46. **Dunn, T. B.,** Normal and pathologic anatomy of the adrenal gland of the mouse, including neoplasms, *J. Natl. Cancer Inst.,* 44, 1323, 1970.
47. **Jayne, E. P.,** A histologic study of the adrenal cortex in mice as influenced by strain, sex and age, *J. Gerontol.,* 18, 227, 1963.
48. **Levine, S. and Treiman, D. M.,** Differential plasma corticosterone response to stress in four inbred strains of mice, *Endocrinology,* 75, 142, 1964.
49. **Wragg, L. E. and Speirs, R. S.,** Strain and sex differences in response of inbred mice to adrenal cortical hormones, *Proc. Soc. Exp. Biol. Med.,* 80, 680, 1952.
50. **Thiessen, D. D. and Nealey, V. G.,** Adrenocortical activity, stress response and behavioral activity of five inbred mouse strains, *Endocrinology,* 71, 267, 1962.
51. **Blake, R. L.,** Regulation of liver tyrosine amino-transferase activity in inbred strains and mutant mice. I. Strain variance in fasting enzyme levels, *Int. J. Biochem.,* 1, 361, 1970.
52. **Treiman, D. M., Fulker, D. W., and Levine, S.,** Interaction of genotype and environment as determinants of corticosteroid response to stress, *Dev. Psychobiol.,* 3, 131, 1970.
53. **Blum, S., Kakihana, R., Shire, J. G. M., and Kessler, S.,** Plasma corticosterone responses to stress in mice: dependence on genotype, gonadal status and maturity, in preparation.
54. **Redgate, E. S. and Eleftheriou, B. E.,** Augmented pituitary adrenal responses to ketamine, an anesthetic with aminergic and hallucinogenic activity, in strains of mice and rabbits susceptible to audiogenic seizures, *Gen. Pharmacol.,* 6, 87, 1975.
55. **Lindberg, M., Shire, J. G. M., Doering, C. H., Kessler, S., and Clayton, R. B.,** Reductive metabolism of corticosterone in mice: differences in NADPH requirement of liver homogenates of males of two inbred strains, *Endocrinology,* 90, 81, 1972.
56. **Shire, J. G. M., Kessler, S., and Clayton, R. B.,** The availability of NADPH for corticosterone reduction in six strains of mice, *J. Endocrinol.,* 52, 591, 1972.
57. **Taylor, H. C. and Waltman, C. A.,** Hyperplasias of the mammary gland in the human being and in the mouse, *Arch. Surg. (Chicago),* 40, 733, 1940.
58. **Thiessen, D. D.,** Population density, mouse genotype and endocrine function in behavior, *J. Comp. Physiol. Psychol.,* 57, 412, 1964.
59. **Doering, C. H., Kessler, S., and Clayton, R. B.,** Genetic variation of cholesterol ester content in mouse adrenals, *Science,* 170, 1220, 1970.
60. **Richardson, M. C. and Schulster, D.,** Corticosteroidogenesis in isolated adrenal cells: effect of ACTH, cAMP and β^{1-24} ACTH diazotised to polyacrylamide, *J. Endocrinol.,* 55, 127, 1972.
61. **Wood, P.,** Responsiveness of adrenal cells to ACTH, *Mouse News Lett.,* 57, 13, 1977.

62. **van Abeleen, J. H. F., van der Kroon, P. H. W., and Bekkers, M. F. J.,** Mice selected for rearing behaviour: some physiological variables, *Behav. Genet.*, 3, 85, 1973.
63. **Shire, J. G. M.,** unpublished observations.
64. **Wahlsten, D. and Anisman, H.,** Shock-induced activity changes, adrenal lipid depletion, and brain weight in mice: a genetic study, *Physiol. Behav.*, 16, 401, 1976.
65. **Taylor, G.,** The Production of Corticosteroids by the Adrenals of various Mouse Strains, and the Effect of Dexamethasone on Thymidine Uptake by Lymphocytes, B.Sc. dissertation, University of Glasgow, 1976.
66. **Stylianopolou, F. and Clayton, R. B.,** Strain-dependent gonadal effects upon adrenal cholesterol ester concentration and composition in C57BL/10J and DBA/2J mice, *Endocrinology*, 99, 1631, 1976.
67. **Stylianopolou, F. and Clayton, R. B.,** Strain-dependent gonadal effects upon the response of adrenal cholesterol esters to ACTH in C57BL/10J and DBA/2J mice, *Endocrinology*, 99, 1638, 1976.
68. **Wood, P.,** personal communication.
69. **McClearn, G. E. and DeFries, J. C.,** *Introduction to Behavioral Genetics*, W. H. Freeman, San Francisco, 1973, 125.
70. **Kakihana, R., Noble, E. P., and Butte, J. C.,** Corticosterone response to ethanol in inbred strains of mice, *Nature (London)*, 218, 360, 1968.
71. **Molne, K.,** Gonadectomy and testosterone substitution in male mice with spontaneous adrenocortical lipid depletion, *Acta Pathol. Microbiol. Scand.*, 76, 35, 1969.
72. **Bartke, A. and Shire, J. G. M.,** Differences between mouse strains in testicular cholesterol levels and androgen target organs, *J. Endocrinol.*, 55, 173, 1972.
73. **McGill, T. E. and Manning, A.,** Genotype and retention of the ejaculatory reflex in castrated male mice, *Anim. Behav.*, 24, 507, 1976.
74. **Bullock, L. P.,** Genetic variations in sexual differentiation and sex-steroid action, in *Genetic Variation in Hormone Systems*, Vol. 1, Shire, J. G. M., Ed., CRC Press, West Palm Beach, Fla., 1979, chap. 4.
75. **Diez, J. A., Sze, P. Y., and Ginsberg, B. E.,** Postnatal development of mouse plasma and brain corticosterone levels: new findings contingent upon the use of a competitive protein-binding assay, *Endocrinology*, 98, 1434, 1976.
76. **Pachciarz, J. A. and Teague, P. O.,** Different responses of two mouse strains to 650 rads and protection by surgical stress, *Proc. Soc. Exp. Biol. Med.*, 148, 1095, 1975.
77. **Taylor, B. A. and Meier, H.,** Mapping the adrenal lipid depletion gene of the AKR/J mouse strain, *Genet. Res.*, 26 307, 1976.
78. **Molne, K. and Brabrand, G.,** Spontaneous adrenocortical lipid depletion in mice. Relationship to general growth, degeneration of adrenal X-zone, and maturation of seminiferous epithelium, *Acta Pathol. Microbiol. Scand.*, 72, 478, 1968.
79. **Solem, J. H.,** The function of the adrenal cortex in mice with spontaneous adrenocortical lipid depletion, *Acta Pathol. Microbiol. Scand.*, 70, 25, 1967.
80. **Brabrand, G. and Molne, K.,** The effect of hypophysectomy on the lipid pattern of the adrenal cortex in mice with spontaneous adrenocortical lipid depletion, *Acta Pathol. Microbiol. Scand.*, 72, 491, 1968.
81. **Molne, K.,** The adrenal weight of mice with spontaneous adrenocortical lipid depletion, *Acta Pathol. Microbiol. Scand.*, 75, 37, 1969.
82. **Molne, K.,** Histometric studies on the adrenal cortex of mice with spontaneous adrenocortical lipid depletion. A comparison with dexamethasone- and ACTH-treated C57BL mice, *Acta Pathol. Microbiol. Scand.*, 75, 51, 1969.
83. **Tuffrey, M., Barnes, R. D., Evans, E. P., and Ford, C. E.,** Dominance of AKR lymphocytes in tetraparental AKR-CBA/T6T6 chimaeras, *Nature (London) New Biol.*, 243, 207, 1973.
84. **Feder, N.,** Solitary cells and enzyme exchange in tetraparental mice, *Nature (London)*, 263, 67, 1976.
85. **Eleftheriou, B. E. and Bailey, D. W.,** Genetic analysis of plasma corticosterone levels in two inbred strains of mice, *J. Endocrinol.*, 55, 415, 1972.
86. **Hawkins, E. F., Young, P. N., Hawkins, A. M. C., and Bern, H. A.,** Adrenocortical function: corticosterone levels in female BALB/c and C3H mice under various conditions, *J. Exp. Zool.*, 194, 479, 1975.
87. **Levine, S. and Treiman, D. M.,** Determinants of individual differences in the steroid response to stress, in *Physiology and Pathology of Adaptation Mechanisms*, Bajusz, E., Ed., Pergamon Press, Oxford, 1969, 171.
88. **Sakellaris, P. C., Peterson, A., Goodwin, A., Winget, C. M., and Vernikos-Danellis, J.,** Response of mice to repeated photoperiod shifts: susceptibility to stress and barbiturates, *Proc. Soc. Exp. Biol. Med.*, 149, 677, 1976.
89. **Mos, L. P.,** Light-rearing effects on factors of mouse emotionality and endocrine organ weight, *Physiol. Psychol.*, 4, 503, 1976.

90. **Nandi, J., Bern, H. A., Biglieri, E. G., and Pierprzyk, J. K.,** In vitro steroidogenesis by the adrenal glands of mice, *Endocrinology,* 80, 576, 1967.
91. **Badr, F. M. and Spickett, S. G.,** Genetic variation in the biosynthesis of corticosteroids in Mus musculus, *Nature (London),* 205, 1088, 1965.
92. **Badr, F. M.,** In vivo secretion of 11-deoxycortisol by mouse adrenals: plasma corticosteroid levels in three strains of mice, *Comp. Biochem. Physiol. B,* 39, 131, 1971.
93. **Wolff, G. L. and Flack, J. D.,** Genetic regulation of plasma corticosterone concentration and its response to castration and allogeneic tumour growth in the mouse, *Nature (London) New Biol.,* 232, 181, 1971.
94. **Stewart, J., Fraser, R., Papaioannou, V. E., and Tait, A.,** Aldosterone production and the zona glomerulosa: a genetic study, *Endocrinology,* 90, 968, 1972.
95. **Papaioannou, V. E. and Fraser, R.,** Plasma aldosterone concentration in sodium deprived mice of two strains, *J. Steroid Biochem.,* 5, 191, 1974.
96. **Dung, H. C. and Swigart, R. H.,** Experimental studies of lethargic mice, *Tex. Rep. Biol. Med.,* 29, 273, 1971.
97. **Dung, H. C.,** Relationship between adrenal cortex and thymic involution in lethargic mutant mice, *Am. J. Anat.,* 147, 255, 1976.
98. **Cartensen, H., Hellman, B., and Larsson, S.,** Biosynthesis of steroids in the adrenals of normal and obese-hyperglycemic mice, *Acta Soc. Med. Ups.,* 66, 139, 1961.
99. **Edwardson, J. A. and Hough, C. A. M.,** The pituitary-adrenal system of the genetically obese (ob/ob) mouse, *J. Endocrinol.,* 65, 99, 1975.
100. **Naeser, P.,** Function of the adrenal cortex in obese-hyperglycemic mice (gene symbol ob), *Diabetologia,* 10, 449, 1974.
101. **Naeser, P.,** Disappearance of ^{3}H-corticosterone from the serum of obese-hyperglycemic mice (gene symbol ob), *Acta Physiol. Scand.,* 93, 10, 1975.
102. **Naeser, P.,** Adrenal function in the diabetic mouse (gene symbol db m), *Acta Physiol. Scand.,* 98, 395, 1976.
103. **Naeser, P.,** Effects of adrenalectomy on the obese-hyperglycemic syndrome in mice (gene symbol ob), *Diabetologia,* 9, 376, 1973.
104. **Naeser, P.,** In vitro release of corticosteroids from adrenal glands of obese-hyperglycemic mice (gene symbol ob), *Acta Physiol. Scand.,* 92, 175, 1974.
105. **Mains, R. E. and Eipper, B. A.,** Molecular weights of adrenocorticotrophic hormone in extracts of anterior and intermediate-posterior lobes of mouse pituitary, *Proc. Natl. Acad. Sci. U.S.A.,* 72, 3565, 1975.
106. **Beloff-Chain, A., Edwardson, J. A., and Hawthorne, J.,** Influence of the pituitary gland on insulin secretion in the genetically obese mouse, *J. Endocrinol.,* 65, 109, 1975.
107. **Beloff-Chain, A., Edwardson, J. A., and Hawthorn, J.,** Corticotrophin-like intermediate lobe peptide as an insulin secretagogue, *J. Endocrinol.,* 74, 28P, 1977.
108. **Jackson, E., Stolz, D., and Martin, R.,** Effect of adrenalectomy on weight gain and body composition of yellow obese mice, (A^y/a), *Horm. Metab. Res.,* 8, 452, 1976.
109. **Dahl, L. K., Heine, M., and Tassinari, C.,** The effects of chronic excess salt ingestion: evidence that genetic factors play an important role in susceptibility to experimental hypertension, *J. Exp. Med.,* 115, 1173, 1962.
110. **Molteni, A. and Brownie, A. C.,** Incidence of salt-induced hypertension in rats from different stocks, *J. Med.,* 3, 193, 1972.
111. **Molteni, A., Nickerson, P. A., Latta, J., and Brownie, A. C.,** Hypertension in rats bearing an adrenocorticotropic hormone-growth hormone-, and prolactin-secreting tumor (MtTF4), *Cancer Res.,* 32, 114, 1972.
112. **Molteni, A., Nickerson, P. A., Gallant, S., and Brownie, A. C.,** Resistance of W/Fu rats to adrenal regeneration hypertension, *Proc. Soc. Exp. Biol. Med.,* 150, 80, 1975.
113. **Hall, C. E., Ayachi, S., and Hall, O.,** Hypertension following adrenal enucleation and its absence during deoxycorticosterone treatment in Long-Evans rats, *Endocrinology,* 92, 1175, 1973.
114. **Hall, C. E., Ayachi, S., and Hall, O.,** Genetic influence on saline consumption and salt hypertension as exhibited by the response of various rat strains and substrains, *Tex. Rep. Biol. Med.,* 33, 509, 1975.
115. **Hall, C. E. and Hall, O.,** Resistance of Fischer 344 rats to deoxycorticosterone hypertension, *Life Sci.,* 20, 1239, 1977.
116. **Hall, C. E., Ayachi, S., and Hall, O.,** Immunity of Fischer 344 rats to salt hypertension, *Life Sci.,* 18, 1001, 1976.
117. **Brownell, K. A., Lee, S. L., Beck, R. P., and Besch, P. K.,** In vitro 17α-hydroxylation of steroids by the adrenals of hypertensive rats, *Endocrinology,* 72, 167, 1963.
118. **Bergon, L. and Brownie, A. C.,** Adrenal mitochondrial and serum corticosteroid studies in rats resistant to adrenal regeneration hypertension, *Endocrinology,* 99, 1080, 1976.

119. **Birmingham, M. K., deNicola, A. F., Oliver, J. T., Traikov, H., Birmingham, M. L., Holzbauer, M., Godden, U., and Sharman, D. F.**, Production of steroids in vivo by regenerated adrenal glands of hypertensive and normotensive rats, *Endocrinology,* 93, 297, 1973.
120. **Engeland, W. C. and Dallman, M. F.**, Neural mediation of compensatory adrenal growth, *Endocrinology,* 99, 1659, 1976.
121. **Fox, R. R. and Crary, D. D.**, Hereditary adrenal hyperplasia in the rabbit: genetics and pathology, *J. Hered.,* 69, 230, 1978.
122. **Rapp, J. P. and Dahl, L. K.**, Mendelian inheritance of 18- and 11β-steroid hydroxylase activities in the adrenals of rats genetically susceptible or resistant to hypertension, *Endocrinology,* 90, 1435, 1972.
123. **Rapp, J. P. and Dahl, L. K.**, Mutant forms of cytochrome P-450 controlling both 18- and 11β-steroid hydroxylation in the rat, *Biochemistry,* 15, 1235, 1976.
124. **Friedman, R. and Iwai, J.**, Genetic predisposition and stress-induced hypertension, *Science,* 193, 161, 1976.
125. **Moll, D., Dale, S. L., and Melby, J. C.**, Adrenal steroidogenesis in the spontaneously hypertensive rat, *Endocrinology,* 96, 416, 1975.
126. **Hartle, D. K., Kapke, G. F., and Baron, J.**, Alterations in the contents of cytochrome P450 and adrenal ferredoxin in adrenals of spontaneously hypertensive rats, *Biochem. Biophys. Res. Commun.,* 77, 953, 1977.
127. **Shire, J. G. M.**, The thyroid gland and thyroid hormones, in *Genetic Variation in Hormone Systems,* Vol. 2, Shire, J. G. M., Ed., CRC Press, Boca Raton, Fla., 1979, chap. 1.
128. **Badr, F. M.**, Genetic variation in prostaglandins, in *Genetic Variation in Hormone Systems,* Vol. 2, Shire, J. G. M., Ed., CRC Press, Boca Raton, Fla., 1979, chap. 3.
129. **Laplante, C., Giroud, C. J. P., and Stachenko, J.**, Lack of appreciable 17α-hydroxylase activity in the normal and regenerated rat adrenal cortex, *Endocrinology,* 75, 815, 1964.
130. **Whitehouse, B. J. and Vinson, G. P.**, Sex and strain differences in the response of rat adrenal tissue to adrenocorticotrophin stimulation in vitro, *J. Endocrinol.,* 71, 65P, 1976.
131. **Stockham, M. A.**, personal communication; quoted in Shire, J. G. M., Endocrine genetics of the adrenal gland, *J. Endocrinol.,* 62, 173, 1974.
132. **Woods, J. W.**, The effects of acute stress and of ACTH upon ascorbic acid and lipid content of the adrenal glands of wild rats, *J. Physiol. (London),* 135, 390, 1957.
133. **Feuer, G.**, Difference in emotional behaviour and in function of the endocrine system in genetically different strains of albino rat, in *Physiology and Pathology of Adaptation Mechanisms,* Bajusz, E., Ed., Pergamon Press, Oxford, 1969, 214.
134. **Stockard, C. R.**, The genetic and endocrinic basis for differences in form and behavior, *Am. Anat. Mem.,* 19, 1, 1941.
135. **Coffin, D. L. and Munson, T. O.**, Endocrine diseases of the dog associated with hair loss: sertoli cell tumor of the testis, hypothyroidism, canine Cushings syndrome, *J. Am. Vet. Med. Assoc.,* 123, 402, 1953.
136. **O'Kelly, J. C.**, The concentrations of lipids in the adrenal cortical tissue of genetically different types of cattle, *Aust. J. Biol. Sci.,* 27, 651, 1974.
137. **Johnston, J. D. and Buckland, R. B.**, Response of male Holstein calves from seven sires to four management stresses as measured by plasma corticoid levels, *Can. J. Anim. Sci.,* 56, 727, 1976.
138. **Eisner, F. F. and Reznichenko, L. P.**, Heritability and recurrence of the adrenocortical function level in cattle, *Genetika,* 13, 430, 1977.
139. **Marple, D. N. and Cassens, R. G.**, Increased metabolic clearance of cortisol by stress-susceptible swine, *J. Anim. Sci.,* 36, 1139, 1973.
140. **Cassens, R. G., Judge, M. D., Sink, J. D., and Briskey, E. J.**, Porcine adrenocortical lipid in relation to striated muscle characteristics, *Proc. Soc. Exp. Biol. Med.,* 120, 854, 1965.
141. **Marple, D. N., Judge, M. D., and Aberle, E. D.**, Pituitary and adrenocortical function in stress-susceptible swine, *J. Anim. Sci.,* 35, 995, 1972.
142. **Aberle, E. D., Riggs, B. L., Alliston, C. W., and Wilson, S. P.**, Effects of thermal stress, breed and stress-susceptibility on corticosteroid binding globulin in swine, *J. Anim. Sci.,* 43, 816, 1976.
143. **Sebranek, J. G., Marple, D. N., Cassens, R. G., Briskey, E. J., and Kastenschmidt, L. L.**, Adrenal response to ACTH in the pig, *J. Anim. Sci.,* 36, 41, 1973.
144. **Smith, C. and Bampton, P. R.**, Inheritance of reaction to halothane-induced anaesthesia in pigs, *Genet. Res.,* 29, 287, 1977.
145. **Rasmussen, B. A. and Christian, L. L.**, H Blood-groups in pigs as predictors of stress susceptibility, *Science,* 191, 947, 1976.
146. **Wingard, D. W.**, Malignant hyperthermia: a human stress syndrome, *Lancet,* 2, 1450, 1974.
147. **Brown, K. I. and Nestor, K. E.**, Implications of selection for high and low adrenal response to stress, *Poult. Sci.,* 53, 1297, 1974.

148. **Edens, F. W. and Siegel, H. S.**, Adrenal responses in high and low ACTH response lines of chickens during acute heat stress. *Gen. Comp. Endocrinol.*, 25, 64, 1975.
149. **Burstein, S.**, Determination of initial rates of cortisol 2α- and 6β-hydroxylation by hepatic microsomal preparations in guinea pigs: effect of phenobarbitol in two genetic types, *Endocrinology*, 82, 547, 1968.
150. **Whipp, G. T., Wintour, E. M., Coghlan, J. P., and Scoggins, B. A.**, Regulation of aldosterone in the guinea-pig: effect of oestrus cycle, pregnancy and sodium status, *Aust. J. Exp. Biol. Med. Sci.*, 54, 71, 1976.
151. **Ghraf, R., Hoff, H. G., Ockenfels, H., and Schrieffers, H,.** Influence of age and sex on the development and differentiation of enzymes involved in the metabolism of steroid hormones in rat liver obtained from two different strains, SpD/UL and FW49, *Res. Steroids*, 5, 249, 1973.
152. **Burstein, S. and Zucker, L. M.**, Genetic differences in hepatic steroid sulfatase activity in two strains of rats differing in their rate of growth, *Endocrinology*, 81, 675, 1967.
153. **Shire, J. G. M.**, Diet interacts with genotype in determining rate of corticosteroid degradation by the liver, *Mouse News Lett.*, 57, 13, 1977.
154. **Hizi, A. and Yagil, G.**, On the mechanism of glucose-6-phosphate dehydrogenase regulation in mouse liver. III. The rate of enzyme synthesis and degradation, *Eur. J. Biochem.*, 45, 211, 1974.
155. **Kramer, R. E. and Colby, H. D.**, Feminization of hepatic steroid and drug metabolizing enzymes by growth hormone in the rat, *J. Endocrinol.*, 71, 449, 1976.
156. **Burstein S.**, Genetic aspects of adrenal and hepatic cortisol 2α- and 6β-hydroxylation in guinea-pigs: developmental pattern and effect of substrate concentration, *Endocrinology*, 86, 851, 1970.
157. **Goldman, A. S. and Klingele, D. A.**, Persistent post-pubertal elevation of activity of steroid 5α-reductase in the adrenal of rat pseudohermaphrodites and correction by large doses of testosterone or DHT, *Endocrinology*, 94, 1232, 1974.
158. **Goldman, A. S. and Shapiro, B. H.**, Correction of developmental defects in adrenal steroid metabolizing enzymes of the genetically male rat pseudohermaphrodite by prolactin, *J. Steroid Biochem.*, 8, 31, 1977.
159. **Maynard, P. V. and Cameron, E. H. D.**, Metabolism of C19 steroids by homogenates of normal rat and mouse tissue, and of the small transplantable rat adrenocortical tumour 494, *J. Endocrinol.*, 52, 20P, 1972.
160. **Lohrenz, F. N., Doe, R. P., and Seal, U. S.**, Idiopathic or genetic elevation of corticosteroid-binding globulin, *J. Clin. Endocrinol. Metab.*, 28, 1073, 1968.
161. **Ohno, S.**, *Sex Chromosomes and Sexlinked Genes*, Springer-Verlag, Berlin, 1967, 1.
162. **Kennedy, P. C., Kendrick, J. W., and Stormont, C.**, Adenohypophyseal aplasia, an inherited defect associated with abnormal gestation in Guernsey cattle, *Cornell Vet.*, 47, 160, 1957.
163. **Holm, L. W., Parker, H. R., and Galligan, S. J.**, Adrenal insufficiency in postmature Holstein calves, *Am. J. Obstet. Gynecol.*, 81, 1000, 1961.
164. **Mains, R. E., Eipper, B. A., and Ling, N.**, Common precursor to corticotropins and endorphins, *Proc. Natl. Acad. Sci. U.S.A.*, 74, 3014, 1977.
165. **Cuson, L., Dupont, A., Kledzik, G. S., Labrie, F., Coy, D. H., and Schally, A. V.**, Potent prolactin and growth hormone releasing activity of more analogues of Met-enkephalin, *Nature (London)*, 268, 544, 1977.
166. **Levine, S. and Levin, R.**, Pituitary-adrenal influences on passive avoidance in two inbred strains of mice. *Horm. Behav.*, 1, 105, 1970.
167. **Chapman, V. M.**, Plasma corticosterone response to stress in two strains of mice and their F1 hybrids, *Physiol. Behav.*, 3, 247, 1968.
168. **Fahringer, E. E., Foley, E. L., and Redgate, E. S.**, Pituitary adrenal response to ketamine and the inhibition of the response by catecholaminergic blockade, *Neuroendocrinology*, 14, 151, 1974.
169. **Shire, J. G. M.**, The forms, uses and significance of genetic variation in endocrine systems, *Biol. Rev.*, 51, 105, 1976.
170. **Daughaday, W.**, A comparison of the X-zone of the adrenal cortex in two inbred strains of mice, *Cancer Res.*, 1, 883, 1941.
171. **Chester-Jones, I.**, The action of testosterone on the adrenal cortex of the hypophysectomized, prepubertally castrated, male mouse, *Endocrinology*, 44, 427, 1949.
172. **Shire, J. G. M. and Hambly, E. A.**, The adrenal glands of mice with hereditary pituitary dwarfism, *Acta Pathol. Microbiol. Scand. Sect. A*, 81, 225, 1973.
173. **Shire, J. G. M.**, Genes, hormones and behavioural variation, in *Genetic and Environmental Influences on Behaviour*, Thoday, J. M. and Parkes, A. S., Eds., Oliver & Boyd, Edinburgh, 1968, 194.
174. **Shire, J. G. M. and Spickett, S. G.**, Genetic variation in adrenal structure: strain differences in quantitative characters, *J. Endocrinol.*, 40, 215, 1968.
175. **Howard, E.**, The representation of the adrenal X-zone in rats, in the light of observations in X-zone variability in mice, *Am. J. Anat.*, 62, 351, 1938.

176. **Smith, P. E. and MacDowell, E. C.,** The differential effect of hereditary mouse dwarfism on the anterior pituitary hormones, *Anat. Rec.,* 50, 85, 1931.
177. **Bartke, A.,** Genetic models in the study of anterior pituitary hormones, in *Genetic Variation in Hormone Systems,* Vol. 1, Shire, J. G. M., Ed., CRC Press, Boca Raton, Fla., 1979, chap. 6.
178. **Cattanach, B. M., Iddon, C. A., Charlton, H. M., Chiappa, S. A., and Fink, G.,** Gonadotrophin-releasing hormone deficiency in a mutant mouse with hypogonadism, *Nature (London),* 269, 338, 1977.
179. **Witorsch, R. J. and Kitay, J. I.,** Pituitary hormones affecting adrenal 5α-reductase activity: ACTH, growth hormone and prolactin, *Endocrinology,* 91, 764, 1972.
180. **Stabler, T. A. and Ungar, F.,** An estrogen effect on 20α-hydroxysteroid dehydrogenase activity in the mouse adrenal, *Endocrinology,* 86, 1049, 1970.
181. **Muller, E.,** Histochemical studies of 3β- and 20α-hydroxysteroid dehydrogenase in the adrenals and ovaries of the nu/nu mouse, *Histochemistry,* 43, 51, 1975.
182. **Westberg, J. A., Bern, H. A., and Barnawell, E. B.,** Strain differences in the response of the mouse adrenal to oestrogen, *Acta Endocrinol. (Copenhagen),* 25, 70, 1957.
183. **McPhail, M. K. and Read, H. C.,** The mouse adrenal, development, degeneration and regeneration of the X-zone, *Anat. Rec.,* 84, 51, 1942.
184. **Voci, V. E. and Carlson, N. R.,** Enhancement of maternal behavior and nest-building following systemic and diencephalic administration of prolactin and progesterone in the mouse, *J. Comp. Physiol. Psychol.,* 83, 388, 1973.
185. **Noirot, E.,** Endocrine studies. H, Behaviour, *Mouse News Lett.,* 36, 27, 1967.
186. **Noirot, E.,** The onset of maternal behavior in rats, hamsters and mice, in *Advances in the Study of Behavior,* Lehrman, D. S., Hinde, R. A., and Shaw, E., Eds., Academic Press, New York, 1972, chap. 4.
187. **Rimoin, D. L. and Richmond, L.,** The pygmy (*pg*) mutant of the mouse: a model of the human pygmy, *J. Clin. Endocrinol. Metab.,* 35, 467, 1972.
188. **Beamer, W. G. and Eicher, E. M.,** Stimulation of growth in the little mouse, *J. Endocrinol.,* 71, 37, 1976.
189. **Dung, H. C.,** Evidence for prolactin cell deficiency in connection with low reproductive efficiency of female torpid mice, *J. Reprod. Fertil.,* 45, 91, 1975.
190. **Chester Jones, I.,** *The Adrenal Cortex,* Cambridge University Press, London, 1957, 109.
191. **Shire, J. G. M.,** Degeneration of the adrenal X-zone in *Tfm* mice with inherited insensitivity to androgens, *J. Endocrinol.,* 71, 445, 1976.
192. **Rapp, J. P.,** Adrenal steroidogenesis and serum renin in rats bred for juxtaglomerular granularity, *Am. J. Physiol.,* 216, 860, 1969.
193. **Rapp, J. P.,** Steroid secretion in vivo in rats bred for high and low juxtaglomerular granularity, *Endocrinology,* 85, 909, 1969.
194. **Rapp, J. P.,** Age-related pathologic changes, hypertension, and 18-hydroxydeoxycorticosterone in rats selectively bred for high and low juxtaglomerular granularity, *Lab. Invest.,* 28, 343, 1973.
195. **Vincent, M., Dupont, J., and Sassard, J.,** Plasma renin activity as a function of age in two new strains of spontaneously hypertensive and normotensive rats, *Clin. Sci. Mol. Med.,* 50, 103, 1976.
196. **Bing, J. and Poulsen, K.,** The renin system in mice. Effects of removal of kidneys or (and) submaxillary glands in different strains, *Acta Pathol. Microbiol. Scand. A,* 79, 134, 1971.
197. **Wilson, C. M., Erdös, E. G., Dunn, J. F., and Wilson, J. D.,** Genetic control of renin activity in the submaxillary gland of the mouse, *Proc. Natl. Acad. Sci. U.S.A.,* 74, 1185, 1977.
198. **McGregor, D. D. and Smirk, F. H.,** Vascular responses in mesenteric arteries from genetic and renal hypertensive rats, *Am. J. Physiol.,* 214, 1429, 1968.
199. **Woolley, G. W.,** Experimental endocrine tumors with special reference to the adrenal cortex, *Recent Prog. Horm. Res.,* 5, 383, 1950.
200. **Ranandive, K. J. and Karande, K. A.,** Pituitaries of spayed mice of different strains: cytology and gonadotrophin content, *J. Endocrinol.,* 48, 449, 1970.
201. **Snell, K. C. and Stewart, H. L.,** Variations in histologic pattern and functional effects of a transplantable adrenal cortical carcinoma in intact, hypophysectomized and newborn rats, *J. Natl. Cancer Inst.,* 22, 1119, 1959.
202. **Lassman, M. N. and Mulrow, P. J.,** Deficiency of deoxycorticosterone binding protein in the hypothalamus of rats resistant to deoxycorticosterone induced hypertension, *Endocrinology,* 94, 1541, 1974.
203. **Stewart, J,.** Genetic studies on the mechanism of action of aldosterone in mice, *Endocrinology,* 96, 711, 1975.
204. **Stewart, J.,** Diuretic responses to electrolyte loads in four strains of mice, *Comp. Biochem. Physiol.,* 30, 977, 1969.
205. **Wilson, T. R.,** Strain and sex differences in gastric ulceration in restrained rats, *Acta Genet. Med. Gemellol.,* 16, 310, 1967.

206. **Sines, J. O.**, Selective breeding for stomach lesions following stress in the rat, *J. Comp. Physiol. Psychol.*, 52, 615, 1959.
207. **Nayudu, P. R. V. and Moog, F.**, The genetic control of alkaline phosphatase activity in the duodenum of the mouse, *Biochem. Genet.*, 1, 155, 1967.
208. **Pla, M., Zákány, J., and Fachet, J.**, H-2 influence on corticosteroid effects on thymus cells, *Fol. Biol. (Prague)*, 22, 49, 1976.
209. **deAsua, L. J., Carr, B., Clingan, D., and Rudland, P.**, Specific glucocorticoid inhibition of growth promoting effects of prostaglandin F2α on 3T3 cells, *Nature (London)*, 265, 450, 1977.
210. **Sibley, C. H. and Tomkins, G. M.**, Mechanisms of steroid resistance, *Cell*, 2, 221, 1974.
211. **Bourgeois, S. and Newby, R. F.**, Diploid and haploid states of the glucocorticoid receptor gene of mouse lymphoid cell lines, *Cell*, 11, 423, 1977.
212. **Hackney, J. F., Gross, S. R., Aronow, L., and Pratt, W. B.**, Specific glucocorticoid binding macromolecules from mouse fibroblasts growing in vitro. A possible steroid receptor for growth inhibition, *Mol. Pharmacol.*, 6, 500, 1970.
213. **Yamamoto, K. R., Gehring, U., Stampfer, M. R., and Sibley, C. H.**, Genetic approaches to steroid hormone action, *Recent Prog. Horm. Res.*, 32, 3, 1976.
214. **Hobart, M. J.**, Immunoglobulins as proteins, in *The Immune System*, Hobart, M. J. and McConnell, I., Eds., J. B. Lippincott, Philadelphia, 1975, 2.
215. **Levisohn, S. R. and Thompson, E. B.**, Tyrosine aminotransferase induction regulation variant in tissue culture, *Nature (London) New Biol.*, 235, 102, 1972.
216. **Thompson, E. B., Aviv, D., and Lippmann, M. E.**, Variants of HTC cells with low tyrosine aminotransferase inducibility and apparently normal glucocorticoid receptors, *Endocrinology*, 100, 406, 1977.
217. **Benedict, W. F., Nebert, D. W., and Thompson, E. B.**, Expression of aryl hydrocarbon hydroxylase induction and suppression of tyrosine aminotransferase induction in somatic-cell hybrids, *Proc. Natl. Acad. Sci. U.S.A.*, 69, 2179, 1972.
218. **Weiss, M. C. and Chaplain, M.**, Expression of differentiated functions of hepatoma cell hybrids: reappearance of tyrosine aminotransferase inducibility after loss of chromosomes, *Proc. Natl. Acad. Sci. U.S.A.*, 68, 3026, 1971.
219. **Ruddle, F. H. and Creagan, R. P.**, Parasexual approaches to the genetics of man, *Annu. Rev. Genet.*, 9, 407, 1975.
220. **Yu, L. Y., Tushinski, R. J., and Bancroft, F. C.**, Glucocorticoid induction of growth hormone synthesis in a strain of rat pituitary cells, *J. Biol. Chem.*, 252, 3870, 1977.
221. **Martial, J. A., Baxter, J. D., Goodman, H. M., and Seeburg, P. H.**, Regulation of growth hormone messenger RNA by thyroid and glucocorticoid hormones, *Proc. Natl. Acad. Sci. U.S.A.*, 74, 1816, 1977.
222. **Seo, H., Vassart, G., Brocas, H., and Refetoff, S.**, Triiodothyronine stimulates specifically growth hormone mRNA in rat pituitary tumor cells, *Proc. Natl. Acad. Sci. U.S.A.*, 74, 2054, 1977.
223. **Samuels, H. H., Horwitz, Z. D., Stanley, F., Casanova, J., and Shapiro, L. E.**, Thyroid hormone controls glucocorticoid action in cultured GH1 cells, *Nature (London)*, 268, 254, 1977.
224. **Marsk, L., Theorell, M., and Larsson, K. S.**, Transfer of blastocysts as applied in experimental teratology, *Nature (London)*, 234, 358, 1971.
225. **Biddle, F. G. and Fraser, F. C.**, Genetics of cortisone-induced cleft-palate in the mouse: embryonic and maternal effects, *Genetics*, 84, 743, 1976.
226. **Bonner, J. J. and Slavkin, H. C.**, Cleft-palate susceptibility linked to histocompatibility-2 (H-2) in the mouse, *Immunogenetics*, 2, 213, 1975.
227. **Francis, B. M.**, Influence of sex-linked genes on embryonic sensitivity to cortisone in three strains of mice, *Teratology*, 7, 119, 1973.
228. **Biddle, F. G. and Fraser, F. C.**, Cortisone-induced cleft-palate in the mouse. A search for the genetic control of the embryonic response trait, *Genetics*, 85, 289, 1977.
229. **Miller, K. K.**, Commercial dietary influences on the frequency of cortisone-induced cleft-palate in C57BL/6J mice, *Teratology*, 15, 249, 1977.
230. **Dostal, M. and Jelinek, R.**, Corticoid-induced cleft-palate as a model system for the distinction of maternal and foetal genomes interacting with exogenous teratogen, *Fol. Biol. (Prague)*, 19, 153, 1973.
231. **Levine, A., Yaffe, S. J., and Back, N.**, Maternal-fetal distribution of radioactive cortisol and its correlation with teratogenic effect, *Proc. Soc. Exp. Biol. Med.*, 129, 86, 1968.
232. **Marsk, L., Ranning, K., and Larsson, K. S.**, ^{3}H corticosterone incorporation in CBA and transferred A/Jax embryos in CBA mothers, *Biol. Neonate*, 24, 49, 1974.
233. **Nguyen, T. T., Rekdal, D. J., and Burton, A. F.**, The uptake and metabolism of ^{3}H corticosterone and fluorimetrically determined corticosterone in fetuses of several mouse strains, *Biol. Neonate*, 18, 78, 1971.
234. **Salomon, D. S. and Pratt, R. M.**, Glucocorticoid receptors in murine embryonic facial mesenchyme, *Nature (London)*, 264, 174, 1976.

235. **Goldman, A. S., Katsumata, M., Yaffe, S. J., and Gasser, D. L.,** Palatal cytosol cortisol-binding protein associated with cleft-palate susceptibility and H-2 genotype, *Nature (London),* 265, 643, 1977.
236. **Wong, M. D. and Burton, A. F.,** Inhibition by corticosteroids of glucose incorporation into fetuses of several strains of mouse, *Biol. Neonate,* 18, 146, 1971.
237. **Belyaev, D. K., Schüler, L., and Borodin, P. M.,** Problems of stress genetics, III. Differential effect of stress on the fertility of mice of different genotypes, *Genetika,* 13, 52, 1977.
238. **Ricardo, N. S. and Miller, J. R.,** Further observations on lg^{ML} (lid-gap Miller) and other open-eye mutants in the house mouse, *Can. J. Genet. Cytol.,* 9, 596, 1967.
239. **Stein, K. F. and Kettyle, C. N.,** Further data on the slit-lid mutant in mice and the effect of cortisone and DOCA on its development, *Teratology,* 8, 51, 1973.
240. **Torday, J. S., Smith, B. T., and Giroud, C. J. P.,** The rabbit fetal lung as a glucocorticoid target tissue, *Endocrinology,* 96, 1462, 1975.
241. **Boiocchi, M., della Torre, G., and della Porta, G.,** Genetic control of endogenous C-type virus production in pancreatic acinar cells of C57BL/He and C57BL/6 mice, *Proc. Natl. Acad. Sci. U.S.A.,* 71, 1892, 1975.
242. **Ringold, G. M., Yamamoto, K. R., Tomkins, G. M., Bishop, J. M., and Varnus, H. E.,** Dexamethasone-mediated induction of mouse mammary tumor virus RNA: a system for studying glucocorticoid action, *Cell,* 6, 299, 1975.
243. **Ringold, G. M., Lasfargues, E. Y., Bishop, J. M., and Varnus, H. E.,** Production of mouse mammary tumor virus by cultured cells in the absence and presence of hormones: assay by molecular hybridization, *Virology,* 65, 135, 1975.
244. **Young, H. A., Scolnick, E. M., and Parks, W. P.,** Glucocorticoid-receptor interaction and induction of murine mammary tumor virus, *J. Biol. Chem.,* 250, 3337, 1975.
245. **Scolnick, E. M., Young, H. A., and Parks, W. P.,** Biochemical and physiological mechanisms in glucocorticoid hormone induction in mouse mammary tumor virus, *Virology,* 69, 148, 1976.
246. **Christian, J. J. and Davis, D. E.,** Endocrines, behavior and population, *Science,* 146, 1550, 1964.
247. **Denton, D. A.,** Evolutionary aspects of the emergence of aldosterone secretion and salt appetite, *Physiol. Rev.,* 45, 245, 1965.
248. **Clark, J. M.,** The effects of selection and human preference on coat-colour gene frequencies in urban cats, *Heredity,* 35, 195, 1975.
249. **Lundin, L. G.,** Evolutionary conservation of chromosomal segments, *Clin. Genet.,* in press.
250. **Funder, J. W., Feldman, D., and Edelman, I. S.,** The roles of plasma binding and receptor specificity in the mineralocorticoid action of aldosterone, *Endocrinology,* 92, 994, 1973.
251. **Funder, J. W., Feldman, D., and Edelman, I. S.,** Glucocorticoid receptors in rat kidney: the binding of tritiated dexamethasone, *Endocrinology,* 92, 1005, 1973.

Chapter 4

GENETIC VARIATIONS IN SEXUAL DIFFERENTIATION AND SEX STEROID ACTION

L. P. Bullock

TABLE OF CONTENTS

I. NORMAL SEXUAL DEVELOPMENT

In mammals, the fetus is phenotypically bipotential with respect to sexual differentiation. However, if male development is to occur, a testis must differentiate and secrete testosterone. In the absence of androgen stimulation, a female phenotype will develop. Thus, abnormal sexual differentiation or abnormal sex steroid action is usually associated with abnormal androgen action, either its absence in males or its presence in females. Abnormalities in female sex hormone action are usually not obvious until after puberty, when problems associated with infertility become apparent.

Although it is ultimately an abnormality in the effects of sex steroids, too much, too little, or an insensitivity that causes defective sexual development, the basis of the defect may arise at any of a number of sites. Thus, before discussing genetic variations in sexual development and sex steroid responsiveness, it is first necessary to discuss normal sexual differentiation. Although sexual differentiation in nonmammalian vertebrates and invertebrates offers many interesting contrasts to that in mammals, this discussion will, for the most part, be limited to mammals.

Normal sexual development is determined by events starting at the time of conception. As the organism differentiates, a set of mechanisms evolves, including the hypothalamus, pituitary, gonad, and target organs, which regulates masculine sexual development (Figure 1). Defects at any one of many points — including abnormal sex chromosomes, organ differentiation, steroid secretion, or tissue response — will result in an abnormality of sexual differentiation and growth. These various topics will be discussed in turn.

A. Genetic Sex

The genetic sex of an individual is determined when the ovum and sperm unite at fertilization.[1,2] In mammals, where the male is the heterogametic sex, genetic sex is determined by the sex chromosome, X or Y, that is present in the sperm. In contrast, in species such as birds, where the female is the heterogametic sex, the ovum carries

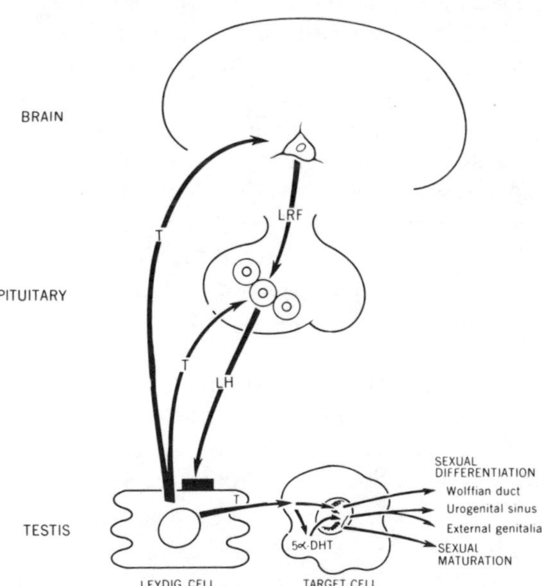

FIGURE 1. Hormonal factors regulating male sexual differentiation. LH-releasing factor (LRF) from the hypothalamus stimulates the release of luteinizing hormone (LH) from the pituitary. This latter hormone stimulates Leydig cells in the testis to secrete androgens, primarily testosterone, which feed back on the hypothalamus and pituitary to reduce the secretion of LRF and LH through a negative feedback mechanism. Testosterone also acts directly, or via conversion to 5α-dihydrotestosterone (DHT), to cause masculine sexual differentiation and growth.

the sex-determining chromosome. Sex chromosomes influence sexual development primarily through their effects on the differentiation of the primitive bipotential gonad. They have little direct influence on secondary sexual characteristics that emerge from other bipotential primordia.

The major function of the Y chromosome in mammals is to induce testicular development.[1,3] This can occur in the presence of multiple X's, as in Klinefelter's syndrome, although testicular development is abnormal.[4] Without some Y-chromosomal material testicular development does not occur. The H-Y antigen has recently received attention for its possible role as a primary determinant of testicular development.[5-7] This histocompatibility antigen was originally recognized by immunologists as being responsible for the rejection of male tissues by females of the same inbred mouse strain. The relationship between the H-Y locus and a testis-determining gene on the Y chromosome is not entirely clear. They are closely linked, and it has been proposed that the two are in fact one and the same.[7] The finding that males with two Y chromosomes have more H-Y antigen than normal males[6] supports the localization of the H-Y gene on the Y chromosome. Additional evidence that the H-Y antigen itself plays a testis-determining role has been obtained from studies of individuals with a discrepancy between gonadal, chromosomal, or phenotypic sex. H-Y antigen was detected in all instances where a testis was present. These phenomena include sex reversal, testicular feminization, and the bovine freemartin, which are discussed in more detail below.

The H-Y antigen appears to have been conserved during evolution, at least to the extent that a similar cross-reactive antigen has been found in humans, mice, rats, guinea pigs, rabbits, birds, and amphibia.[6] In birds, females are heterogametic, ZW. In amphibia, the heterogametic sex in *Rana pipiens* is the male, but in *Xeonopus laevis* it is the female. The presence of a cell surface component cross-reacting with antiserum to mouse H-Y antigen is present in the heterogametic sex in both birds and amphibia. From results obtained in the nonmammalian species, it has become apparent that the H-Y antigen should more correctly be described as the director of differentiation of the heterogametic gonad. The presence of H-Y antigen in heterogametic females, androgen-insensitive mice and humans, and eight-cell mouse embryos[6] indicates that its expression is not dependent on androgen action. Interestingly, with the possible exception of genes affecting stature and spermatogenesis, there is little evidence for the presence of other genes on the Y chromosome of man.[1,8]

The sex chromosome requirement for ovarian differentiation varies between species. In women with an XO sex chromosome complement (Turner's syndrome), ovaries do not develop.[9] In contrast, ovaries not only develop in XO mice, but they are functional.[10] The X chromosome contains genetic information coding for a wide variety of functions.[1] According to the Lyon hypothesis, genetic imbalance between individuals with different numbers of X chromosomes is avoided by the early inactivation of all but one X chromosome.[11] Inactive X's appear as condensed chromatin (Barr bodies), along the inner nuclear membrane. The nuclear sex of an individual refers to the presence or absence of these Barr bodies in normal females and males, respectively. Although this inactivation is generally thought to be a random phenomenon, there are some instances where random inactivation does not appear to have taken place (see O^{hv} below). Once inactivation has occurred, the same X chromosome is inactivated in all descendants of that cell. Control of X chromosome inactivation is not well understood, although it has been proposed that it is regulated by a site on a maternal autosome in the mouse.[12-15]

B. Gonadal Sex

Gonadal sex is primarily determined by the chromosomal sex of the individual. During early embryonic life, the gonad develops in an identical fashion in both sexes and has the potential to develop into either an ovary or a testis.[16] It is formed by primordial germ cells, that have migrated from the endoderm of the yolk sac, along with coelomic epithelium and underlying mesenchyme of the gonadal ridge. Testes differentiate from this undifferentiated primordium earlier than do ovaries. During testicular development, primary sex cords proliferate in the medulla and germ cells, migrating from the cortical area, are incorporated into developing seminiferous tubules. Leydig cells differentiate from the surrounding mesenchyme and, when stimulated by chorionic gonadotropin, initiate testosterone biosynthesis. This results in male differentiation of genital ducts and external genitalia. The medulla of the testis continues to enlarge, and the cortex regresses as testicular differentiation proceeds. In the absence of a Y chromosome, differentiation of an ovary will occur. Primary germ cells replicate in the peripheral embryonic cortex, but medullary tissue regresses.

The gonadal differentiation and sexual development of birds[2,17] present an interesting contrast to those of mammals. The female is the heterogametic sex (ZW) and expresses the H-Y antigen,[6] whereas the male is homogametic (ZZ) and the neutral phenotype. In genetic males both gonads differentiate as testes. In contrast, in genetic females an ovary differentiates from the left gonad and an oviduct from the left Müllerian duct, but the right gonad remains undifferentiated and the right Müllerian and Wolffian ducts regress. Removal of the left gonad in females will result in a type of sex reversal. Immediately after removal of the left gonad the plumage changes to the male or neutral type. As the right gonad differentiates into a testis or ovotestis, the type of plumage will depend on the amount of ovarian tissue present. Androgen production from the newly differentiated gonad is usually sufficient to cause growth of the comb. The development of testicular tissue in the right gonad of the female bird has not been explained. It would be interesting to know if H-Y antigen or its receptors, which are necessary for the development of ovarian tissue in birds, are abnormal in this tissue.

C. Genital Sex

In contrast to gonadal sex, genital sex and secondary sexual characteristics are hormonally determined.[18] The primordia of both male (Wolffian duct) and female (Müllerian duct) internal duct systems are present early in fetal life. The Wolffian duct differentiates into epididymis, vas deferens, seminal vesicles, and the ejaculatory duct. Müllerian ducts are precursors to Fallopian tubes, uterus, and the anterior portion of the vagina. In mammals, gonoducts and external genitalia have an inherent tendency to feminize unless acted upon by some masculinizing influence. The opposite is true in birds, where the neutral sex is male. Abnormal secretion of, or treatment with, androgenic steroids during mammalian development may result in genital sex that is inconsistent with gonadal sex.

The fetal testis plays an important dual role in genital duct development. Müllerian inhibiting substance[19] is secreted from fetal Sertoli cells and causes regression of female ductal elements. Without inhibition by this testicular protein, the Müllerian duct would remain and differentiate, since no further stimulus is needed. Androgens from fetal Leydig cells are required for Wolffian duct development. Without androgenic stimulation, this primitive tissue will spontaneously regress. The stimulus for testicular androgen secretion during the time of male differentiation comes from placental gonadotropins. However, as pregnancy continues and the concentration of these hormones falls, it is necessary for fetal gonadotropins to take over if adequate ductal and genital growth are to occur in utero.[20]

The primordia of the external genitalia of both sexes are similar and have the ability to differentiate in either a male or a female direction. Androgen stimulation is necessary for male differentiation to occur, resulting in the formation of the penis, the penile urethra, and the scrotum. In its absence, external genitalia will develop into female organs: the clitoris, labia minora, and labia majora. Once female structures have differentiated, with the exception of clitoral hypertrophy, they cannot be induced to form the homologous male structures, even under the influence of large doses of androgen.

Both testosterone and its 5α-reduced metabolite, dihydrotestosterone, are important in mediating the differentiation of masculine genital sex (Figure 1). In studies of fetal tissues from man (Figure 2) and animals, Wilson et al.[21-23] found that in the urogenital tubercle and urogenital sinus testosterone was metabolized to dihydrotestosterone, and this latter steroid was the major intranuclear, and thus active androgen. In contrast, in the Wolffian ducts testosterone was not metabolized and was itself retained in nuclei. 5α-Reductase activity, reducing testosterone to dihydrotestosterone, did not appear in ductal tissue until after male differentiation had occurred. In contrast to the importance of testosterone in mediating some fetal differentiation, in the adult dihydrotestosterone is concentrated in nuclei and is the active androgen in all male secondary sex tissue. The study of males with 5α-reductase deficiency (see below) has contributed significantly to our understanding of the roles of testosterone and dihydrotestosterone in normal male sexual differentiation.

II. GENETIC DEFECTS IN SEXUAL DEVELOPMENT

A. Defects in Genetic and Gonadal Sex

1. Abnormal Sex Chromosome Complement

Many examples of abnormalities in sex chromosome constitution have been described in man and animals.[1,2,24] Genotypes vary from XO (Turner's syndrome) to conditions with multiple X's or Y's. The presence of more than one X is incompatible with normal maturation of male germ cells.[24,25] Similarly, evidence of hypogonadism may be more frequent in XYY then in normal males. The etiology of these defects is not well understood and is probably variable. Extensive discussion of these abnormalities is beyond the scope of this chapter.

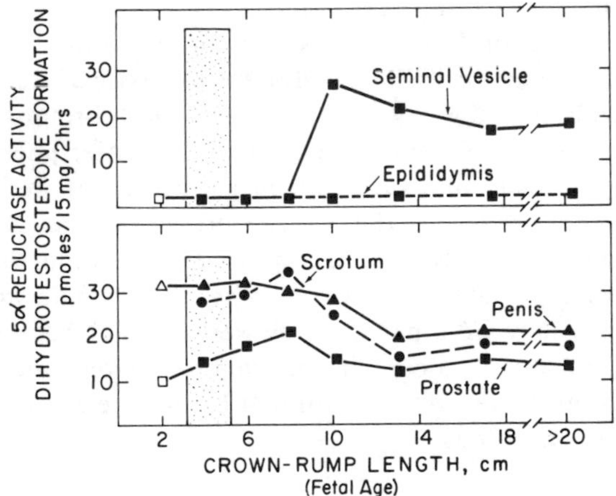

FIGURE 2. 5α-Reductase activity in urogenital tracts of male human embryos as a function of age. Enzyme activity was evaluated by the formation of 5α-dihydrotestosterone from testosterone. Tissues in the upper panel are derived from the Wolffian ducts, and in the lower panel from the urogenital sinus (prostate), urogenital swelling (scrotum), and urogenital tubercule (penis). Stippled bar represents the period of masculine genital differentiation. (From Siiteri, P. K. and Wilson J. D., *J. Clin. Endocrinol. Metab.*, 38, 113, 1974. With permission.)

The best-studied animal models of an abnormal sex chromosome complement are the calico male cat (XXY)[26-28] and the XO mouse.[1,10] In most instances the XXY condition in animals is probably not recognized. However, in the cat, where yellow and black are coat color alleles on the X chromosome, the presence of both colors in a male cat indicates the presence of two X chromosomes. In these cats the testes are small and spermatogenesis is usually decreased. As mentioned above, the effects of XO differ in the mouse and human. In the mouse functioning ovaries develop; streak gonads are found in the human. This suggests that additional unrecognized factors on the X chromosome influence ovarian development.

In contrast to the above examples of deleterious changes in sex chromosome complement of individuals, there are several mammalian species in which an adaptive change in the sex chromosome mechanism has evolved.[1,29] One interesting example is the mole-vole (*Ellobius lutescens*).[30] In this animal both males and females have an XO chromosome constitution in soma and germ cells. Despite the apparent absence of a Y chromosome, the presence of the H-Y antigen has been detected in XO males but not in XO females. During evolution of this species, the H-Y gene has apparently been linked with the male X. The detection of H-Y antigen in XO males gives further support to the testis-organizing function of the H-Y antigen.

2. *Abnormalities in H-Y Antigen*

There are no proven examples of abnormalities of H-Y antigen production, but there are several instances in which such a situation probably exists. In humans, occasional patients have been described with streak gonads, a female phenotype, and a normal male XY karyotype.[24] The syndrome is inherited as an X-linked recessive or male-limited autosomal dominant trait. The absence of testes and subsequent lack of masculine development is probably due to abnormal H-Y antigen. Cases of imperfect testicular development and some true hermaphrodites, where an ovary and testis develop together, may also represent an abnormality in this protein. Continued studies of H-Y antigen in cases of gonadal abnormalities should be extremely interesting. A gene affecting H-Y expression is discussed below.

The sex ratio in the wood lemming, *Myopus schisticolor* Lilljeborg, reflects an interesting biological phenomenon.[6] Not only is there an overabundance of females in the wild population, but somatic cells in females are of two genetic types, XX and XY. However, females with an XY genotype have an XX sex chromosome complement in germ cells and produce only X-bearing egg cells. This latter phenomenon is thought to be the result of selective nondisjunction in germ cells of the fetal ovary, with a doubling of the X and the loss of the Y. The presence of an XY karyotype in the absence of testes appears to contradict the concept that in mammals the Y chromosome carries a testis-determining factor. However, when XY female wood lemmings were typed for H-Y antigen they were negative, as were normal XX females. In contrast, XY males were H-Y positive. To explain this enigma, Silvers and Wachtel[6] have proposed the presence of an X-linked mutation that blocks the expression of H-Y antigen in the XY female wood lemming.

3. *Absence of Müllerian Inhibiting Substance*

There have been occasional case reports concerning man[24] and animals[31,32] in which the presence of Müllerian derivatives, a uterus and Fallopian tubes, have been found in an individual with otherwise normal male development. The condition is inherited as an autosomal or sex-linked recessive and is probably due to insufficient production of Müllerian inhibiting substance by fetal testes. Recent advances[19] in the study of Müllerian inhibiting substance should allow us to learn more about the physiology of this protein.

4. Sex Reversal

The presence of a female karyotype but a male phenotype with testes has been called sex reversal. This abnormality has been described in a number of different species, including amphibians, goats, pigs, mice, and man.[33] This condition has been most extensively studied in the mouse and has been associated with a mutant gene, *Sxr*.[34] Despite extensive cytological studies, results from early investigations gave no evidence of a Y chromosome. Thus, in 1971, Cattanach et al.[34] described the mutation in the mouse as a sex-limited, dominant mutation carried by normal males and expressed in genotypic females. However, the possibility that a small male-determining region of the Y chromosome was present elsewhere in the genome was not excluded. Recent studies by Bennett et al.[35] indicate that this may be the case. Serological studies detected H-Y antigen (discussed above) in *Sxr* XX males. These results suggest that a portion of the Y chromosome carrying male and H-Y-determining factors is present in *Sxr* animals. Thus, a translocation between the Y and the X or an autosomal chromosome that cannot be detected cytologically has apparently occurred in *Sxr* mice. Different factors may be involved in sex-reversed goats[2] and pigs,[36] since this defect is apparently inherited as an autosomal recessive.

Both the seminiferous tubules[34] and Leydig cells[33] are abnormal in *Sxr* XX mice. Germ cells are present in seminiferous tubules in fetal and early postnatal life, but are lost progressively with age. Thus, in adult *Sxr* XX mice, testes are small and contain well-formed seminiferous tubules that have Sertoli cells but lack germ cells. Plasma FSH concentrations are twice the normal level, but less than castrate levels. Despite high plasma concentrations of LH, there is little histochemical and ultrastructural evidence of Leydig cell response. Plasma testosterone concentrations are correspondingly low. These findings are consistent with a Leydig cell defect involving an early step in LH action.[33]

Results from studies of *Sxr* XX male mice have given support to several biological theories. The fact that spermatogenesis is absent in *Sxr* XX mice, yet present in *Sxr* XO and *Sxr* XY mice,[35] reinforces the proposal that two X chromosomes are incompatible with normal male germ cell differentiation. However, spermiogenesis in *Sxr* mice is not completely normal, suggesting that the Y was not translocated intact and supporting the localization of some genes affecting spermatogenesis on the Y chromosome. The detection of H-Y antigen[35] in these mice supports its role as a testis-organizing factor. The *Sxr* gene has been combined with the *Tfm* gene for androgen insensitivity and the O^{hv} gene (see below) to yield further information on the control of X inactivation and differentiation in androgen-responsive cells.[37-39]

5. The Bovine Freemartin

In cattle, the sexual development of a female in the presence of a male twin is often abnormal.[18,40] The ovary in affected females may vary from that containing only a few seminiferous tubules to one resembling a small testis. Derivatives of Müllerian ducts are usually absent, and there is some evidence of androgen-dependent masculinization of the remainder of the genital tract, including the external genitalia and the presence of some portion of Wolffian ducts. Although testosterone from the male twin could account for the masculinization of the genital tract, it would not explain the differentiation of testicular components in the ovary. Since freemartins were known to be XX/XY chimeras, it was thought that the associated testicular differentiation was due to cellular exchange. Ohno[3] proposed that in the gonad H-Y antigen from XY cells induced associated XX cells to undergo testicular differentiation, and he used the results from studies of the virilized freemartin gonad to support this theory. He recently reported the presence of H-Y antigen in this organ.[41] Interestingly, chimerism from chorionic fusion also occurs in man and marmosets, yet conditions similar to the bovine freemartin have not been detected in instances of heterosexual dizygotic twins. This could be due to species differences in the degree of chimerism that occurs in the affected ovary or the time during differentiation at which cellular exchange takes place.

B. Defects in the Biosynthesis of Androgens

1. Defects at the Level of the Hypothalamus and Pituitary

These defects have been best described in the human.[4,20] They include deficiencies in secretion of releasing factors from the hypothalamus and the synthesis and release of luteinizing hormone (LH) from the pituitary. The LH deficiency may be isolated or exist in combination with deficiencies of other pituitary hormones. In utero chorionic gonadotropin stimulates the testes to secrete androgens, so that normal male differentiation occurs even in affected males. However, the concentration of this placental hormone eventually falls and, without fetal LH to maintain the androgenic milieu, normal intrauterine genital growth does not take place. Gonadotropin deficiency may also become apparent postnatally when the normal hormonal increase does not occur at puberty. In these instances, affected males and females will remain sexually immature. The etiology and genetic factors that result in decreased gonadotropins are variable and not completely understood. There is evidence that in some instances of hypothalamic disorders there is autosomal dominant inheritance.[4] Defects in animals are discussed in depth in Volumc I, chapter 6 by Bartke.[99]

2. Defects in the Synthesis of Sex Hormones

a. Defective Testicular and Adrenal Enzymes

Steroid hormones of all classes are derived from common precursors before diverging to form unique products of widely varying biologic actions (Figure 3). An enzyme defect may have divergent effects, depending on its position in the biosynthetic pathway. The testis contains enzymes (A to E, Figure 3) necessary for the synthesis of sex steroids only, but the adrenal contains enzymes for androgen as well as for glucocorticoid and mineralocorticoid production. Decreased activity of enzymes A to E will result in male pseudohermaphroditism. Newborn males have ambiguous genitalia due to deficient testicular androgen production in utero. Defective function of the remaining enzymes, necessary for corticosteroid production, will result in adrenal hyperplasia due to increased secretion of ACTH through the negative feedback mechanism. This is associated with excessive androgen production by the adrenal due to the buildup of precursor steroids. Often this adrenal androgen production is sufficient to cause prenatal masculinization in females and precocious puberty in males.

There are numerous examples of defective synthesis of sex hormones in humans.[24] Enzyme defects involving only androgens are inherited as male-limited autosomal

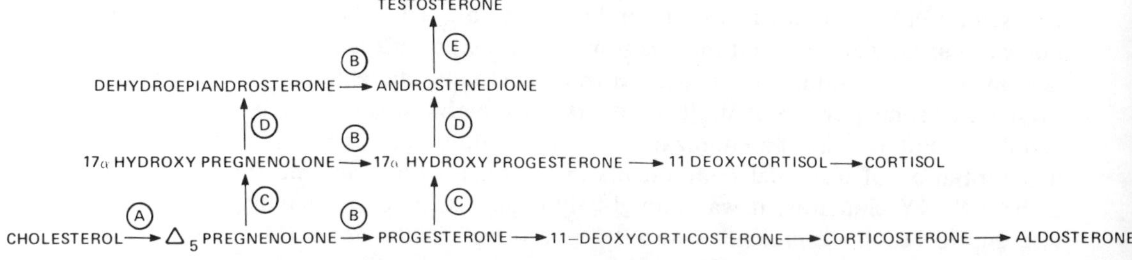

FIGURE 3. Biosynthetic pathway for testicular and adrenal steroids. Defects in enzymes A to E cause male pseudohermaphrodism. Abnormalities in the other enzymes result in excessive androgen production by the adrenal due to the buildup of precursor steroids. A = cholesterol desmolase; B = 3β-hydroxysteroid dehydrogenase; C = 17α-hydroxylase; D = 17,20-desmolase; E = 17β-hydroxy-oxidoreductase.

dominant or X-linked recessive traits, whereas the remaining abnormalities are transmitted as autosomal recessives. An inherited defect in 17α-hydroxylase has been reported in inbred Jersey cattle.[42] Affected animals evidenced decreased vigor as well as impaired fertility and sterility.

b. The vet *Rat*

This mutation was originally described by Stanley et al.[43] and named *vet* due to the nature of the testes (vestigial testes) in affected animals. The recessive mutation results in animals that are male pseudohermaphrodites with a female phenotype, an XY karyotype, and a chromatin-negative nuclear sex. In more extensive studies, Bardin et al.[44] reported that, although the only Wolffian duct derivative present was a rudimentary microscopic epididymis, tissues in these animals were, nevertheless, androgen responsive. This defect in masculinization was associated with castrate levels of LH, but undetectable plasma testosterone concentrations, suggesting a defect in the response of the Leydig cells. Subsequent histochemical and electron-microscopic studies of testes indicated the presence of unstimulated immature Leydig cells. Administration of hCG of proven biological potency had no effect on morphology or testosterone secretion from these vestigial cells. It was proposed that *vet* rats had an inherited defect of the LH receptor. The resulting failure of Leydig cell differentiation and subsequent androgen biosynthesis would result in the development of the *vet* rat as a male pseudohermaphrodite.

Recently a male pseudohermaphrodite has been described that may be the human counterpart of the *vet* rat.[45] The patient had a female phenotype and a XY genotype. Plasma concentrations of LH were elevated, FSH was normal, and testosterone was low. Testes and Wolffian ducts were present, but no Müllerian structures were seen. Hyalinized seminiferous tubules contained normal Sertoli cells and occasional immature germ cells. No Leydig cells could be identified by either light or electron microscopy.

C. Abnormalities at the End Organ

To understand the functional importance of abnormalities in androgen action at the end organ it is first necessary to understand the general mechanism of steroid action. This is similar for all three classes of sex steroids. Since no abnormalities are known for estrogen and progesterone, the discussion will focus on androgen action.[46] Testosterone, the major circulating androgen, enters the target tissue, where in many cases it is metabolized to 5α-dihydrotestosterone by 5α-reductase. This metabolite is prominent in reproductive tissues and skin derivatives. However, in other target organs, such as kidney, testis, and brain, 5α-reductase activity is low and testosterone is the active androgen. Metabolism is not required for activation of estradiol or progesterone. The active steroid is bound by specific intracellular receptors and the complex transferred into the nucleus where it binds to chromatin at specific acceptor sites. This initiates a series of metabolic steps resulting in the synthesis of specific RNAs, proteins, and ultimately organ growth. There are, thus, several points at which a defect could affect target organ responsiveness.

1. 5α-Reductase Deficiency

The importance of the metabolism of testosterone to 5α-dihydrotestosterone for androgen action has been difficult to evaluate due to the lack of mutants. Evidence for its role in differentiation and growth of some sexual tissue has recently been obtained by the identification of a syndrome of 5α-reductase deficiency in humans that results in a form of incomplete male pseudohermaphroditism (Figure 4).[47,48] This defect is inherited as an autosomal recessive. At birth, affected males have ambiguous genitalia,

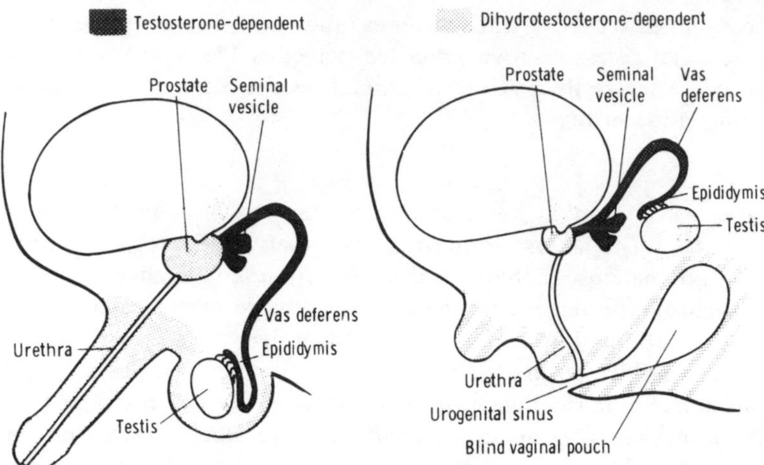

FIGURE 4. Evidence for the roll of testosterone and 5α-dihydrotestosterone in sexual differentiation. Genitalia from normal (left) and 5α-reductase-deficient (right) males are depicted. In affected males, differentiation of testosterone-dependent but not dihydrotestosterone-dependent tissue occurs. (From Imperato-McGinley, J. and Peterson, R. E., *Am. J. Med.*, 61, 251, 1976. With permission.)

although internal structures derived from Wolffian ducts are normally differentiated. Testes are located in the inguinal canal or labia. At puberty there is marked virilization, including some phallic growth. Spermatogenesis, although somewhat abnormal, may be complete. Not all masculine features develop normally; however, the prostate remains small, there is little beard, and there is no temporal recession of the hairline or acne. Studies of androgen metabolic clearance rates, production rates,[49] and metabolism by cultured fibroblasts[50] have confirmed the absence of 5α-reductase in affected individuals.

The abnormalities in these patients confirm the suggestion of Wilson et al.[21-23] that differentiation is mediated by testosterone in some male secondary sex tissues and by 5α-dihydrotestosterone in others. They also provide some inferential information on the mechanism of androgen action. Partially purified androgen receptors will bind both testosterone and dihydrotestosterone,[46,51,52] implying that both steroids are potentially active. Although in normal accessory sex tissues the action of testosterone cannot be evaluated due to its rapid metabolism to dihydrotestosterone, in tissues that normally lack 5α-reductase, such as mouse kidney, both testosterone and dihydrotestosterone (exogenous) are active.[44] One might expect that testosterone would be similarly active in tissues with 5α-reductase deficiency. However, the absence of prostate growth and certain other androgen responses in affected patients suggest that steroid response may be regulated by other factors in addition to specific cytoplasmic receptors and steroid-metabolizing enzymes.

Despite their having been recognized for some time, little is known about the molecular nature of the enzyme defects resulting in abnormal androgen action. This is primarily due to the lack of suitable experimental models. Several examples of alterations in steroid action or response for which the genetic mechanisms are known will be discussed below. This in-depth knowledge has been gained primarily through the use of animal models.

2. *Androgen Insensitivity (Testicluar Feminization)*

a. *Description of the Defect*

One of the best-described genetic defects in steroid action is that of androgen insensitivity or testicular feminization (reviewed in References 44 and 53). This defect has been described in man, mouse, rat, and is probably also seen in the cow and rabbit.[54] The mutant gene (*Tfm*) is X-linked in the mouse[55] and human,[56] and probably so in rats. It is transmitted by the female to one half of her sons, which differentiate as androgen-insensitive male pseudohermaphrodites. Affected individuals have a female phenotype, despite an XY karyotype and a chromatin-negative nuclear sex. There is a short blind vagina that usually opens somewhat later than normal. In rodents the characteristic female nipple line is present. Small, bilateral inguinal or abdominal testes are the only evidence of a reproductive tract. The androgen insensitivity of fetal anlagen results in the absence of Wolffian duct derivatives. The lack of Müllerian derivatives is consistent with normal testicular production of Müllerian inhibiting substance. In mice, rats, and most human patients[56,57] this syndrome has been associated with the absence of an effective androgen receptor. 5α-Reductase activity is not deficient, but is similar to that in females. Recently, evidence has been reported for another form of androgen insensitivity in some humans who have normal androgen binding but an absence of nuclear androgen retention.[58] Most of the following section will summarize studies done on *Tfm* rats and mice, due to the large body of information available on these animals.

Although affected animals do not have prostate or seminal vesicles, androgen response has been examined by a variety of investigators, using tissues such as kidney, brain, submaxillary gland, and preputial gland, which require androgens for growth but not differentiation. Response to both endogenous and exogenous androgens has been evaluated, using behavior, tissue weight, a wide variety of sexually dimorphic enzymes, and RNA, DNA, and protein synthesis. Generally the basal level of the various endpoints was similar in *Tfm* and female litter mates. Although the *Tfm* rat was insensitive to physiological doses of androgens, some androgenic response could be elicited by the administration of pharmacologic doses of androgen.[59] This usually required a 20- to 100-fold greater dose than that needed to stimulate a response in normal rats. In addition, studies by Goldman[60] suggested that some masculinization of the urogenital sinus and hypothalamus-pituitary may have occurred in *Tfm* rats in utero. In contrast, despite the use of large doses of androgens, no response could be elicited in *Tfm*/Y mice. The difference in the degree of androgen insensitivity associated with the two genetic defects represented by the rat and mouse corresponds with the range of androgen insensitivity, from complete to partial, that has been reported for the multiple *Tfm* mutations that have occurred in the human population. The absence of even an intranuclear response in *Tfm*/Y mice[61] supports the hypothesis that the *Tfm* mutation produces a pretranscriptional regulatory defect.

Despite the known occurrence of androgen insensitivity in three species and its probable presence in several others, there is no evidence for a similar situation involving estrogen or progesterone in any species. It would be surprising, however, if such mutations had not occurred. An explanation for the apparent absence of such individuals is that insensitivity to either estrogen or progesterone is lethal to the developing embryo. This possibility is supported by the recent reports of the estrogen dependence of mouse preimplantation embryos[62] and the presence of estrogen receptors in rabbit blastocysts.[63] In addition, there is evidence for the role of ovarian steroids in placental development and weight,[64,65] and progesterone[66]- and estrogen[67]-binding proteins in fetal membranes. Additional study of tissues from spontaneously aborted fetuses for the detection of these abnormalities could be rewarding.

b. Molecular Nature of the Defect

The nature of the defect involved in androgen insensitivity was suggested by the absence in *Tfm* animals of specific in vivo[44,68] and in vitro[69] androgen uptake by nuclei of various tissues that are normally androgen responsive. One explanation for this inability to concentrate androgens at the active site in the cell was that cytoplasmic androgen receptors were defective. This hypothesis has been confirmed by numerous investigators using a variety of techniques. In early studies, analysis of multiple tissues from both the *Tfm* rat and mouse indicated a complete absence of androgen receptors[53,70] (Figure 5). However, later investigations using more sensitive techniques did detect small amounts of this protein in the pituitary of *Tfm* rats,[71] and kidney[72,73] and brain/hypothalamus[74,75] of *Tfm*/Y mice. The androgen receptor in *Tfm* animals had normal or only slightly reduced affinity for androgens. Thus, the androgen insensitivity of both *Tfm* rats and mice can be correlated with an inadequate concentration of effective androgen receptors. The apparent normality of the receptors that have been detected suggests an abnormality in a regulatory rather than a structural gene.

Studies of androgen binding in human patients with clinical evidence of androgen insensitivity have used cultured human skin fibroblasts. In most instances, a decrease in binding capacity has been found.[56,57] Recently a second group of patients has been identified.[58] Although these patients show clinical evidence of androgen insensitivity, specific dihydrotestosterone-binding in whole fibroblasts and purified nuclei was evaluated as normal. This suggests that an abnormality in receptor-chromatin interaction or gene transcription may exist.

c. Use of Tfm Animals

Androgen-insensitive rats and mice have been extremely valuable in both genetic and biological studies concerning the role of androgens in tissue differentiation.[53] The abnormal androgen biosynthesis in *Tfm* rodents has been used to characterize the partial androgen dependence of some Leydig cell testosterone-biosynthesizing enzymes.[44,53] In addition, as a result of studies using the *Tfm* rat, Purvis et al.[76] proposed that an intact

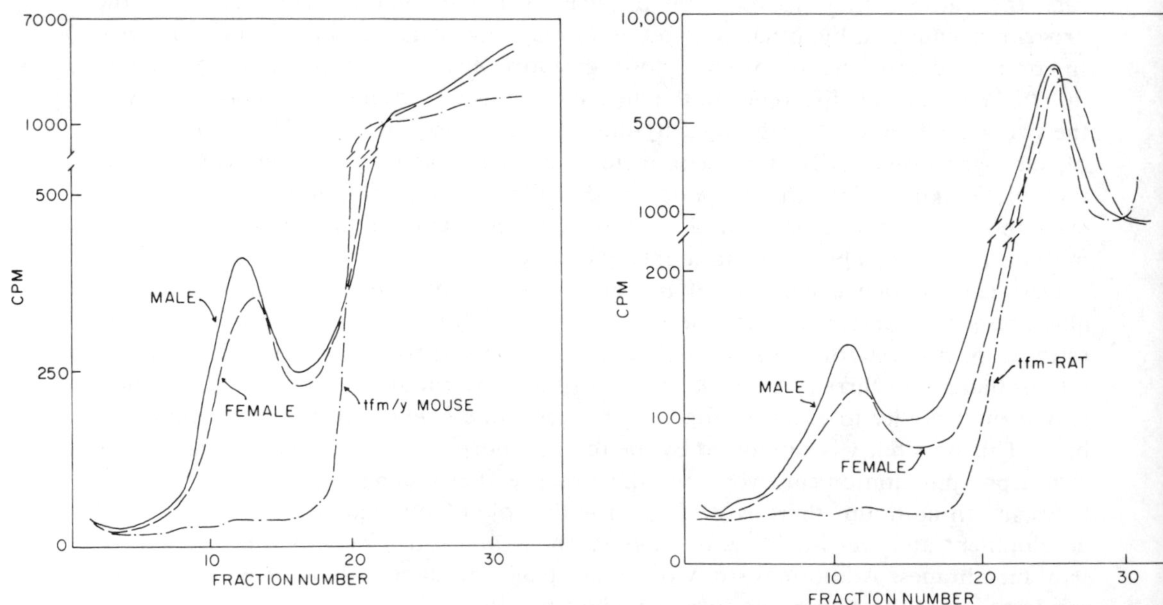

FIGURE 5. ^{3}H-androgen binding in tissues from normal male, female, and androgen-insensitive *tfm* rodents. ^{3}H-testosterone was incubated with mouse kidney cytosol (left), and ^{3}H-dihydrotestosterone was incubated with rat preputial gland cytosol (right) and sedimented through sucrose gradients. In each tissue, the smaller peak, sedimenting in about fraction 12, represents specific, high-affinity androgen binding. The absence of specific androgen binding in tissues from *tfm* animals is in marked contrast to that present in normal male and females. (From Bullock, L. P. and Bardin, C. W., *J. Clin. Endocrinol. Metab.*, 35, 935, 1972. With permission.)

androgen response is also necessary for normal induction of LH receptors in Leydig cells. The absence of the final stages of spermatogenesis in *Tfm* rodents was thought to be a reflection of the androgen dependence of sperm per se. However, in the report by Lyon et al.[77] that fertile *Tfm*-bearing sperm can develop in male mice, chimeric for androgen-resistent and normal genotypes, suggests that the androgen dependence of germ cells may be mediated through testicular somatic cells. The detection of H-Y antigen in *Tfm* mice and humans[6] supports the concept that expression of the H-Y locus is directly related to the presence of the Y chromosome and not induced by androgens. The gene for sex reversal, *Sxr*, and *Tfm* have been combined in normal and XO mice to confirm the role of androgens in ovarian,[78,79] testicular,[80] and accessory sex tissue[37,38] differentiation and function.

Female mice carrying the *Tfm* gene on one of their X chromosomes manifest a wide range of androgen responsiveness[81] and renal androgen receptor concentrations.[53] These data support the Lyon hypothesis of random X-inactivation and are further evidence of the direct role of the *Tfm* gene and the androgen receptor in regulating androgen response. Ohno et al.[82] used data from female mice carrying the *Tfm* and O^{hv} (discussed below) genes to estimate the number of progenitor cells of renal proximal tubules to be from four to six.

Tfm/Y mice have also been used in studies of steroid action. In normal mice, progestins simulate androgen action, whereas no response is elicited in *Tfm*/Y mice.[53] This insensitivity, coupled with the absence of cytoplasmic or nuclear binding of progestins in *Tfm*/Y mice, strengthens the hypothesis that the androgenic effects of progestins are mediated via the androgen receptor. In drug studies, the response of female litter mates to androgens was indicated by the enhancement of kidney microsomal activation of some potential carcinogens,[83] the induction of renal chloroform toxicity,[84] and an alteration in the activity of some hepatic microsomal drug-metabolizing enzymes.[85] The absence of response in *Tfm*/Y mice suggested that these responses also require a functional androgen receptor. In contrast, when other endpoints, which were thought to be affected by androgens, were used, *Tfm*/Y mice responded normally. These include the erythropoietic response to either 5α- or 5β-dihydrotestosterone,[53] adrenal X-zone degeneration,[86] and compensatory renal hypertrophy.[87] The normal response of the *Tfm*/Y mouse suggests that, in these instances, the role of androgen may be secondary or that the androgen effects are mediated through a mechanism that does not require the same androgen receptor that is present in accessory sex tissue.

3. The Seabright Bantam

Similar to the early interpretation of the *Tfm* syndrome, the Seabright bantam was originally thought to represent an example of abnormal or excessive estrogen secretion by the testis, since the plumage was henny, or of the female type, in both sexes.[17] However, it was subsequently determined that castration of the male resulted in the development of normal male plumage, and administration of androgen to the capon caused female-type feathering. This unexpected response was shown to be due to a single autosomal dominant gene, *Hf*, which changed the response of feather follicles so that female-type plumage was produced in response to androgens.[27] This type of response is not unique to the Seabright bantam, as large doses of testosterone have been reported to feminize the plumage of the ovariectomized female silver pheasant.[17]

III. OTHER GENETIC CONTROLS OF STEROID RESPONSE

A. Genetic Regulation of β-glucuronidase

The best understanding of the genetic control of an androgenic response is that of mouse kidney β-glucuronidase. This is due primarily to the work of Paigen and his colleagues, using inbred strains of mice.[88] The response of β-glucuronidase to androgen stimulation is inherited as a single Mendelian trait, which is regulated by the *Gur* locus. *Gur* represents one of the first known mammalian regulatory elements that governs the response of an enzyme to a physiologic stimulus. It is epistatic to genes regulating the variation in response that are associated with differences in the potencies of inducing agents. *Gur* is tightly linked to the glucuronidase structural gene, *Gus*, on mouse chromosome 5 and acts in a cis manner through a nondiffusible factor to regulate the rate of glucuronidase synthesis. There are two alleles, Gur^a and Gur^b, which are inherited in a codominant manner. In Gur^a mice the glucuronidase response to androgen has a short lag and a rapid rise to maximal enzyme activity (Figure 6).[89] The response in Gur^b mice has a longer lag and a slower rise to maximum enzyme activity, which is only about one fourth that of the first group (Figure 6). Swank et al.[90] recently reported that hypophysectomy markedly decreases the androgen-stimulated increase in the rate of synthesis and subsequent activity of glucuronidase, but not other renal androgen-responsive enzymes. Thus, it is possible that pituitary hormones may also have a role in regulating this enzyme.

There are other known genetic factors that influence final glucuronidase activity in mouse kidney.[88] These include the alleles of the structural gene *Gus*, the temporal locus *Gut*, which controls glucuronidase activity during development, and the *Eg* locus, which regulates intracellular processing of glucuronidase. Continued studies of the genetic control of glucuronidase activity will help define and understand the functional units of the mammalian chromosome.

B. The O^{hv} Gene

A controlling element or set of genes on the X chromosome that regulates the inactivation of the X chromosome has been described.[12-15] Recently, Ohno and his collaborators[38] reported a mutation, O^{hv}, which they believe to be an allele of these control-

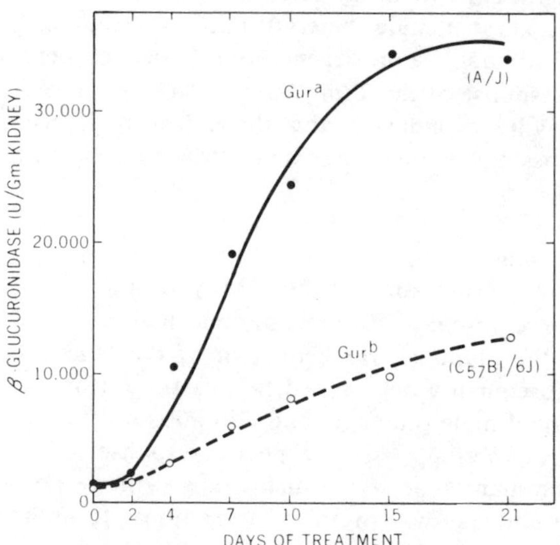

FIGURE 6. Regulation of mouse kidney β-glucuronidase by the Gur locus. Inbred mice, homozygous for Gur^a (A/J) or Gur^b ($C_{57}BL/6J$) were given daily doses of testosterone (2 mg). The points show the mean activity in five animals. (From Bardin, C. W., Bullock, L. P., Gupta, C., and Brown, T., *Int. Congr. Series No. 40a, Endocrinol.*, 1976, 481. With permission.)

ling element genes. The X chromosome that carries O^{hv} is preferentially activated. If the gene for androgen insensitivity, *Tfm*, is coupled with O^{hv}, it should result in the development of a greater number of unresponsive cells and thus, secondarily, affect the androgen responsiveness of heterozygous *Tfm*/+ organisms. This theory was supported by results that were obtained by using coat color, androgen responsiveness of kidneys, and differentiation of the Wolffian duct and urogenital sinus in sex-reversed *Sxr*, O^{hv} mice.[38,82]

C. Tissue Culture and Steroid Responsive Cell Lines

A great deal of information about the mechanism of steroid action has been gained through the approach advanced by Yamamoto and his colleagues[91] (in collaboration with Tomkins, who began this study prior to his death) using a glucocorticoid-sensitive cell line that normally dies in the presence of steroid (see chapter 3).[100] A variety of dexamethasone-resistant clones have been developed. Not only have some clones been shown to lack a cytoplasmic glucocorticoid receptor, similar to the lack of androgen receptor in *Tfm* mutants, but a number of other alterations in the mechanism of steroid activation of a cell have been described. These include impaired nuclear transfer, increased nuclear transfer, and cells (deathless) that have no defects in either receptor binding or nuclear transfer, but are, nevertheless, steroid resistant. The defect associated with clones having altered nuclear transfer is thought to represent changes in that portion of the receptor needed for chromatin binding. The defect associated with deathless mutants has not yet been defined.

Although a similar system has not been developed using sex-steroid-responsive cells, some steroid-dependent cell lines are available. The greatest success has been achieved with cells derived from tumors. One of the best-known androgen-dependent tumors is the mouse mammary adenocarcinoma, Shionogi carcinoma 115. Recently, the development of both androgen-dependent and autonomous, androgen-independent cell lines of this tumor has been reported.[92] The MCF-7 human breast cancer cell line has been reported to contain receptors for estrogens, androgens, progestins, and glucocorticoids[93,94] and is, thus, potentially useful. Sex-steroid-dependent cell lines have also been established from a variety of other tumors.[95-97] The establishment of long-term cell lines from normal tissue is much more difficult. One such line, mouse fibroblast L-929 cells, has been reported to have androgen, estrogen, and glucocorticoid receptors.[98] Short-term cultures of human skin fibroblasts have been used to evaluate androgen binding and response,[50,58] but continuous cell lines have not been developed. Currently, the opportunity for in-depth study of defects in sex steroid responsiveness is limited by the absence of an identifiable, inducible gene product or usable cellular response. Once this is overcome, studies similar to those of Gehring and Tomkins[73] should enhance our ability to elucidate genetic control of sex steroid action.

REFERENCES

1. **Ohno, S.**, *Sex Chromosomes and Sex Linked Genes*, Springer-Verlag, New York, 1967.
2. **Mittwock, U.**, *Genetics of Sex Differentiation*, Academic Press, New York, 1973.
3. **Ohno, S.**, Major regulatory genes for mammalian sexual development, *Cell*, 7, 315, 1976.
4. **Paulsen, C. A.**, The testes, in *Textbook of Endocrinology*, Williams, R. H., Ed., W. B. Saunders, Philadelphia, 1974, 323.
5. **Ohno, S.**, A hormone-like action of H-Y antigen and gonadal development of XY/XX mosaic males and hermaphrodites, *Hum. Genet.*, 35, 21, 1976.
6. **Silvers, W. K. and Wachtel, S. S.**, H-Y antigen: behavior and function, *Science*, 195, 956, 1977.

7. **Wachtel, S. S., Ohno, S., Koo, G. C., and Boyse, E. A.,** Possible role of H-Y antigen in the primary determination of sex, *Nature (London),* 257, 235, 1975.
8. **McKusick, V. A. and Ruddle, F. H.,** The status of the gene map of the human chromosomes, *Science,* 196, 390, 1977.
9. **Ross, G. T. and VandeWiele, R. L.,** The ovaries, in *Textbook of Endocrinology,* Williams, R. H., Ed., W. B. Saunders, Philadelphia, 1974, 368.
10. **Cattanach, B. M.,** XO mice, *Genet. Res.,* 3, 487, 1962.
11. **Lyon, M. F.,** X-chromosome inactivation and developmental patterns in mammals, *Biol. Rev.,* 47, 1, 1972.
12. **Brown, S. W. and Chandra, H. S.,** Inactivation system of the mammalian X-chromosome, *Proc. Natl. Acad. Sci. U.S.A.,* 70, 195, 1973.
13. **Cattanach, B. M., Pollard, C. E., and Perez, J. N.,** Controlling elements in the mouse X-chromosome. I. Interaction with the X-linked genes, *Genet. Res.,* 14, 223, 1969.
14. **Cattanach, B. M., Perez, J. N., and Pollard, C. E.,** Controlling elements in the mouse X-chromosome. II. Location in the linkage map, *Genet. Res.,* 15, 183, 1970.
15. **Cattanach, B. M.,** Controlling elements in the mouse X-chromosome. III. Influence upon both parts of an X divided by rearrangement, *Genet. Res.,* 16, 293, 1970.
16. **Jost, A.,** Embryonic sexual differentiation, in *Hermaphroditism, Genital Anomalies and Related Endocrine Disorders,* Jones, H. W. and Scott, W. W., Eds., Williams & Wilkins, Baltimore, 1971, 16.
17. **Parkes, A. S. and Emmens, C. W.,** Effect of androgens and estrogens on birds, *Vitam. Horm. (N.Y.),* 2, 361, 1944.
18. **Jost, A., Vigier, B., Prepin, J., and Perchellet, J. P.,** Studies on sex differentiation in mammals, *Rec. Prog. Horm. Res.,* 29, 1, 1973.
19. **Josso, N., Picard, J.-Y., Tran, D.,** Antimuellerian hormone, *Rec. Prog. Horm. Res.,* 33, 117, 1977.
20. **Smith, D. W.,** Micropenis and its management, in *Morphogenesis and Malformation of the Genital System,* Blandau, R. J. and Bergsma, D., Eds., Alan R. Liss, New York, 1977, 147.
21. **Siiteri, P. K. and Wilson, J. D.,** Testosterone formation and metabolism during male sexual differentiation in the human embryo, *J. Clin. Endocrinol. Metab.,* 38, 113, 1974.
22. **Wilson, J. D.,** Testosterone uptake by the urogenital tract of the rabbit embryo, *Endocrinology,* 92, 1192, 1973.
23. **Wilson, J. D. and Lasnitzki, I.,** Dihydrotestosterone formation in fetal tissues of the rabbit and rat, *Endocrinology,* 89, 659, 1971.
24. **Grumbach, M. M. and VanWyk, J. J.,** Disorders of sex differentiation, in *Textbook of Endocrinology,* Williams, R. H., Ed., W. B. Saunders, Philadelphia, 1974, chap. 8.
25. **Lyon, M. F.,** Sex chromosome activity in germ cells, in *Physiology and Genetics of Reproduction,* Part A, Coutinho, E. M. and Fuchs, F., Eds., Plenum Press, New York, 63, 1974.
26. **Centerwall, W. R. and Benirschke, K.,** An animal model for the XXY Klinefelter's syndrome in man: tortoise shell and calico male cats, *Am. J. Vet. Res.,* 36, 1275, 1975.
27. **Hutt, F. B.,** *Animal Genetics,* Ronald Press, New York, 1964, 159, 432.
28. **Thuline, H. C. and Norby, D. E.,** Spontaneous occurrence of chromosome abnormality in cats, *Science,* 134, 554, 1961.
29. **Fredga, K.,** Unusual sex chromosome inheritance in mammals, *Philos. Trans. R. Soc. London,* 259, 15, 1970.
30. **Nagai, Y. and Ohno, S.,** Testis-determining H-Y antigen in XO males of the mole-vole *(Ellobius lutescens), Cell,* 10, 729, 1977.
31. **Biggers, J. D. and McFeely, R. A.,** Intersexuality in domestic mammals, *Adv. Reprod. Physiol.,* 1, 29, 1966.
32. **Dain, A. R.,** Intersexuality in a cocker spaniel dog, *J. Reprod. Fertil.,* 39, 365, 1974.
33. **Chung, K. W., Blackburn, W. R., Bullock, L. P., Santen R. J., and Bardin, C. W.,** Leydig cell structure-function relationships in the mouse with XX-sex reversal, in *The Testis in Normal and Infertile Men,* Troen, P. and Nankin, H. R., Eds., Raven Press, New York, 1977, 45.
34. **Cattanach, B. M., Pollard, C. E., and Hawkes, S. G.,** Sex-reversed mice: XX and XO males, *Cytogenetics,* 10, 318, 1971.
35. **Bennett, D., Mathieson, B. J., Scheid, M., Yanagisawa, K., Boyse, E. A., Wachtel, S., and Cattanach, B. M.,** Serological evidence for H-Y antigen in Sxr, XX sex-reversed phenotypic males, *Nature (London),* 265, 255, 1977.
36. **Hard, W. L. and Eisen, J. D.,** A phenotypic male swine with a female karyotype, *J. Hered.* 56, 254, 1965.
37. **Drews, U.,** Direct and mediated effects of testosterone: the development of intersexes in sex reversed mosaic mice, heterozygous for testicular feminization, *Anat. Embryol.* 146, 325, 1975.
38. **Drews, U., Blecher, S. R., Owen, D. A., and Ohno, S.,** Genetically directed preferential X-activation seen in mice, *Cell,* 1, 3, 1974.

39. **Drews, U. and Drews, U.**, Metabolic cooperation between tfm and wild-type cells in mosaic mice after induction of DNA synthesis, *Cell*, 6, 475, 1975.
40. **Short, R. V.**, The bovine freemartin — a new look at an old problem, *Philos. Trans. R. Soc. London*, 259, 141, 1970.
41. **Ohno, S., Christian, L. C., Wachtel, S. S., and Koo, G. C.**, Hormone-like role of H-Y antigen in bovine freemartin gonad, *Nature (London)*, 261, 597, 1976.
42. **Cupps, P. T., Laben, R. C., and Huff, R. L.**, Steroid metabolism in an inbred strain of Jersey cattle, *J. Dairy Sci.*, 53, 79, 1970.
43. **Stanley, A. J., Gumbreck, L. G., and Allison, J. E.**, Male pseudohermaphroditism in the laboratory Norway rat, *Rec. Prog. Horm. Res.*, 29, 43, 1973.
44. **Bardin, C. W., Bullock, L. P., Sherins, R. J., Mowszowicz, I., and Blackburn, W. R.**, Androgen metabolism and mechanism of action in male pseudohermaphroditism: a study of testicular feminization, *Rec. Prog. Horm. Res.*, 29, 65, 1973.
45. **Berthezene, F., Forest, M. G., Grimaud, J. A., Claustrat, B., and Mornex, R.**, Leydig-cell agenesis: a cause of male pseudohermaphroditism, *N. Engl. J. Med.*, 295, 969, 1976.
46. **Mainwaring, W. I. P.**, The mechanism of action of androgens, in *Monographs on Endocrinology*, Vol. 10, Springer-Verlag, New York, 1977.
47. **Imperato-McGinley, J. and Peterson, R. E.**, Male pseudohermaphroditism: the complexities of male phenotypic development, *Am. J. Med.*, 61, 251, 1976.
48. **Walsh, P. C., Madden, J. D., Harrod, M. J., Goldstein, J. L., MacDonald, P. C., and Wilson, J. D.**, Familial incomplete male pseudohermaphroditism, type 2. Decreased dihydrotestosterone formation in pseudovaginal perineoscrotal hypospadias, *N. Engl. J. Med.*, 291, 944, 1974.
49. **Peterson, R. E., Imperato-McGinley, J., Gautier, T., and Sturla, E.**, Male pseudohermaphroditism due to steroid 5α-reductase deficiency, *Am. J. Med.*, 62, 170, 1977.
50. **Wilson, J. D.**, Dihydrotestosterone formation in cultured human fibroblasts. Comparison of cells from normal subjects and patients with familial incomplete male pseudohermaphroditism, type 2, *J. Biol. Chem.*, 250, 3498, 1975.
51. **Heyns, W., Verhoeven, G., and de Moor, P.**, A comparative study of androgen binding in rat uterus and prostate, *J. Steroid Biochem.*, 7, 987, 1976.
52. **Verhoeven, G.**, *A Comparative Study of the Androgen Receptor Apparatus in Rodents*, ACCO (Academic Publishing), Leuven, Belgium, 1974.
53. **Bullock, L. P. and Bardin, C. W.**, Androgen-insensitive animals as a tool for understanding the mode of androgen action, in *Androgens and Anti-androgens*, Martini, L. and Motta, M., Eds., Raven Press, New York, 1977, 91.
54. **Shaver, E. L.**, Two cases of intersex in rabbits, *Anat. Rec.*, 159, 127, 1966.
55. **Lyon, M. F. and Hawkes, S. G.**, X-linked gene for testicular feminization in the mouse, *Nature (London)*, 227, 1217, 1970.
56. **Meyer, W. J., III, Migeon, B. R., and Migeon, C. J.**, Locus on human X chromosome for dihydrotestosterone receptor and androgen insensitivity, *Proc. Natl. Acad. Sci. U.S.A.*, 72, 1469, 1975.
57. **Kaufman, M., Straisfeld, C., and Pinsky, L.**, Male pseudohermaphroditism presumably due to target organ unresponsiveness to androgens, *J. Clin. Invest.*, 58, 345, 1976.
58. **Amrhein, J. A., Meyer, W. J., III, Jones, H. W., Jr., and Migeon, C. J.**, Androgen insensitivity in man: evidence for genetic heterogeneity, *Proc. Natl. Acad. Sci., U.S.A.*, 73, 891, 1976.
59. **Sherins, R. J. and Bardin, C. W.**, Preputial gland growth and protein synthesis in the androgen-insensitive male pseudohermaphroditic rat, *Endocrinology*, 89, 835, 1971.
60. **Goldman, A. S.**, Recent studies on the intersexual programming of the genetic rat male pseudohermaphrodite, in *Int. Symp. Intersexuality Animal Kingdom*, Springer-Verlag, Heidelberg, 1975, 422.
61. **Janne, O., Bullock, L. P., Bardin, C. W., and Jacob, S. T.**, Early androgen action in kidney of normal and androgen insensitive (tfm/y) mice, *Biochim. Biophys. Acta*, 418, 330, 1976.
62. **Gupta, J. S., Dey, S. K., and Dickmann, Z.**, Evidence that "embryonic estrogen" is a factor which controls the development of the mouse preimplantation embryo, *Steroids*, 29, 363, 1977.
63. **Bhatt, B. M. and Bullock, D. W.**, Binding of oestradiol to rabbit blastocysts and its possible role in implantation, *J. Reprod. Fertil.*, 39, 65, 1974.
64. **Csapo, A., Dray, F., and Erdos, T.**, The biological effects of injected antibodies to estradiol-17β and to progesterone in pregnant rats, *Endocrinology*, 97, 603, 1975.
65. **Pijnenborg, R., Robertson, W. B., and Brosens, I.**, The role of ovarian steroids in placental development and endovascular trophoblast migration in the golden hamster, *J. Reprod. Fertil.*, 44, 43, 1975.
66. **Schwarz, B. E., Milewich, L., Johnston, J. M., Porter, J. C., and MacDonald, P. C.**, Initiation of human parturition. V. Progesterone binding substance in fetal membranes, *Obstet. Gynecol.*, 48, 685, 1976.
67. **McCormack, S. A. and Glasser, S. R.**, A high-affinity estrogen-binding protein in rat placental trophoblast, *Endocrinology*, 99, 701, 1976.

68. **Goldstein, J. L. and Wilson, J. D.,** Studies on the pathogenesis of the pseudohermaphroditism in the mouse with testicular feminization, *J. Clin. Invest.,* 51, 1647, 1972.
69. **Drews, U., Itakura, H., Dofuku, R., Tettenborn, U., and Ohno, S.,** Nuclear DHT-receptor in tfm/y kidney cell, *Nature (London), New Biol.,* 238, 216, 1972.
70. **Bullock, L. P. and Bardin, C. W.,** Androgen receptors in testicular feminization, *J. Clin. Endocrinol. Metab.,* 35, 935, 1972.
71. **Naess, O., Haug, E., Attramadal, A., Aakvaag, A., Hansson, V., and French, F.,** Androgen receptors in the anterior pituitary and central nervous system of the androgen "insensitive" (tfm) rat: correlation between receptor binding and effects of androgens on gonadotropin secretion, *Endocrinology,* 99, 1295, 1976.
72. **Attardi, B. and Ohno, S.,** Cytosol androgen receptor from kidney of normal and testicular feminized (tfm) mice, *Cell,* 2, 205, 1974.
73. **Gehring, U. and Tomkins, G. M.,** Characterization of a hormone receptor defect in the androgen-insensitivity mutant, *Cell,* 3, 59, 1974.
74. **Attardi, B., Geller, L. N., and Ohno, S.,** Androgen and estrogen receptors in brain cytosol from male, female, and testicular feminized (tfm) mice, *Endocrinology,* 98; 864, 1976.
75. **Fox, T. O.,** Androgen- and estrogen-binding macromolecules in developing mouse brain: biochemical and genetic evidence, *Proc. Natl. Acad. Sci., U.S.A.,* 72, 4303, 1975.
76. **Purvis, K., Calandra, R., Naess, O., Attramadal, A., Torjesen, P. A., and Hansson, V.,** Do androgens increase Leydig cell sensitivity to luteinizing hormone? *Nature (London),* 265, 169, 1977.
77. **Lyon, M. F., Glenister, P. H., and Lamoreux, M. L.,** Normal spermatozoa from androgen-resistant germ cells of chimaeric mice and the role of androgen in spermatogenesis, *Nature (London),* 258, 620, 1975.
78. **Lyon, M. F. and Glenister, P. H.,** Evidence from Tfm/O that androgen is inessential for reproduction in female mice, *Nature (London),* 247, 366, 1974.
79. **Ohno, S., Christian, L., and Attardi, B.,** Role of testosterone in normal female functions, *Nature (London), New Biol.,* 243, 119, 1973.
80. **Lyon, M. F.,** Role of X and Y chromosomes in mammalian sex determination and differentiation, *Helv. Paediatr. Acta Suppl.,* 34, 7, 1974.
81. **Tettenborn, U., Dofuku, R., and Ohno, S.,** Noninducible phenotype exhibited by a proportion of female mice heterozygous for the X-linked testicular feminization mutation, *Nature (London), New Biol.,* 234, 37, 1971.
82. **Ohno, S., Geller, L. N., and Kan, J.,** The analysis of Lyon's hypothesis through preferential X-activation, *Cell,* 1, 175, 1974.
83. **Bakshi, K., Brusick, D., Bullock, L., and Bardin, C. W.,** Hormonal regulation of carcinogen metabolism in mouse kidney, in *Origins of Human Cancer,* Cold Spring Harbor Laboratory, New York, 1977, 347.
84. **Hill, R. N.,** Differential toxicity of chloroform in the mouse, in *Conf. on Aquatic Pollutants and Biological Effects with Emphasis on Neoplasia,* Vol. 298, Kraybill, H. F., Dawe, C. J., Harshburger, J. C., and Tardiff, R. G., Eds., N.Y. Academy Sci., N.Y., 1977, 170.
85. **Brown, T. R., Bardin, C. W., and Greene, F. E.,** Hormonal control of cytochrome P-450 dependent ethylmorphine N-demethylase activity of the mouse, in *Pharmacology of Steroid Contraceptive Drugs,* Garattini, S. and Berendes, H. W., Eds., Raven Press, New York, 1977.
86. **Shire, J. G. M.,** Degeneration of the adrenal X-zone in tfm mice with inherited insensitivity to androgens, *J. Endocrinol.,* 71, 445, 1976.
87. **Malt, R. A., Ohno, S., and Paddock, J. K.,** Compensatory renal hypertrophy in the absence of androgen binding, *Endocrinology,* 96, 806, 1975.
88. **Paigen, K., Swank, R. T., Tomino, S., and Ganschow, R. E.,** The molecular genetics of mammalian glucuronidase, *J. Cell. Physiol.,* 85, 379, 1975.
89. **Bardin, C. W., Bullock, L. P., Gupta, C., and Brown, T.,** Genetic factors which modulate androgen action, in *Int. Congr. Series No. 402, Endocrinol.,* Vol. 1, James, V. H. T., Ed., Excerpta Medica, Amsterdam, 1976, 481.
90. **Swank, R. T., Davey, R., Joyce, L., Reid, P., and Macey, M. R.,** Differential effect of hypophysectomy on the synthesis of β-glucuronidase and other androgen-inducible enzymes in mouse kidney, *Endocrinology,* 100, 473, 1977.
91. **Yamamoto, K. R., Gehring, U., Stampfer, M. R., and Sibley, C. H.,** Genetic approaches to steroid hormone action, *Rec. Prog. Horm. Res.,* 32, 3, 1976.
92. **Stanley, E. R., Palmer, R. E., and Sohn, U.,** Development of methods for the quantitative in vitro analysis of androgen-dependent and autonomous Shionogi carcinoma 115 cells, *Cell,* 10, 35, 1977.
93. **Horwitz, K. B., Costlow, M. E., and McGuire, W. L.,** MCF-7: a human breast cancer cell line with estrogen, androgen, progesterone, and glucocorticoid receptors, *Steroids,* 26, 785, 1975.

94. **Lippman, M. G., Huff, K. K., and Bolan, G.,** Glucocorticoid and progesterone interaction in human breast cancer in long term tissue culture, in *Biochemical Actions of Progesterone and Progestins,* Vol. 286, Gurpide, E., Ed., N. Y. Academy Sci., 1977, 101.
95. **Farookhi, R. and Sonnenschein, C.,** Estrogen-binding parameters of cytoplasmic and nuclear receptors in an established rat endometrial cell line and tumor, *Endocr. Res. Commun.,* 3, 1, 1976.
96. **Norris, J. S. and Kohler, P. O.,** The coexistence of androgen and glucocorticoid receptors in the DDT_1 cloned cell line, *Endocrinology,* 100, 613, 1977.
97. **Sonnenschein, C., Posner, M., Sahr, K., Farookhi, R., and Brunelle, R.,** Estrogen sensitive cell lines: establishment and characterization of new cell lines from estrogen-induced rat pituitary tumors, *Exp. Cell Res.,* 84, 399, 1974.
98. **Jung-Testas, I., Bayard, F., and Baulieu, E. E.,** Two sex steroid receptors in mouse fibroblasts in culture, *Nature (London),* 259, 136, 1976.
99. **Bartke, A.,** Genetic models in the study of anterior pituitary hormones, in *Genetic Variation in Hormone Systems,* Vol. 1, Shire, J. G. M., Ed., CRC Press, Boca Raton, Fla., 1979, chap. 6.
100. **Shire, J. G. M.,** Corticosteroids and adrenocortical function in animals, in *Genetic Variation in Hormone Systems,* Vol. 1, Shire, J. G. M., Ed., CRC Press, Boca Raton, Fla., 1979, chap. 3.

Chapter 5

REPRODUCTION IN DOMESTIC MAMMALS

R. B. Land and W. R. Carr

TABLE OF CONTENTS

I. INTRODUCTION

Genetic variation in reproductive performance has long been recognized, yet the physiological control of this variation is only now beginning to be understood. This understanding is relevant to both the geneticist and the physiologist; on the one hand it is an essential step in gene action and a possible means of estimating genetic merit, and on the other, genetic variation presents the opportunity for the quantitative investigation of physiological systems by studying a wide range of normal animals without resorting to artificial stimulation or suppression.

Genetic variation may be easily recognized as differences between species or between breeds within species when they are kept in the same environment. Within individual populations, genetic variation can also be recognized by the extent to which unrelated individuals tend to be less alike than related ones. The extent to which related individuals resemble each other may be assessed by comparing offspring with their parents or groups of offspring from different parents (see Falconer).[1] To consider genetic variation separately from environmental variation is to some extent artificial, for the two together control the development of the phenotype of an individual. The extent to which genetic and environmental variation act through the same physiological pathways will be considered, for this has a bearing on the use of "physiological traits" to predict phenotypic merit. The benefits of being able to do so will be discussed, together with the contribution that physiological predictors of genetic merit may make to the design of genetic improvement schemes. Emphasis will also be given to evidence that neither the genes that control quantitative variation in reproductive performance nor all the physiological pathways which express this control are sex limited.

The main species of domestic animals vary considerably in their reproductive endocrinology as might be expected — what is surprising is their frequent similarities. In this chapter, only sheep, cattle, and pigs will be considered. Their differences and similarities are outlined briefly. Most genetic studies within species have been carried out in sheep and the majority of the chapter is concerned with the results and interpretation of these studies. Before discussing variation, a summary of the information on the physiological control of reproduction in domestic mammals will be presented. Reference is then given to the limited data from studies within other species, to the effects of sex, and finally to the implications of this work.

II. CONTROL MECHANISMS

The same pituitary gonadotropins, follicle-stimulating hormone (FSH), and luteinizing hormone (LH) stimulate the gonads of both sexes of all mammals. In addition to the production of gametes in response to this stimulus, the gonads also produce steroid hormones which in turn "feedback" and control the release of gonadotropins. These relationships form the basis of an equilibrated buffered system that leads to the ovulation of the "usual" number of eggs per ovulation and the "usual" number of sperm; the basic elements of this system are summarized in Figure 1. The study of genetic variation in the endocrinology of reproduction is the study of variation in these control systems.

Gonadotropin release from the pituitary gland is influenced in part by the stimulus of gonadotropin-releasing factor (LRF) from the hypothalamus and in part by the modification of the gland's response to this stimulus by the action of gonadal steroids. The net result of these two control mechanisms can be studied by examining the concentration of gonadotropins in peripheral plasma. However, plasma concentration is not a function of secretion alone, it is also a function of the catabolism of the hormones. Furthermore, these hormones, especially LH, tend to be released in a pulsatile manner, and it would be reasonable to assume that the study of plasma concentration may give an accurate indication of the presence or absence of a pulse, but not necessarily of the amount released. The relative importance of the size and the frequency of pulses is not known, and indeed this is an example of the sort of problem which lends itself to a genetic-physiological approach; the relationship between genetic differences in pulse rate, for example, and the output from the physiological system, say number of eggs shed, could be readily tested. The extent to which variation in the concentration of gonadotropins in peripheral plasma causes variation in ovarian activity lends itself to genetic analysis.

One cannot, however, make any fundamental conclusions from the study of plasma gonadotropins alone for, as mentioned earlier, plasma concentrations are only one component of the equilibria associated with release; it is therefore necessary to consider these equilibria further. Changes in "sensitivity to negative feedback" are often impli-

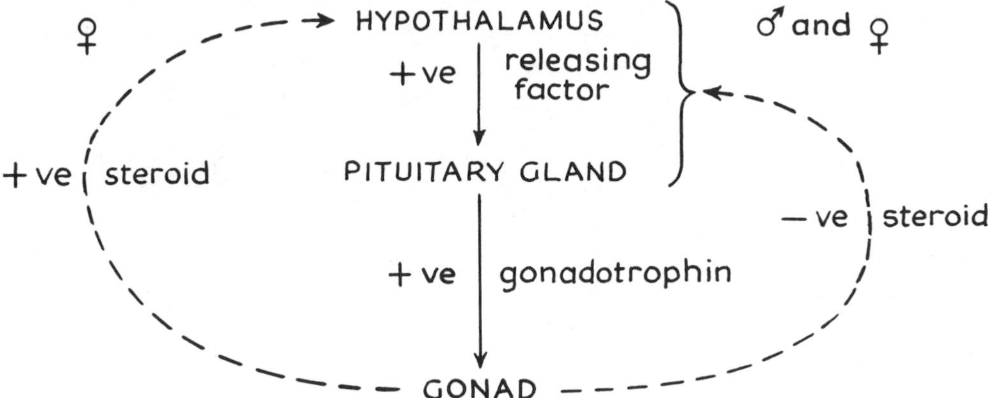

FIGURE 1. Diagrammatic representation of the main components of the hormonal stimulation of the ovaries and testes (–) and its feedback control (- - -).

cated in the interpretation of data, but the term tends to be used in a descriptive sense without a specific physiological meaning. Different levels of gonadotropins in the presence of similar steroid patterns could be ascribed to differences in sensitivity to negative feedback, and so could similar gonadotropins in the presence of different steroid patterns. Operationally the term may be considered to imply that a differential response to feedback arises from differences in the repressive action of the steroids rather than a change in the unmodulated level of synthesis and release, but in many experiments the data do not allow these to be separated. It is often necessary to check whether the conclusion " . . . arose from changes in sensitivity to negative feedback" is really supported by the data.

The equilibria controlling gonadal stimulation are not stable. Indeed, puberty may be associated with a change in sensitivity to negative feedback; the mature individual tolerates a higher level of gonadal activity and steroid output before it reduces gonadal stimulation. Despite the question of whether this arises from a true change in sensitivity to negative feedback, or from a higher primary signal strength which enables the post-puberal animal to maintain the same gonadal stimulus despite the stronger feedback stimulus, the instability of the equilibria adds an extra dimension to the study of genetic variation in reproductive endocrinology.

III. COMPARISONS AMONG SPECIES

A study of interspecific genetic variation can often give insight into differences found within a species and aid in their understanding. Caution, however, is required, as most information is based on results from radioimmunoassays, and different workers using different reagents can obtain vastly different results. Protein hormones are often species specific, and comparison of activities can be meaningless. FSH, for instance, prepared from bovine pituitary glands in a highly purified form[2] can achieve a potency of 45 times that of the NIH-FSH sheep reference standard when measured by bioassay, whereas a similar preparation from human pituitary glands[3] has a potency of 630 times the NIH standard. However, comparative studies of changes which occur in the hormone levels of females during estrus, pregnancy, and anestrus and of the male in and out of the breeding season are possible, as these do not depend so much on the interpretation of biological activity in different species. By contrast, steroid hormones are not species specific, so that although different methods may give differing results, comparisons among species within method are valid.

Peripheral blood serum or plasma levels of hormones provide, by far, the major source of our knowledge of the changes which occur in the hormones associated with reproduction. Development of the radioimmunoassay and competitive protein binding methods in recent years has enormously increased our knowledge, as the very low levels of most hormones in peripheral blood are below the sensitivity of most bioassay techniques.

It was soon obvious that a large preovulatory discharge of LH occurred in different breeds of cattle, sheep, and pigs. This is often referred to as positive feedback (Figure 1).[4-7] The general nature of the surge was the same for the three species, but the peak concentration relative to the baseline levels of LH immediately before the estrus surge varied. Sows gave an increase of about 6 times,[8] ewes about 100 to 200 times,[6] and cows 10 to 50 times.[4,5] Limited information is available regarding plasma FSH levels at estrus, but there appears to be a slight increase in levels at estrus in the three species, with sows and ewes showing a further increase at about day 2 of the estrous cycle.[9-11]

Examination of the estrogens and progesterone at different stages of the estrous cycle again shows a similar pattern of behavior in the three species. The complex feedback relationship between the pituitary gonadotropins and the gonadal steroids already discussed makes it difficult to consider them in isolation. The luteotropic action of LH would be expected to increase blood progesterone levels, and a large increase in progesterone occurs during the luteal phase of the cycle. In sows, plasma progesterone increases from levels of 1 ng/mℓ or less during estrus to 30 to 50 times that at mid-cycle.[8] Ewes show a similar pattern, although the mid-cycle increase is about tenfold,[12] and in cows the mid-cycle increase is even less, about sixfold.

Estrogen levels in peripheral blood are very low in the three species and approach the sensitivity of the methods available. Studies of the preovulatory estrogen rise suggest that sows produce the greatest amount of estrogen, giving concentrations in peripheral plasma around 60 to 70 pg/mℓ.[8] The highest plasma concentration in cattle was much lower,[13] of the order of 15 to 25 pg/mℓ. In ewes[14] the increase was to 13 pg/mℓ. For cattle and sheep the increase from basal levels was said to be about three times, compared to about six times in the pig.

The species with the highest ovulation rate has the highest concentration of estrogen in peripheral plasma and presumably secretes, as expected, the greatest amount of estrogens preceding ovulation. Positive feedback to the hypothalamus and pituitary, however, results in stimulation of a smaller secretion of LH, suggesting that the hypothalamo-pituitary axis is less sensitive in the more prolific species. It will be seen whether this relationship may also apply within a species.

Insufficient information is known about the feedback control of the pulsatile release of LH in the luteal phase of the cycle to determine whether the higher secretion of progesterone in sows has an additional suppressing effect on basal levels or indeed affects the preovulatory surge. Observations in ewes suggest that the secretion of estradiol during the luteal phase is in the same range as that occurring before the LH surge and emphasize that it may be the inhibitory effect of luteal progesterone rather than an inadequacy of estrogen which prevents the positive feedback of estrogen during the luteal phase.[15]

During pregnancy the steroid hormones behave somewhat differently in the three species. Plasma progesterone depends on nutrition and the number of fetuses in the sheep[16,17] and varies from 2 to 3 ng/mℓ in early pregnancy to about 10 to 20 ng/mℓ at day 130 to 140, finally dropping to very low levels at parturition. The levels are significantly affected by the number of lambs interacting with the nutritional state, both large numbers of lambs and inadequate nutrition being associated with higher progesterone concentrations. With such a low frequency of twinning in cattle, an effect of the number of fetuses has not been reported; the greater milk progesterone concentration of higher yielding cows, however, indicates that nutrition may affect progesterone levels in cattle as in sheep.[18] Donaldson et al.[19] showed that plasma progesterone levels rose initially, declined during mid pregnancy, and then increased to maximum levels before falling to very low levels at parturition. The levels rise from very low levels at estrus (1 ng/mℓ) to about 6 to 12 ng/mℓ at day 28. By day 200, concentrations slightly below this are obtained.[20]

In sows, plasma progesterone drops from high levels in early pregnancy (22 ng/mℓ) to about 13 ng/mℓ at day 30 and thereafter drops slowly until parturition.[7,21] In this respect the sow is more similar to the cow than the sheep, and it is doubtful whether there is any clear relationship with species litter size except very early in pregnancy when the very much higher levels in the pig are a clear indication of the substantially greater numbers of corpora lutea.

Most of the interest in levels of estrogens during late pregnancy must lie in their role at parturition. Robertson and his colleagues have studied these in all three species and thus provide good comparative data. Although the time scales differ, there is a sharp increase in plasma estrogens, reaching a peak just before parturition in the sow,[21] the ewe,[22] and the cow.[23] Unconjugated estrogens in the blood start rising about 40 days before parturition in the pig and the cow, reaching 3 to 5 ng/mℓ, whereas in the ewe the levels start increasing about 40 hr before parturition, reaching a peak of about 0.5 ng/mℓ. As with progesterone, the sow and the cow appear to behave similarly and there appears to be no correlation with the number of fetuses in each species.

Studies on the male animal have been largely confined to LH, FSH, and testosterone. Seasonal breeding in sheep may result in different profiles at different times of the year.[24] Levels of LH remain at about 1 ng/mℓ, with pulsatile spikes occurring at levels of up to 9 ng/mℓ, the number of spikes increasing in the breeding season (January compared with August). The LH spikes were followed by increased blood concentration of testosterone, which had basal levels of 1 ng/mℓ but could rise to over 20 ng/mℓ. Schanbacher and Ford,[25] however, report no effect of season on either size or frequency of LH pulses between May and September, although basal levels are reduced in the former month. Unpublished results by the present authors tend to confirm the results of Sanford et al.[24] The problem of seasonal effects interacting with those of breed is discussed later. FSH levels remained relatively constant, except in the period immediately before the breeding season, when there were appreciable increases in levels.[26]

In bulls, a similar pulsatile release of LH has been reported,[27] with basal and peak levels of testosterone and LH very similar to those reported in the ram. Very limited information is available in pigs; Ellendorff and his colleagues,[28] working with miniature Gottingen boars, reported a basal level of LH of about 0.8 ng/mℓ with spikes of about 2 ng/mℓ, but these spikes did not appear to initiate testosterone release as in the other two species. Although variable, the testosterone mean levels were found to be around 5 ng/mℓ.[28] Further studies are therefore required before it is possible to say whether the characteristics of gonadotropin and testosterone release of the pig differ from those of sheep and cattle.

The comparison of the three domestic species gives an indication of the variation in reproductive characteristics and may also indicate possible relationships between one characteristic and another. Of these, the overall range is of considerable interest, for it shows the extent of the physiological variation which is compatible with successful reproduction. The relationships, however, must be treated with caution, for it must be remembered that there may be marked exceptions to general trends. Among the three species, for example, higher plasma estrogen concentrations tend to be associated with higher litter sizes, but the knowledge that man with a similar litter size to cattle may have a plasma estrogen concentration 1000 times greater puts such an association into perspective. It is within species, and more especially within populations, that causative associations can best be studied. By far, the majority of such studies have been conducted in sheep, and these will now be considered.

IV. VARIATION AMONG SHEEP

A. Lambs

The first report of genetic variation in mammalian plasma gonadotropins was the paper of Thimonier et al.,[29] presented to the Society for the Study of Fertility. In addition to the demonstration of genetic variation, this study also showed that this variation was not sex limited and that it is expressed at an early age. It is unfortunate that the demonstration of these three fundamental facts was not pursued more thoroughly, but it is nevertheless worthy of reassessment. The study was based on the comparison of lambs of both sexes of breeds of sheep with different ovulation rates, the Romanov and the Prealpe, and the cross between them. Under conditions similar to those of this experiment, the Romanov would be expected to shed 2.7 eggs, the Prealpe 2.0, and the crossbred 2.4.[30] At that time little was known of the pulsatile nature of LH release, plasma ovine FSH assays were not available, and single blood samples were taken at weekly intervals from 4 to 11 weeks of age. Despite the deficiencies in experimental design, the study of males showed that the rate of increase of LH concentrations over this period was higher in the crossbred than in the pure Prealpe lambs (Figure 2). In the females the concentration increased in the Prealpe lambs over this period and declined in the Romanovs but did not change linearly in the crosses. Further studies have since clarified the evolution of hormonal equilibria. In a more extensive study of male lambs of various breeds, Blanc et al.[31] found that the concentration of LH in the plasma of Romanov lambs had fallen by 11 weeks of age to a level below that of Ile de France and Prealpe lambs, whereas at 5 weeks of age the mean concentration had been more than twice as high (4.8 vs. 2.2 ng/mℓ). Courot et al.[32] studied Ile de France lambs to a greater age and found that the concentration of LH in peripheral plasma also reached a peak in this breed, but not until about 12 weeks of age. One can now combine this information to illustrate the differences in the change in LH concentration before puberty in lambs of different breed types, and this is represented diagrammatically in Figure 3. The different breeds go through their peak concentrations at different ages. In the early lamb study of Thimonier et al.,[29] the peak for crossbred females would have taken place during the sampling period, thus obscuring any linear time trends. The female peak occurs at an earlier age than the male one; Foster et al.[33] have shown that gonadal negative feedback starts at a later age in females than in males. This diagrammatic representation can now be used as a basis for the discussion of later studies.

Bindon and Turner[34] reported that young males of three strains of Merino selected for differing fecundity had different levels of LH at 30 days of age, which were ranked in the same order as adult fecundity. The differences had however disappeared by 100 days. Knowing the late puberty of Merinos, the age scale in Figure 3 would be changed and the difference at 30 days may correspond to the early difference at 3 to 4 weeks of age in the model, the similarity of the different strains corresponding to studies at about 10 weeks of age. Between-breed studies, based on the Romanov and the Finnish Landrace (which has similar characteristics to the Romanov), are also compatible with the model. The higher LH concentration of Finnish Landrace lambs than those of other breeds[35] would correspond to a study between the ages of 4 and 9 weeks. Likewise, the similarity of Finnish Landrace lambs and crosses to others of less prolific breed types[36,37] could have arisen from the ages of the lambs chosen for study. Echternkamp and Laster[36] studied females at 9, 13, and 17 weeks of age, when the hormone concentration of the different types would not be expected to be ranked with the ovu-

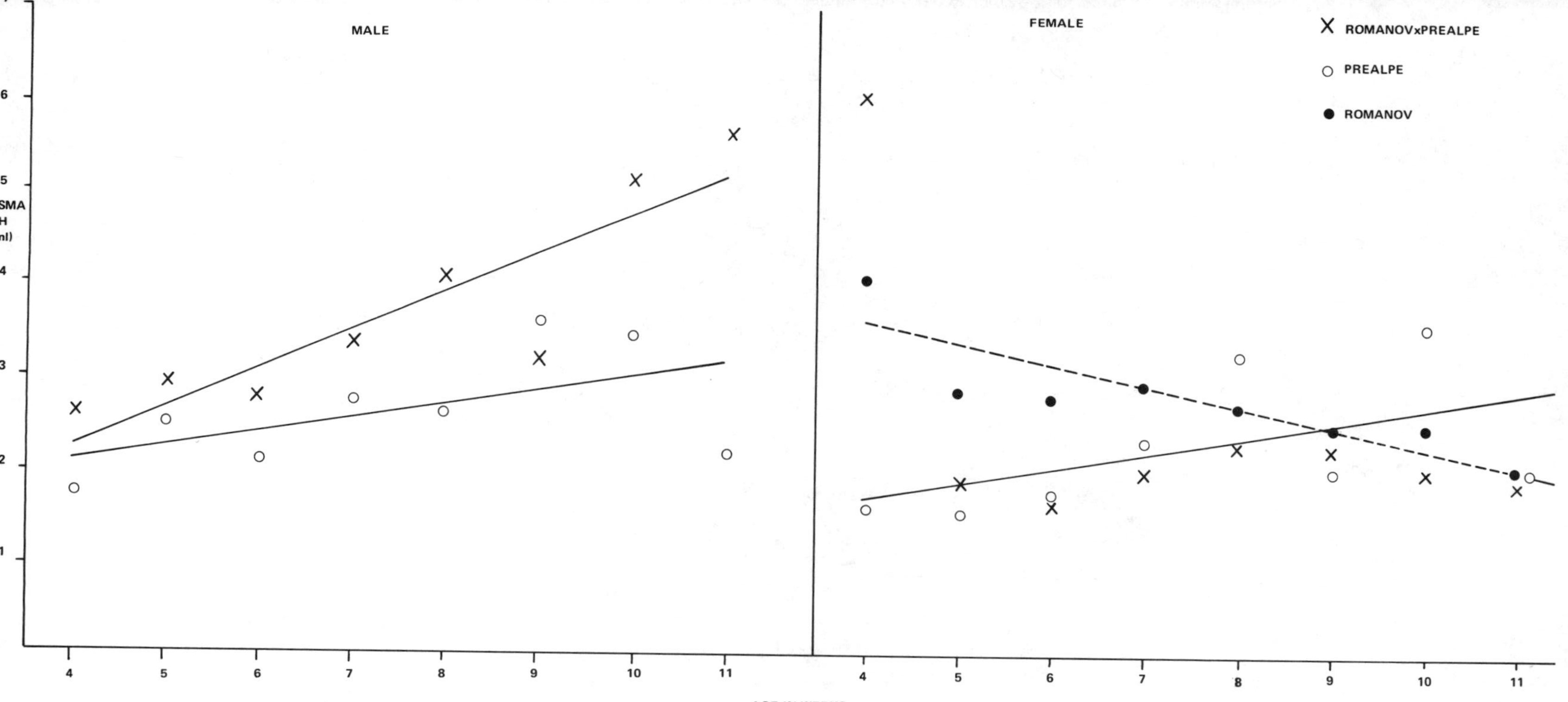

FIGURE 2. The concentration of LH in the peripheral plasma of male and female Romanov, Prealpe, and crossbred lambs from 4 to 11 weeks of age.

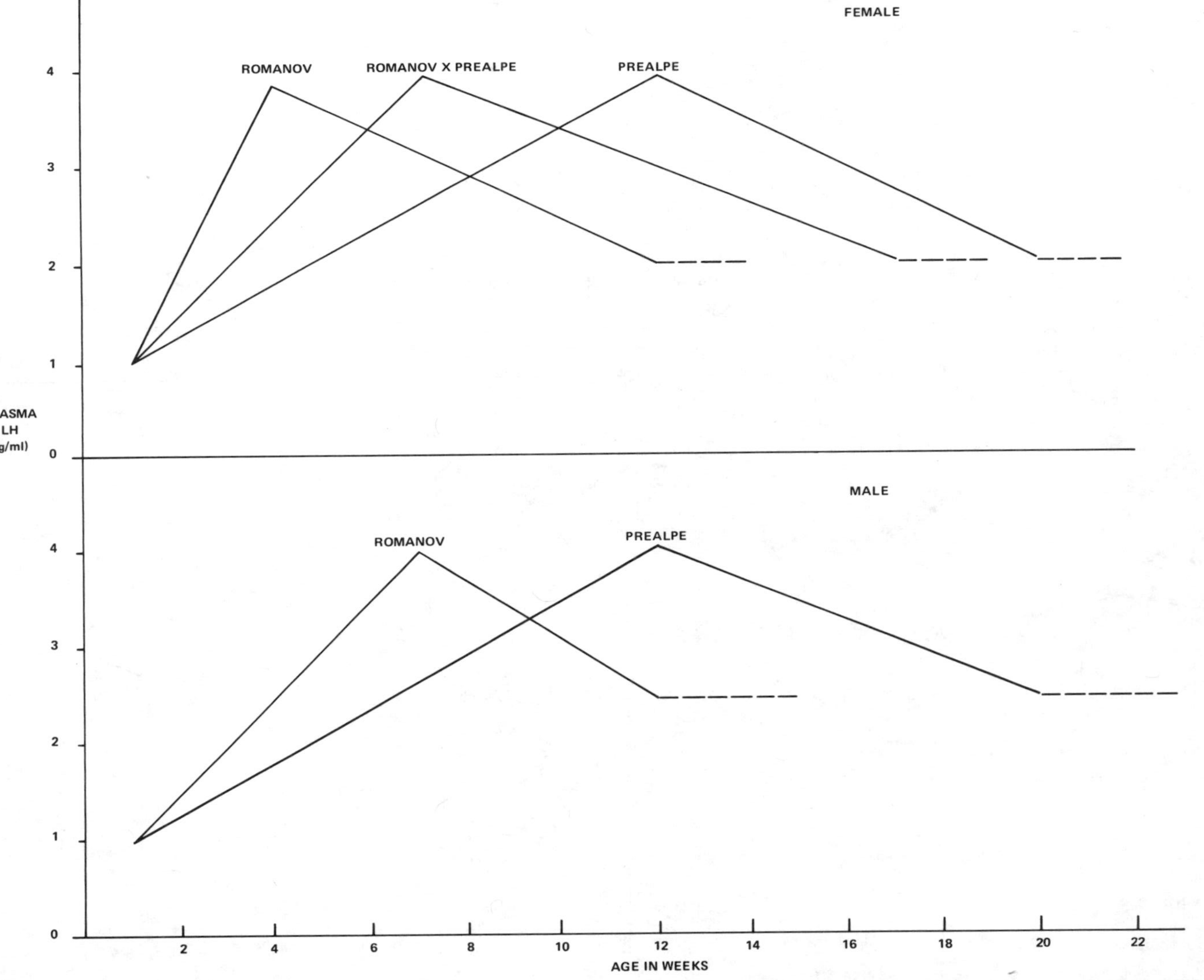

FIGURE 3. Diagrammatic representation of genetic variation in plasma LH concentration of male and female lambs.

lation rate. Hanrahan et al.[37] would have missed any differences occurring between the ages of 3 and 9 weeks of those chosen for study. The data of Blanc et al.[31] show no differences between Romanov and other lambs at 3 weeks of age or at 9, despite the twofold difference at 5 weeks. The later studies show how carefully experiments have to be designed to study variation in a rapidly changing situation. Thimonier et al.[29] and Bindon and Turner[34] were fortunate to have demonstrated the presence of variation in their early studies.

More recently, there have been preliminary reports of variation in the concentration of FSH in the plasma of young lambs. Findlay and Bindon[38] found it to be higher in female lambs of highly prolific strains, but not in males. Again, as with LH, the concentration of FSH may vary with age, and this report of a sex difference may be simply a function of the age chosen for study. Further studies may clarify this.

B. Criteria for Selection

The possibility that hormone levels in young males may be used to predict the genetic merit of their daughters has aroused great interest. If sheep breeds with high reproductive merit have high LH concentration at a certain age, the hypothesis has been put forward that selection within a breed on the basis of hormonal levels may lead to a causally correlated change in reproductive merit. Put in physiological terms, variation in LH concentration may be associated with variation in reproductive merit.

One must however be wary of the chance association of traits, and the presence of between breed associations does not necessarily mean that the same association also holds within breeds. In this respect the study of Bindon and Turner[34] is of particular importance for two of the strains studied originated from the same base population of Merino sheep; direct selection for the number of lambs born changed the equilibria of gonadotropin secretion, and hence it can be argued that the reverse would also happen. The probability of chance fixation of alleles controlling the two traits during the process of selection is less than in the case of different breeds which may have passed through small "bottlenecks" and become "fixed" for two unrelated traits.

Given that the genetic differences in the age changes in LH concentration are associated with the adult reproductive merit of the breed or strain type, how useful may they be as selection criteria to improve adult performance? Is the rate of response to indirect selection through the use of a predictive trait likely to be greater than that to direct selection for the desired trait itself? The merits of indirect selection in general are discussed by Falconer,[1] but with traits such as reproduction which are sex limited and only recognizable in mature animals, the advantages are likely to be greater than with traits of the growing animal. The possibility of using predictive physiological criteria to facilitate selection among both sexes and with a shorter generation interval is discussed by Land.[39]

The merits of indirect selection for the desired trait are dependent upon the selection intensity per unit of time (i/L) which can be applied to the predictive trait (p) and to the desired trait (d), the heritabilities of the two traits (h_p^2 and h_d^2), and the genetic correlation between them (r_A). Indirect selection is superior to direct selection when $i_p/L_p \cdot h_p \cdot r_A$ is greater than $i_d/L_d \cdot h_d$. One could therefore estimate these parameters and compare the rates of response under the two alternative selection procedures, but as a guide the removal of sex limitation with no change in the generation interval would increase the selection intensity per year twofold; hence, with the additional benefits of a reduction in the generation interval, it is reasonable to assume that the annual selection intensity would be two to three times as great. When $h_p r_A$ is greater than ⅓ to ½ h_d, indirect selection would therefore be beneficial. This, however, assumes that the genetic correlation remains constant, and it is here that the physiological understanding of the control of LH release in the lamb is of particular relevance. To return to Figure

3, the critical difference between the high and low fertility breed types is the age of maximum LH concentration so that the selection of, say, Prealpe males at 10 weeks of age would bring the peak to an earlier age, but then no further progress would be made. The genetic correlation would gradually decline to nought. If the physiological mediation of a statistical correlation is understood, the opportunities for using it wisely can be seen to be considerably greater.

The physiological variables underlying the correlation between lamb plasma LH concentration and adult merit among breed or strain types indicate that the genetic correlation within breed types is likely to change. The big variations in some plasma levels due to pulsatile release also indicate that the genetic correlation is likely to be very low within populations or at least dependent upon very many estimates of plasma LH concentrations. Using the Mean Squares from the Analysis of Variance of plasma LH in the lamb, published by Carr and Land,[35] to calculate the intraclass correlation, the correlation between successive LH measures is found to be 0, 0.2, and 0.1 at the four ages studied. Pooling the components gives an overall estimate of 0.12, showing that on an average only 1.4% of the variation in the concentration of LH on one occasion was related to that at the next. The relation between a single LH concentration and any measure of reproductive performance is therefore trivial and of no predictive merit. There are two possible ways of increasing this correlation: to take repeated samples of plasma or to overcome the pulsatile release. In that the objective is to develop a simple criterion for the assessment of reproductive performance, the second of these alternatives has been pursued more actively. In particular, LRF has been used to stimulate LH release, but few data have been published.

As with the basic LH studies described earlier, the study of genetic variation in LH release in response to an exogenous LRF stimulus has been based on the comparison of different breeds and crosses. The philosophy has usually been to give a dose of LRF which was large enough to overcome the normal pattern of release, but small enough to give an estimate of the response to LRF over the normal physiological range. Therefore, two aspects of the response had to be studied. First, the order of magnitude of the dose which would meet the above requirements, and second, the time interval between the introduction of exogenous LRF and the presence, if any, of genetic variation in plasma LH concentration. Early studies were based on the comparison of Scottish Blackface and Finnish Landrace lambs of both sexes, using a continuous blood sampling system. The mean response of ram lambs of the two breeds[40] to 5 μg LRF is given in Figure 4. It can be seen that the rate of decline of the mean log-transformed concentration of plasma LH is linear and that it is similar in the two breeds, but that the absolute concentration over a period from 20 min through to the end of the study 150 min after injection was greater in the Finn than the Blackface lambs. It was concluded that it would be possible to detect the difference in response by the use of acute samples at set times after the injection of LRF.

The next stage of the investigation was based on such an acute sampling technique, and, in addition, in order to estimate genetic effects more specifically, environmental, including maternal effects, were minimized by studying lambs born from the same breed of mother over the same period of time and on the same farm, but sired by males expected to have different characteristics. Scottish Blackface ewes were allocated at random to Finnish Landrace or Tasmanian Merino sires. Donald et al.[41] reported that the litter size of the two breeds was 2.3 and 1.2, respectively, i.e., the Tasmanian Merino lowered the reproductive performance of its crossbred offspring relative to that of purebred Blackfaces, whereas the Finnish Landrace raised it. Any differences between the two crosses must be genetic sire effects.

Lambs were bled at 30, 45, 60, and 75 min after injection of 5 or 10 μg at 3, 7, 12, and 18 weeks of age. The mean log response of lambs of both sexes of the two types

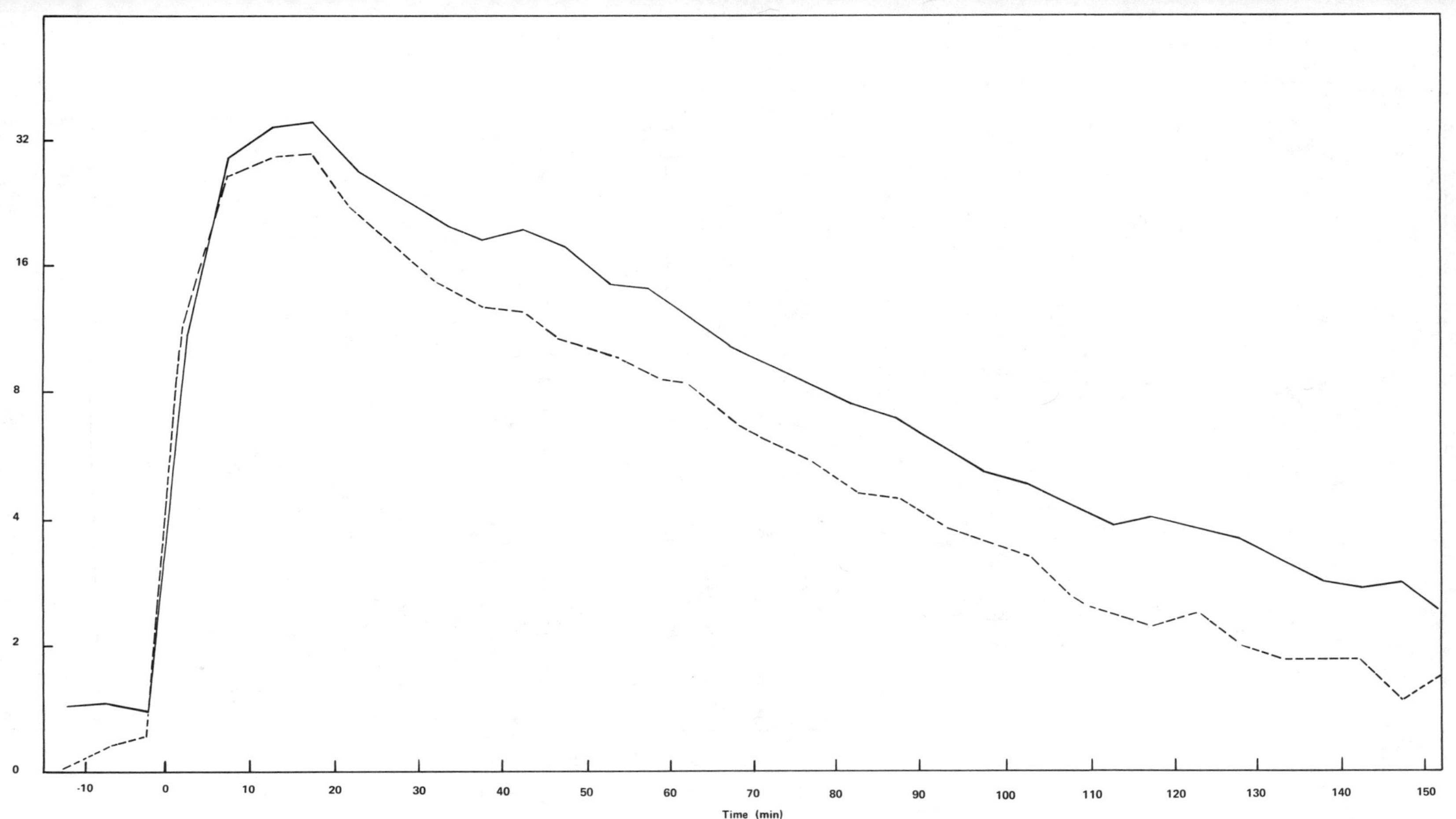

FIGURE 4. The concentration of LH in the peripheral plasma of Finn and Blackface male lambs following the injection of 5 μg of LRF at 12 weeks of age.

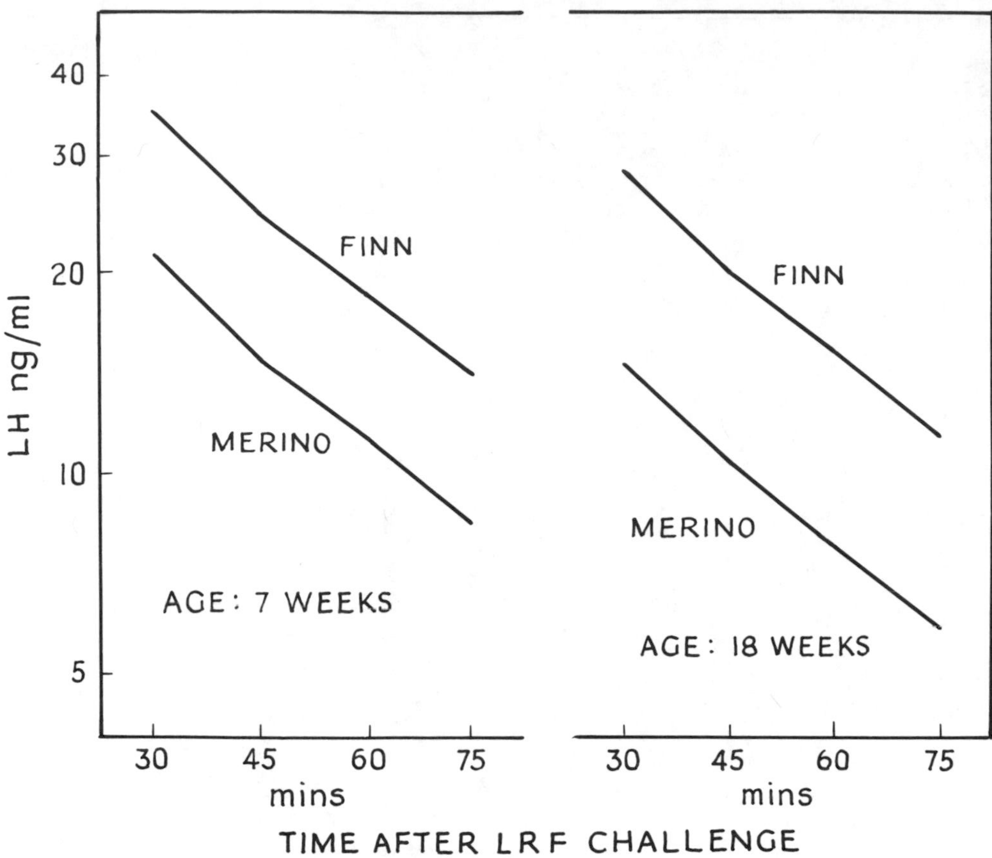

FIGURE 5. The response of Finn × Blackface and Merino × Blackface lambs to the injection of LRF at 7 and 18 weeks of age as measured by the concentration of LH in peripheral plasma.

is illustrated in Figure 5, at 7 and 18 weeks of age. As with the more complex laboratory experiment described earlier, this farm trial revealed differences in the mean concentration of LH, while the rate of decline in concentration was similar. The repeatability between lambs within crosses was estimated to be 0.5. With 25% of the variation on one occasion in common with that 3 weeks later or earlier, the response to LRF is a more consistent trait than a single estimate of the natural plasma concentration.

The response to LRF may be a suitable means of assessing lamb LH "status", which in turn may be correlated with adult reproductive performance. The extent to which this difference arises from basic differences in pituitary characteristics or whether it is "self-induced" via feedback from the gonads is of interest. It may be argued that from a practical point of view, the only concern is the magnitude of the genetic correlation within the population to be improved, but we have already seen that the understanding of the physiological pathways underlying a correlation may enable it to be used more widely. Galloway and Pelletier[42] have shown that the response to LRF is affected by sexual maturation (although they did use very large doses based on body weight) and suggest that this may be the result of the modification of the sensitivity of the pituitary gland to LRF by testicular steroids. Sire effects on rates of sexual development could therefore interact with, and hence contribute to, the present observed differences. These effects have to be investigated. The correlation could therefore arise either from the primary characteristics of the pituitary gland or the secondary characteristics arising from steroid modification by feedback from the gonads.

C. Characteristics of Adults

The comparative study of genetic variation in the development of adult characteristics has received less attention than the study of single genetic types through puberty and the comparison of mature males and females. Since sheep are seasonal breeders, puberty in both sexes is influenced by daylength in the higher latitudes where most sheep research has been conducted.

1. Males

The concentration of LH in both plasma and the pituitary gland has been shown to increase from 10 to 70 days of age in both spring- and autumn-born lambs, but the rate of rise was observed to be greater in the spring-born rams.[32] The rate of testis growth, the concentration of LH in the pituitary gland, and the total content of the gland were, however, greater in the autumn-born group. Even when the peak LH concentration at 70 days was passed, the concentration continued to be affected by the season of birth. The concentration was lower in 125-day-old autumn-born lambs measured in February than in 125-day-old spring-born lambs measured in July. It is likely that the autumn-born, but not the spring-born, lambs would have established the ability to mate and to inseminate by 150 days of age. The seasonal association of high rates of testis growth and low rates of increase in plasma LH concentration and vice versa contrasts with the genetic association of high rates of testis growth with high LH concentrations.[35] The seasonal and genetic variation in reproductive activity is apparently not mediated through similar changes in endocrine pathways. The positive genetic association between plasma LH concentration and rate of testis growth is readily understandable in terms of the observation of Courot,[43] in which LH increases the rate of testis growth of hypophysectomized ram lambs. The seasonal differences in the characteristics of the lambs are compatible with the seasonal variation in adult performance. Lincoln,[44] for example, shows that males on short daylength have high testosterone, large testes, and low LH, relative to those which have been on long days for some time. Lincoln, et al.[26] show that high plasma FSH concentration is synchronized with high LH and precedes the testis diameter and testosterone peak. One could explain the seasonal effect if there were a time lag between gonadotropin stimulation and its effect on the testis and vice versa, but this does not help to explain the seasonal effect on the testis growth—plasma LH relationship, unless undetected perinatal elevation of gonadotropins led to a higher autumn growth rate. Alternatively the possibility that the difference could be an artifact should not be neglected. The sampling procedure of Courot et al.[32] was relatively crude, and the mean levels reported could reflect differences in the amplitude or the frequency of pulse releases. Pulse frequency, therefore, could be higher in the autumn-born than in the spring-born lambs, so that if this is the main determinant of gonadal stimulation, it could be higher in autumn- than spring-born lambs.

A further difference between the two types of variation is that genotype but not the environment affected the age of the maximum LH concentration. The genetic variation could be argued to be associated with differences in the effects of gonadal feedback on gonadotropin release, with highly prolific animals maintaining the stimulus in the presence of large testes, and this is supported by the fact that hemicastration has a much greater effect on males of low prolificacy than in males of high prolificacy.[45] Although testosterone has less of an effect on LH release in rams on short days than in those on long days,[46] such a difference in the characteristics of gonadotropin release could not account for both the higher testosterone and lower LH observed on short days[44] nor the seasonal variation in the plasma concentration of LH in castrate males.[47] Further understanding will probably be dependent upon experimental tests, and the contemporary study of lambs of different breeds and different ages should help to separate genetic and environmental effects.

Seasonal variation in reproductive activity complicates the study of adults themselves as well as the attainment of puberty. The plasma concentration of LH changes rapidly and severalfold over a very short period of time. In unpublished work, the present authors have examined plasma LH levels in pure and crossbred rams of differing genetic characteristics in January, May, and July. The presence of frequent and apparently random pulses makes the results difficult to interpret. In general, more pulses were detected in January and July than in May, and mean plasma LH levels were highest in July. However there was considerable variation in the manner in which the different breed groups behaved at different times of the year. Differences among breeds on any occasion could, therefore, arise from either the timing of the response to seasonal changes or the magnitude of synchronous responses. The comparison of Finnish Landrace and Suffolk rams every 8 weeks over a period of 14 months[48] showed an earlier, although not statistically significant, seasonal rise in plasma LH concentration in the Suffolk rams, but there were no marked differences in the amplitude of the changes or the mean overall concentration. The similar LH concentrations however were associated with higher testosterone concentrations in the Finnish Landrace rams. Again, evidence revealed that rams of the breed of high female prolificacy may be able to tolerate higher gonadal steroid concentrations without depressing their plasma LH concentration.

Greater gonadotropic signal strength in rams of breeds where ewes have high levels of performance could, therefore, be associated with higher rates of testis growth, earlier prepubertal peak LH concentration, and the ability to withstand higher plasma concentrations of plasma steroids.

2. Females

Variation in the reproductive endocrinology of adult females has been studied more extensively than that of males, but there are few studies of juveniles.

Quantitative physiological studies show that the concentration of LH during the estrous cycle is similar in breeds of sheep shedding from 1.1 to 2.6 eggs.[30,36,55] Bindon et al.[30] extended this conclusion to show that the concentration of plasma FSH was also similar. The only trait found to be associated with ovulation rate by Land et al.[55] and Bindon et al.[30] was the duration of the interval between the onset of estrus and the preovulatory discharge of LH. This was about 8 hr in the breeds of low ovulation rate, compared to about 17 hr in the high ovulation rate Romanovs, but the characteristics of the discharge of LH were considered to be too late to influence the associated ovulation and too early to influence the subsequent ovulation.

The independence of the concentration of gonadotropins during the estrous cycle and the ovulation rate was not expected, and it was considered that variation in pulsatile release characteristics may not have been detected by the sampling techniques used. As mentioned earlier, frequent small pulses could give the same overall mean concentration as infrequent large ones, but their physiological effect may be very different. Frequent sampling techniques have, therefore, been used to study the detailed characteristics of LH release on different days of the estrous cycle. The comparison of Finnish Landrace, Scottish Blackface, and Tasmanian Merino ewes (ovulation rates 3.0, 1.3, and 1.0, respectively), using a system of continuous blood collection, indicated that the mean LH concentration may be inversely related to the ovulation rate of the breed type.[56] Examples of LH plasma levels measured during day 13 of the estrous cycle for one typical animal of each breed are shown in Figure 6. Each point represents a 12-min sample for a continuous collection over a period of 5 hr 36 min. Even at these relatively low levels of LH there is a tendency for frequent pulsatile release, and when the proportion of samples falling within three ranges of LH concentration are examined, the breed distributions (Table 1) again suggest that plasma LH

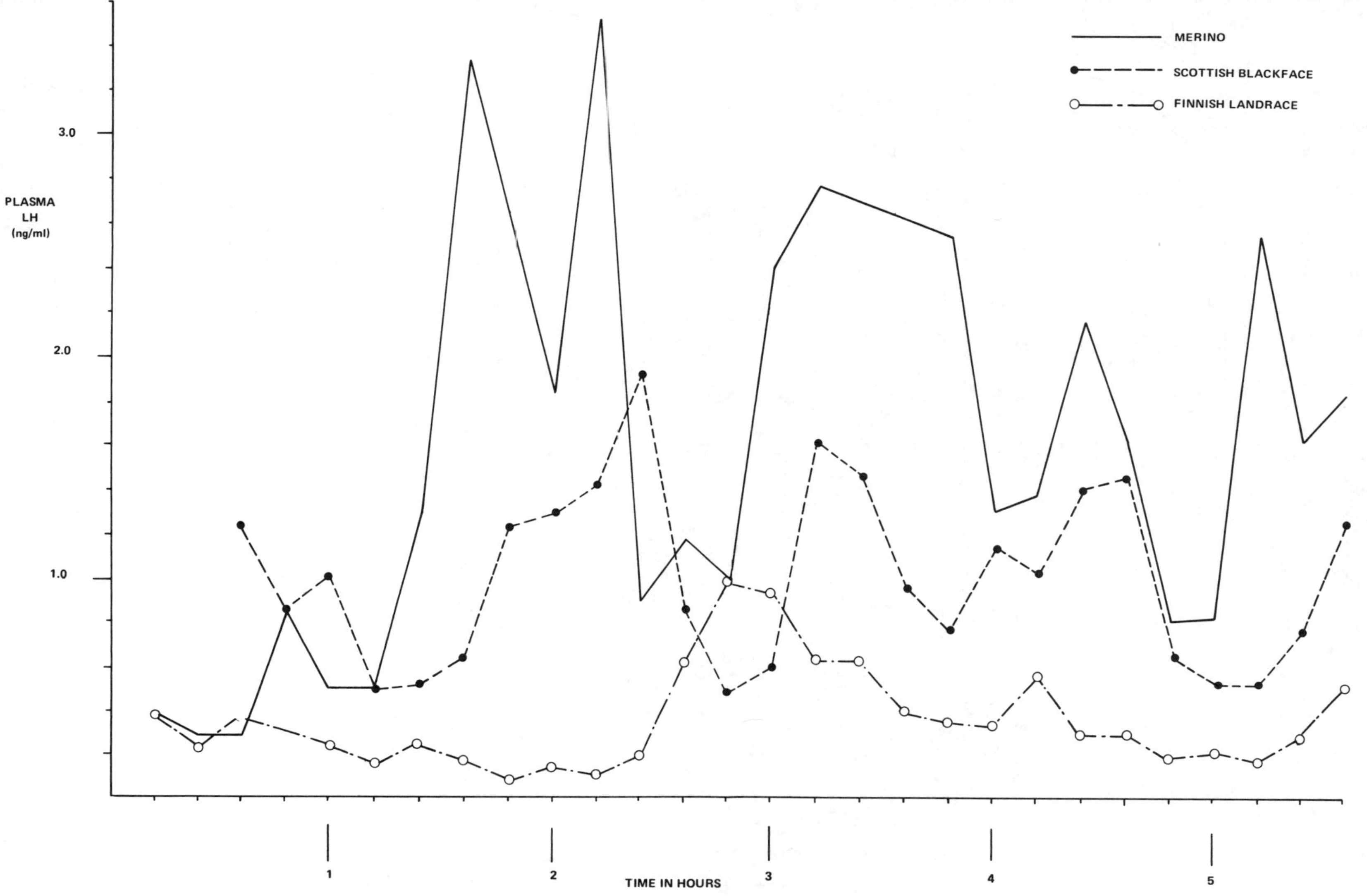

FIGURE 6. The concentration of LH in the peripheral plasma of individual ewes of the Finn, Blackface, and Tasmanian Merino breeds over a period of 5 hr 30 min on day 13 of the estrous cycle.

TABLE 1

The Distribution of the Plasma Concentration of LH over a Period of 5 to 6 hr for Blackface, Finn, and Merino Females on Day 13 of the Estrous Cycle

Breed	No. of animals	Samples per animal	% samples (ng/mℓ plasma) Below 1.0	1.0—2.0	Above 2.0
Merino	5	28	46	37	17
Blackface	7	28	70	25	5
Finn	6	28	89	9	2

concentration may rank inversely with ovulation rate. In the absence of variation in gonadotropin stimulation, differences in ovulation rate may be associated with variation in steroid feedback. The basic problem, however, has been the difficulty of measuring normal levels of estrogen in the peripheral plasma of the ewe during the estrous cycle.

The longer time interval between the onset of estrous and the discharge of LH in highly prolific ewes was the first indication that differences in the effects of steroid feedback may be the key variation in ovulation rate. Castrated Finnish Landrace ewes showed estrous earlier than Blackfaces in response to a single intramuscular injection of 50 μg estradiol benzoate, but had a longer interval to the discharge of LH and much lower peak concentrations.[57] Both higher behavioral sensitivity and lower LH discharge sensitivity, therefore, appear to contribute to the longer interval in intact ewes of the highly prolific breed types studied. The reduction in the concentration of LH in peripheral plasma (the negative feedback effect) may also have been greater in the Blackface ewes, indicating greater sensitivity to both the positive and negative feedback effects of estrogen on LH release, but the experiment was not designed to test this. Seasonal and genetic variation in the negative effects of estrogen may therefore have been similar — anestrous and lowly prolific ewes were more sensitive —, but the positive effects contrasted, anestrous and highly prolific ewes were both less sensitive. Further indirect evidence for the presence of genetic variation in the relative sensitivity of behavioral and gonadotropin release centers in the hypothalamus comes from the incidence of silent ovulations in different breeds: given that sheep ovulate, the probability of highly prolific ewes also showing estrous is higher than for ones of low prolificacy.[58] Direct evidence would be of greater value.

Bindon et al.[30] report that variation in the concentration of "total estrogens" in the peripheral plasma is not associated with variation in the prolificacy of ewes of different breeds. The comparison of two breeds, Finnish Landrace and Scottish Blackface, indicated that the concentrations of estradiol did not differ significantly.[59] Further analysis of these data showed that the difference of 0.061 pg/mℓ between the two breeds relative to the least squares fitted a mean of 1.70 pg/mℓ and had a standard error of 0.135. It has since been shown that estrogen, like LH, is released in a pulsatile manner during the estrous cycle,[60] so that the high variability of single daily samples is to be expected. Further complications in comparisons of this type are that the concentrations observed are close to the lower limit of detection of the methods available and, secondly, that the important difference is the percentage difference, which is dependent upon knowledge of the threshold below which estradiol does not have a feedback effect and of the measured estradiol which is of extra-ovarian origin. It is also possible that the relationship between the concentration of estradiol and its effect on the release of LH is not linear. In a comparable situation, the concentration of estradiol in a castrated ram was 1.1 pg/mℓ. If this were the "true blank", the difference between the breeds would be up to 55% in favor of the Finnish Landrace. With a nonlinear relationship between estradiol and ovulation rate, the difference in effective feedback could be anything.

Alternative approaches to the feedback problem have used the measurement of estrogen secretion rates. This has been made possible by the collection of timed samples of ovarian venous blood from animals with ovarian cervical autotransplants.[61] Wheeler[62] used this technique to estimate the rate of ovarian estradiol production in Tasmanian Merino and Merino × Finn ewes of similar age and in similar physiological states (i.e., with a corpus luteum which had been maintained for 90 days). The analysis of variance of animal means showed that the mean secretion rate of the Finn crosses (0.99 ± 0.17 ng/min) was significantly greater than that of the pure bred Merinos (0.37 ± 0.09 ng/min, $p<0.05$), indicating a threefold difference in the rate of estrogen production. That high ovulation rate animals can "tolerate" more estrogen is undoubtedly true; Finnish Landrace ewes continued to ovulate despite the injection of 25 μg of estradiol benzoate on each of days 3 to 14 of the estrous cycle, whereas only one third of the comparable Blackface ewes did so.[62] In terms of the number of corpora lutea observed, the exogenous estrogen reduced the ovarian activity of the Blackfaces by 70% compared to a reduction of 25% for the Finns.

Variation in the fertility of sheep has also been reported to be associated with the different alleles at the hemoglobin locus. Sheep carrying the B allele gave birth to more lambs than those carrying the A allele,[49] a difference reported to increase as the conditions and overall level of performance increased. In the reverse situation under adverse conditions, the performance of individuals carrying the A allele may exceed that of those with the B,[50] and an extreme example of this is the markedly greater ability of homozygous AA animals to reproduce when grazing Yarloop subterranean clover ("estrogenic" clover). Obst et al.[51] reported that whereas 100% of AA sheep conceived, only 33% BB sheep did so on a Yarloop-dominated sward ($p<0.01$), but that there was no difference between them on a primarily grass sward. "Estrogenic" clover infertility has been reported to arise from abnormal LRF release;[52] LRF but not estrogen induced the release of LH.

The association between the hemoglobin allele and the PMS-induced ovulation rate is less clear. Pant and Pandey[53] report that the response of BB homozygotes of the Indian Bikaneri breed exceeded that of heterozygotes, which in turn exceeded that of those homozygous for the A allele. In Welsh Mountain sheep, however, Trounson et al.[54] reported the responses of the three genotypes to be similar. The difference between these two sets of data may arise from the different environments or from different genes carried by the two breeds. Further studies are needed to differentiate between these two possibilities. The data are, however, compatible with the conclusions from laboratory animal studies where the genetic correlation between the number of eggs shed at natural ovulation and following PMS treatment may be low. The association between hemoglobin type and fertility may arise from tight linkage, the hemoglobin genes being linked with different alleles at the neighboring "fertility" locus in different populations. It would, however, be necessary to argue that each population has passed through bottleneckes for the linkage disequilibrium to be generated and that the linkage is extremely close for the disequilibrium to be maintained. At present therefore it would seem likely that the two effects are pleiotropic.

The comparison of different breeds suggests a negative relationship between hypothalamic sensitivity to estrogen and the number of eggs shed. Comparisons with data discussed earlier indicate that this may be a general phenomenon. Pigs with their high ovulation rates had relatively smaller positive, preovulatory LH discharges than sheep or cattle with their low ovulation rates, just as the sheep of a highly fertile breed had relatively smaller discharge than those of a breed of lower fertility. Within breeds of sheep, those homozygous for the HbA allele have smaller litter sizes, yet higher fertility against a background of exogenous estrogen than those homozygous for HbB; greater sensitivity of HbA sheep to estrogen would lead to both lower litter size under "normal" conditions and the maintenance of the positive discharge of LH under the adverse estrogenic "environment".

Is the variation among breeds of sheep of a similar physiological nature to that among seasons? Scaramuzzi and Baird[64] conclude from the observation of a lower frequency of LH pulses during anestrus than during the estrous cycle that anestrus sheep are more sensitive to negative feedback from endogenous estrogen. They do not however test this hypothesis, and their observations are equally compatible with a reduction in primary drive, although their interpretation is supported by the observed depression of the concentration of LH in the peripheral plasma of castrated ewes implanted with estrogen during anestrus but not during the breeding season.[65]

Evidence to the contrary is presented by Wheeler et al.;[66] when the maintained corpora lutea of ewes with ovarian autotransplants were regressed during anestrum, the gonadotropic stimulation was so weak that a possible increase in estrogen secretion was not detected. Such a reduction in primary drive during anestrus would also account for the absence of discharges of LH during anestrus[57] and avoid the difficulty of accounting for increased sensitivity to negative feedback and decreased sensitivity to positive feedback encountered by Scaramuzzi and Baird.[64]

Genetic and environmental variation may therefore be controlled, at least in part, by different endocrinological variation — less frequent pulses during ovarian inactivity but no correlation between pulse frequency and ovarian activity given that they are cyclic. The possibility that genetic variation in female reproduction arises primarily from change in sensitivity to negative feedback while seasonal environmental variation arises primarily from changes in primary drive is therefore similar to the relationship considered earlier for males. If this is correct, the similar variation in males and females supports the contention that the control of reproductive activity is not sex limited.

D. Perspective

Genetic variation in the relationships between the primary gonadotropin signal and the negative effects of gonadal activity on the strength of this signal has been demonstrated. Possibly the next step in the physiological study of this variation is to try to assess the relative importance of the primary drive to effects of feedback and of variation in characteristics of the hypothalamus and the pituitary gland, especially the extent to which this is intrinsic or modified by steroids. In both cases, however, answers are unlikely to be all one or the other. It may be a question of gradually collecting data rather than designing specific experiments to give complete answers. Some information, however, is available from experiments in which the number of variables has been reduced.[67]

The response to LRF of castrated females of breeds of sheep with differing gonadotropin/steroid relationships was examined at three different times of the year. There were no marked differences between the Finnish Landrace, Scottish Blackface, and Tasmanian Merino ewes examined, nor were there any marked differences between seasons. The basic ability of the pituitary gland to release LH may therefore be quantitatively similar in each breed and in each season, suggesting the variation described earlier to be either hypothalamic or gonadal.

The characteristics of the unmodulated release of prolactin was studied in castrated rams of the three breeds mentioned earlier (Finnish Landrace, Scottish Blackface, and Tasmanian Merino) and was found to be similar. All three breeds showed maximum prolactin concentration before the longest day, despite the fact that seasonal variation in gonadal activity differs. The anestrus season of Blackfaces is symmetrical about the longest day, that of Merinos about a month earlier, and that of Finns about a month later.[58] Similarly, testis growth of Merino males occurs earlier in the season than that of Finns.[68] That reproduction varies seasonally is a genetic characteristic of sheep, and that the timing of this variation differs in the absence of differences in hypothalamic/pituitary activity suggests that this genetic variation arises from differences in gonadal feedback. The study of the effects of steroids on LRF release, LRF-binding in the pituitary gland, and the "firing" of sites, given that they are bound, may all be very rewarding.

V. VARIATION AMONG CATTLE AND PIGS

Twin and breed comparative studies have been reported for cattle, but the authors are not aware of any published studies of genetic variation within pigs.

A. Response of Bulls to LRF

The release of LH following the injection of 250 μg LRF to young postpuberal bulls was found to be a characteristic of the individual.[69] Subsequent studies of the response of twin bulls showed that twins are more alike than unrelated animals, the intraclass correlation being 0.98 and 0.96 on two occasions.[70] With such a high correlation most of the variation in the LH response to LRF may be controlled genetically, but the contribution of long-term environmental effects, pre- as well as postnatal, must be assessed before this can be concluded.

B. Testosterone and Bull Fertility

A genetic correlation between a bull's response to LRF and its fertility would obviously be of great interest. That it might be possible to predict a bull's fertility and that the prediction may have a genetic basis is indicated by the report that Africander cross bulls are both more fertile than Brahman crosses (77 vs. 61%) and have a higher frequency of testosterone pulses (3.7 vs. 2.5 per 24 hr, $p<0.01$).[71]

C. Bovine Placental Hormones

The only genetic variation in the endocrinology of pregnancy within a species of domestic mammals has been reported in cattle. Terqui et al.[72] first reported that a calf may be able to influence its own milk supply. Large or numerous fetuses were observed to be associated with high maternal plasma estrogen concentrations, which are known to stimulate mammary development and milk production. Bolander et al.[73] considered the concentration of placental lactogen in maternal serum to be associated with fetal mass. They also showed that maternal placental lactogen levels are higher in dairy than in beef breeds. A new expression of genetic variation has been revealed; the evolutionary association of fetal and mammary development is intriguing and the practical implications are considerable. Taylor et al.[74] have shown that bulls which sire high-yielding daughters may depress the yield of their mates and vice versa. We now have the beginning of the physiological framework to investigate this correlation and to consider the development of improved criteria for the selection of dairy bulls. The study of genetic variation in reproductive physiology may have implications outside reproduction.

VI. THE EFFECT OF SEX

The simplest and most obvious genetic variation in reproductive endocrinology is that of sex, and an earlier chapter deals with some inherited sexual abnormalities.[76] Despite the obvious differences between males and females, the degree of similarity underlying the difference is considerable, if not surprising.

The genes controlling female sexual characteristics are inherited through both sexes, as are those carrying male characteristics. The same gonadotropic hormones control reproduction in both sexes. Genetic variation in reproductive performances of males is mediated in a similar way to that of females. The genes for sexually dimorphic characters are not necessarily either sex linked or sex limited.[75] Once the male/female switch has been set, the same genetic control system can effect the quantitative determination of the reproductive characteristics of both sexes. Small endocrinological differences gradually magnify to give the gross differences between males and females. Once the sex of the gonad is determined, sex steroids are determined, and it is they that determine secondary sexual characteristics. The observed endocrinological differences between males and females are not, therefore, primary genetic effects, but secondary, effected through the action of hormones of an earlier stage of differentiation. Some of the differences are nevertheless worthy of note.

The positive feedback release of LH by estrogen is only present in females, and the negative effects are common to both sexes. Gonadectomy affects plasma LH concentration in the young male lamb, but not in the female. The latter difference, however, arises from differences in gonadal steroid production rather than differences in the hypothalamus or pituitary gland of the two sexes[33] so that this too is a clear example of sexual differentiation without sex-limited gene action. Lambs of both sexes pass through a peak of LH concentration well before puberty, and the age ranking of different breeds is common to both sexes.

It must be acknowledged that the recent report of Karsch et al.,[65] showing the characteristics of LH in peripheral plasma of castrated ewes to remain constant throughout the year, indicates a contrast with the observation of Pelletier and Ortavant[47] that seasonal variation in LH of the castrated ram was similar to that of the intact male (albeit about a higher mean), but this has yet to be substantiated.

VII. PRESENT SITUATION AND FUTURE PROSPECTS

The inheritance of the variation discussed is little understood. Neither selection for an endocrine component of the physiology of reproduction nor conventional quantitative genetic analyses of variation in such a component in a random bred population have been reported for domestic animals.

The physiology of the variation observed is similarly little understood. The fact that one is reduced to talking in terms of "primary gonadotropic signal strength" or "sensitivity to negative feedback", or even worse that much of the evidence does not even discriminate between these sources of variation, illustrates the primitive level of understanding. Before being too despondent, however, it is revealing to consider how much progress has been made. Until recently, genetic variation in gonadotropic stimulation was taken as the differences in gonadal activity, which could not be accounted for by variation in gonadal response to exogenous gonadotropins. It has been less than 10 years since the first assays for gonadotropins in peripheral plasma were described. During this time, the importance of the feedback control of gonadotropin release has been realized and the theory that the control of reproduction is not sex limited has been proposed. The study of the physiological expression of genetic variation may well provide the link between cellular and quantitative genetics.

While statistical techniques for the analysis of genetic variation have been available for some time, it is only recently that the first steps in understanding the biochemistry of gene action and protein synthesis have been made. Along with this, following the development of the radioimmunoassay and radioreceptor assays, theories of hormone action, and some knowledge of their receptor sites, are being developed. The use of animals with different levels of activity of the same physiological pathways presents the opportunity to study the control of these rates. Structural genes may be essential, as gonadotropins are essential for ovulation, but neither tell us anything about the determination of a particular level of activity. In order to understand this determination, this homeostasis of development, it is necessary to understand the mechanism of action of regulator genes and the feedback control of gonadotropin release.

The relevance of these studies to animal breeding should not be neglected, and it may be no coincidence that most of the developments have come from workers in this field. Improvement depends on the intelligent exploitation of variation; the understanding of variation may facilitate this process.

REFERENCES

1. **Falconer, D. S.,** *Introduction to Quantitative Genetics,* Ronald Press, New York, 1960, 1.
2. **Papkoff, H., Gospodarowicz, D., and Li, C. H.,** Purification and properties of ovine follicle stimulating hormone, *Arch. Biochem. Biophys.,* 120, 434, 1967.
3. **Roos, P.,** Human follicle stimulating hormone, *Acta Endocrinol. (Copenhagen) Suppl.,* 59, 131, 1968.
4. **Schams, D. and Karg, H.,** Radioimmunologi che LH Bestimmung im Blutserum vom rindunter besonderer Berucksichtigung des Brunstzyklus, *Acta Endocrinol. (Copenhagen),* 61, 96, 1969.
5. **Carr, W. R.,** Radioimmunoassay of luteinizing hormone in the blood of Zebu cattle, *J. Reprod. Fertil.,* 29, 11, 1972.
6. **Goding, J. R., Catt, K. J., Brown, J. M., Kaltenbach, C. C., Cumming, I. A., and Mole, B. J.,** Radioimmunoassay for ovine luteinizing hormone. Secretion of luteinizing hormone during estrus and following estrogen administration in the sheep, *Endocrinology,* 85, 133, 1969.
7. **Tillson, S. A., Erb, R. E., and Niswender, G. D.,** Comparison of luteinizing hormone and progesterone in blood and metabolites of progesterone in urine of domestic sows during estrus and early pregnancy, *J. Anim. Sci.,* 30, 795, 1970.
8. **Henricks, D. M., Guthrie, H. D., and Handlin, D. L.,** Plasma oestrogen, progesterone and luteinizing hormone levels during the estrous cycle in pigs, *Biol. Reprod.,* 210, 1972.
9, **L'Hermite, M., Niswender, G. D., Reichert, L. E., Jr., and Midgley, A. R., Jr.,** Serum follicle stimulating hormone in sheep as measured by radioimmunoassay, *Biol. Reprod.,* 6, 325, 1972.
10. **Akbar, A. M., Reichert, L. E., Jr., Dunn, T. G., Kaltenbach, C. C., and Niswender, G. D.,** Serum levels of follicle stimulating hormone during the bovine estrous cycle, *J. Anim. Sci.,* 39, 360, 1974.
11. **Rayford, P. L., Brinkley, H. J., Young, E. P., and Reichert, L. E.,** Radioimmunoassay of porcine FSH, *J. Anim. Sci.,* 39, 348, 1974.
12. **Stabenfeldt, G. H., Holt, J. A., and Ewing, L. L.,** Peripheral plasma progesterone levels, during the ovine estrous cycle, *Endocrinology,* 85, 11, 1969.
13. **Henricks, D. M., Dickey, J. F., and Hill, J. R.,** Plasma estrogen and progesterone levels in cows prior to and during estrus, *Endocrinology,* 89, 1350, 1971.
14. **Yuthasastrarosol, P., Palmer, W. M., and Howland, B. E.,** Luteinizing hormone, oestrogen and progesterone levels in peripheral serum of anoestrous and cycle ewes as determined by radioimmunoassay, *J. Reprod. Fertil.,* 43, 57, 1975.
15. **Baird, D. T. and Scaramuzzi, R. J.,** Changes in the secretion of ovarian steroids and pituitary luteinizing hormone in the periovulatory period in the ewe; the effect of progesterone, *J. Endocrinol.,* 70, 237, 1976.
16. **Bassett, J. M., Oxborrow, T. J., Smith, I. D., and Thorburn, G. D.,** The concentration of progesterone in the peripheral plasma of the pregnant ewe, *J. Endocrinol.,* 45, 449, 1969.
17. **Sheva Y., Black, W. J. M., Carr, W. R., and Land, R. B.,** The effects of nutrition on the reproductive performance of Finn × Dorset ewes. I. Plasma progesterone and LH concentration during late pregnancy, *J. Reprod. Fertil.,* 45, 283, 1975.

18. **Carr, W. R., Taylor, S. C. S., and Booth, J. B.**, unpublished data, 1977.
19. **Donaldson, L. E., Bassett, J. M., and Thorburn, G. D.**, Peripheral plasma progesterone concentration of cows during puberty, oestrous cycles, pregnancy and lactation and the effects of undernutrition or exogenous oxytocin on progesterone concentration, *J. Endocrinol.*, 48, 599, 1970.
20. **Carr, W. R.**, unpublished data, 1977.
21. **Robertson, H. A. and King, G. J.**, Plasma concentrations of progesterone, oestrone, oestradiol-17β and oestrone sulphate in the pig at implantation, during pregnancy and at parturition, *J. Reprod. Fertil.*, 40, 133, 1974.
22. **Robertson, H. A. and Smeaton, T. C.**, The concentration of unconjugated oestrone, oestradiol-17α and oestradiol-17β in the maternal plasma of pregnant ewe in relation to the initiation of parturition and lactation, *J. Reprod. Fertil.*, 35, 461, 1973.
23. **Robertson, H. A.**, Changes in the concentration of unconjugated oestrone, oestradiol-17α and oestradiol-17β in the maternal plasma of the pregnant cow in relation to the initiation of parturition and lactation, *J. Reprod. Fertil.*, 36, 1, 1974.
24. **Sanford, L. M., Winter, J. S. D., Palmer, W. M., and Howland, B. E.**, The profile of LH and testosterone secretion in the ram, *Endocrinology*, 95, 627, 1974.
25. **Schanbacher, B. D. and Ford, J. J.**, Seasonal profiles of plasma luteinizing hormone, testosterone and estradiol in the ram, *Endocrinology*, 99, 752, 1976.
26. **Lincoln, G. A., Peet, M. J., and Cunningham, R. A.**, Seasonal and circadian changes in the episodic release of follicle stimulating hormone, luteinizing hormone and testosterone in rams exposed to artificial photoperiods, *J. Endocrinol.*, 72, 337, 1977.
27. **Katongole, C. B., Naftolin, F., and Short, R. V.**, Relationship between blood levels of luteinizing hormone and testosterone in bulls, and the effects of sexual stimulation, *J. Endocrinol.*, 50, 457, 1971.
28. **Ellendorff, F., Parvizi, N., Pomerontz, D. K., Hartjen, A., Konig, A., Smidt, D., and Elsaesser, F.**, Plasma luteinizing hormone and testosterone in the adult male pig: 24 hours fluctuations and the effect of copulation, *J. Endocrinol.*, 67, 403, 1975.
29. **Thimonier, J., Pelletier, J., and Land, R. B.**, The concentration of plasma LH in male and female lambs of high and low prolificacy breed types, *J. Reprod. Fertil.*, 31, 498, 1972.
30. **Bindon, B. M., Blanc, M. R., Pelletier, J., Terqui, M., and Thimonier, J.**, Preovulatory gonadotrophin and ovarian steroid patterns in 4 French sheep breeds of differing fecundity, *J. Reprod. Fertil.*, in press, 1977.
31. **Blanc, M. R., Courot, M., Pelletier, J., and Thimonier, J.**, Étude de la puberté et de la saison sexuelle chez les races prolifiques et leurs croisements avec des races francaises, in *Journées de la Récherche Ovine et Caprine*, INRA-ITOVIC, Paris, 1975, 18.
32. **Courot, M., de Reviers, M. M., and Pelletier, J.**, Variations in pituitary and blood LH during puberty in the male lamb. Relation to time of birth, *Ann. Biol. Anim. Biochim. Biophys.*, 15, 509, 1975.
33. **Foster, D. L., Cook, B., and Nalbandov, A. V.**, Regulation of Luteinizing Hormone (LH) in the fetal and neonatal lamb: effect of castration during the early post-natal period on levels of LH in sera and pituitaries of neonatal lambs, *Biol. Reprod.*, 6, 253, 1972.
34. **Bindon, B. M. and Turner, H. N.**, Plasma LH of the prepubertal lamb: a possible early indicator of fecundity, *J. Reprod. Fertil.*, 39, 85, 1974.
35. **Carr, W. R. and Land, R. B.**, Plasma luteinizing hormone levels and testis diameters of ram lambs of different breeds, *J. Reprod. Fertil.*, 42, 325, 1975.
36. **Echternkamp, S. E. and Laster, D. B.**, Plasma LH concentrations for prepubertal, postpubertal anoestrous and cyclic ewes of varying fecundity, *J. Anim. Sci.*, 42, 444, 1976.
37. **Hanrahan, J. P., Quirke, J. F., and Gosling, J. P.**, Genetic and non-genetic effects on plasma LH in lambs at 4- and 8-weeks of age, *J. Reprod. Fertil.*, in press, 1977.
38. **Findlay, J. K. and Bindon, B. M.**, Plasma FSH in Merino lambs selected for fecundity, *J. Reprod. Fertil.*, 46, 515, 1976.
39. **Land, R. B.**, Genetic variation and improvement, in *Reproduction in Domestic Animals*, 3rd ed., Cole, H. H. and Cupps, P. T., Eds., Academic Press, New York, 1977, 577.
40. **Carr, W. R., Land, R. B., and Sales, D. I.**, The effect of gonadotrophin releasing hormone (GnRH) on plasma levels of luteinizing hormone (LH) in lambs of breeds with high and low ovulation rates, *Ann. Biol. Anim. Biochim. Biophys.* 16, 167, 1976.
41. **Donald, H. P., Read, J. L., and Russell, W. S.**, A comparative trial of crossbred ewes by Finnish Landrace and other sires, *Anim. Prod.*, 10, 413, 1968.
42. **Galloway, D. B. and Pelletier, J.** Influence of age on the pituitary response of male lambs to synthetic LH-RH injection, *Horm. Metab. Res.*, 6, 240, 1974.
43. **Courot, M.**, Établissement de la Spermatogénése chez l'agneau (*Ovis aries*): Étude Éxperiméntale de son Contrôle Gonadotrope; Importance des Cellules de la Lignée Sertolienne. These de Doctorat d'étât es—sciences naturelles, univérsité, Paris, 1971.

44. **Lincoln, G. A.**, Seasonal variation in the episodic secretion of luteinizing hormone and testosterone in the ram, *J. Endocrinol.*, 69, 213, 1976.
45. **Land, R. B. and Carr, W. R.**, Testis growth and plasma LH concentration following hemicastration and its relation with female prolificacy in sheep, *J. Reprod. Fertil.*, 45, 495, 1975.
46. **Pelletier, J. and Ortavant, R.**, Photoperiodic control of LH release in the ram. II. Light-androgens interaction, *Acta Endocrinol. (Copenhagen)*, 78, 442, 1975.
47. **Pelletier, J. and Ortavant, R.**, Photoperiodic control of LH release in the ram. I. Influence of increasing and decreasing photoperiods, *Acta Endocrinol. (Copenhagen)*, 78, 435, 1975.
48. **Schanbacher, B. D. and Lunstra, D. D.**, Seasonal changes in sexual activity and serum levels of LH and testosterone in Finnish Landrace and Suffolk rams, *J. Anim. Sci.*, 43, 644, 1976.
49. **Evans, J. V. and Turner, H. N.**, Haemoglobin types and reproductive performance in Australian Merino sheep, *Nature (London)*, 207, 396, 1965.
50. **Agar, N. S., Evans, J. V., and Roberts, J.**, Red blood cell potassium and haemoglobin polymorphism in sheep, a review, *Anim. Breeding Abstr.*, 40, 407, 1972.
51. **Obst, J. M., Seamark, R. F., and McGowan, C. J.**, Haemoglobin type and fertility of Merino ewes grazing oestrogenic (Yarloop Clover) pastures, *Nature (London)*, 232, 497, 1971.
52. **Findlay, J. K., Buckmaster, J. M., Chamley, W. A., Cumming, I. A., Hearnshaw, H., and Goding, J. R.**, Release of luteinizing hormone by oestradiol 17β and a gonadotrophin releasing hormone in ewes affected with clover disease, *Neuroendocrinology*, 11, 57, 1973.
53. **Pant, H. C. and Pandey, M. D.**, Influence of haemoglobin type on the induced ovulation rate in sheep, *Nature (London)*, 256, 738, 1975.
54. **Trounson, A. O., Willadsen, S. M., Moor, R. M., and Tucker, E. M.**, Haemoglobin type and superovulation in ewes, *Nature (London)*, 262, 329, 1976.
55. **Land, R. B., Pelletier, J., Thimonier, J., and Mauleon, P.**, A quantitative study of genetic differences in the incidence of oestrus, ovulation and plasma luteinizing hormone concentrations in the sheep, *J. Endocrinol.*, 58, 305, 1973.
56. **Carr, W. R. and Land, R. B.**, unpublished observations, 1975.
57. **Land, R. B., Wheeler, A. G., and Carr, W. R.**, Seasonal variation in the oestrogen induced LH discharge of ovariectomized Finnish Landrace and Scottish Blackface ewes, *Ann. Biol. Anim. Biochim. Biophys.*, 16, 521, 1976.
58. **Wheeler, A. G. and Land, R. B.**, Seasonal variation in oestrus and ovarian activity of Finnish Landrace, Scottish Blackface and Tasmanian Merino ewes, *Anim. Prod.*, 24, 363, 1977.
59. **Scaramuzzi, R. J. and Land, R. B.**, Estradiol levels during the estrous cycle: a comparison of 3 breeds of different fecundity, *Theriogenology*, 6, 606, 1976.
60. **Baird, D. T., Swanston, I., and Scaramuzzi, R. J.**, Pulsatile release of LH and secretion of ovarian steroids in sheep during the luteal phase of the estrous cycle, *Endocrinology*, 98, 1490, 1976.
61. **Baird, D. T., Land, R. B., Scaramuzzi, R. J., and Wheeler, A. G.**, Functional assessment of the autotransplanted uterus and ovary in the ewe, *Proc. R. Soc. London, Ser. B.*, 92, 463, 1976.
62. **Wheeler, A. G.**, Seasonal and Breed Variation in the Reproductive Activity of the Ewe, Ph.D. thesis, University of Edinburgh, Edinburgh, 1975.
63. **Land, R. B.**, The sensitivity of the ovulation rate of Finnish Landrace and Blackface ewes to exogenous oestrogen, *J. Reprod. Fertil.*, 48, 217, 1976.
64. **Scaramuzzi, R. J. and Baird, D. T.**, Ovarian steroid secretion in sheep during anoestrus, in *Sheep Breeding*, Thomas, G. J., Robertson, D. E., and Lightfoot, R. J., Eds., West Australian Institute of Technology, Perth, 1976, 330.
65. **Karsch, F. J., Legan, S. J., and Ryan, K. D.**, The feed-back effects of ovarian steroids on gonadotrophin release, in *Proc. Univ. of Nottingham, 26th Easter School: Control of Ovulation*, Butterworths, London, 1977, 137.
66. **Wheeler, A. G., Baird, D. T., Land, R. B., and Scaramuzzi, R. J.**, Seasonal variation in oestrus, the secretion of oestrogen and progesterone and LH levels prior to ovulation in the ewe, *J. Reprod. Fertil.*, 51, 427, 1977.
67. **Land, R. B. and Carr, W. R.**, unpublished data, 1977.
68. **Islam, A. B. M. M. and Land, R. B.**, Seasonal variation in testis diameter and sperm output of rams of breeds of differing prolificacy, *Anim. Prod.*, 25, 311, 1977.
69. **Thibier, M.**, Effect of synthetic gonadotrophin releasing hormone (GnRH) on circulating luteinizing hormone (LH) and testosterone in young postpubertal bulls, *Acta Endocrinol. (Copenhagen)*, 81, 636, 1976.
70. **Thibier, M.**, Influence of genotype on peripheral luteinizing hormone (LH) and testosterone (T) levels in young twin bulls, in *Proc. 8th Int. Congr. Animal Reproduction and Artificial Insemination*, Kracow, 1, 261, 1976.
71. **Post, T. B. and Christensen, H. R.**, Testosterone variability and fertility in bulls, *Theriogenology*, 6, 615, 1976.

72. **Terqui, M., Delouis, C., Thimonier, J., and Ortavant, R.,** Relations entre les oestrogens au cours de la gestation, le poids à la naissance, et al croissance ultérieure des veaux de race charolaise, *C. R. Acad. Sci.,* 280, 2789, 1975.
73. **Bolander, F. F., Jr., Ulberg, L. C., and Fellows, R.,** Circulating placental lactogen levels in dairy and beef cattle, *Endocrinology,* 99, 1273, 1976.
74. **Taylor, St. C. S., Monteiro, L. S., Murray, J., and Osmond, T. J.,** personal communication, 1977.
75. **Land, R. B.,** The expression of female sex-limited characters in the male, *Nature (London),* 241, 208, 1973.
76. **Bullock, L. P.,** Genetic variations in sexual differentiation and sex steroid action, in *Genetic Variation in Hormone Systems,* Vol. 1, Shire, J. G. M., Ed., CRC Press, Boca Raton, Fla., 1979, chap. 4.

Chapter 6

GENETIC MODELS IN THE STUDY OF ANTERIOR PITUITARY HORMONES

A. Bartke

TABLE OF CONTENTS

I. INTRODUCTION

Secretions of the anterior pituitary play a pivotal role in endocrine integration. Thyroid-stimulating hormone (TSH) and adrenocorticotropic hormone (ACTH) provide a major regulatory input for the function of the thyroid gland and the adrenal cortex, respectively. Luteinizing hormone (LH) and follicle-stimulating hormone (FSH) affect different compartments of the male and female gonads to control the production of both gametes and sex steroids. Growth hormone (GH) is indispensable for postnatal growth and development and exerts a number of metabolic effects in the adult. Prolactin (PRL), in addition to its role in the regulation of the mammary gland, exerts a variety of seemingly unrelated effects on numerous target organs. Comparative studies of the effects of PRL in fish, amphibians, reptiles, birds, and various groups of mammals provide fascinating material for speculations on the evolution of the endocrine system in vertebrates.[1]

Genetic variations in the structure and function of the anterior pituitary provide valuable material for studying the physiology of the adenohypophyseal hormones and permit the obtaining of information that would be difficult or impossible to acquire using more conventional approaches, such as surgical ablation of endocrine glands, replacement therapy with hormones, or pharmacological manipulations of hormone release and action. Furthermore, the study of genetic variation in endocrine function is of considerable importance in understanding the normal variation in hormone levels and in responsiveness to hormones in human populations. The significance of hereditary variations and genetic models in the study of the endocrine system was recently reviewed by Shire.[2]

Much of the work in the field of endocrine genetics was done using laboratory mice (*Mus musculus*), undoubtedly due to the availability of numerous mutations and inbred strains and the relatively short generation time in this species. Most studies involved examining the consequences of hereditary hormone deficiency, correlating hormone levels with hormone-dependent physiological characteristics in inbred strains, or comparing various parameters of endocrine function in lines selected for different reproductive performance. The genetic control of the structure of adenohypophyseal hormones received little attention, but Seavey et al.[3] described two allelic forms of bovine GH. Studies on the hereditary differences in the responses of the pituitary to hypothalamic releasing hormones have been initiated only recently.[4]

This chapter will illustrate the applicability of genetic models to the study of the adenohypophyseal hormones. The author wishes to apologize to those whose work, relevant to this subject, is not mentioned due to limitations of space or to inadvertent omissions.

II. PRIMARY HORMONE DEFICIENCY IN HEREDITARY DWARF MICE

In 1929, Snell[5] described a recessive mutation in the laboratory mouse which caused severe retardation of postnatal growth and named it dwarf, *dw*. Animals homozygous for this condition (*dw/dw*) have normal body weight at birth, but after the first week of life their growth rate becomes progressively retarded and adult dwarf mice rarely exceed one third of the body weight of their normal littermates.[6] The pituitaries of hereditary dwarf mice are extremely small and lack the acidophilic cells which are the source of GH.[7-12] The results of examining dwarf mouse pituitaries for the content of GH by bioassay,[13] polyacrylamide disc electrophoresis,[14] or radioimmunoassay[15] indicate that GH is either entirely absent or present in extremely small amounts. Surprisingly, immunoreactive GH was detected in the peripheral serum of hereditary dwarf mice, although in amounts significantly smaller than those found in the normal littermates.[15] It is possible that the results of radioimmunoassay determinations of mouse GH represent a sum of biologically active GH and some unidentified substance(s) which cross react with the antibody employed in this assay. The responsiveness of target tissues to GH is apparently not affected by the *dw* mutation, because parabiotic union of a hereditary dwarf mouse with a normal littermate results in rapid growth of the dwarf partner.[16] Furthermore, treatment of dwarf mice with crude pituitary extracts[17,18] or with various preparations of GH[19-22] also produces a pronounced growth response. This indicates that the retarded growth of *dw/dw* mice is due to GH deficiency. The elegant experiments of Carsner and Rennels[23] provided conclusive evidence that the deficiency of GH in dwarf mice is due to a defect in pituitary rather than hypothalamic function. These investigators have shown that transplantation of the pituitary gland from a normal mouse into the *sella turcica* of a hypophysectomized dwarf results in resumption of near-normal growth. Conversely, growth ceased in normal mice which had their pituitaries removed and replaced by pituitaries from dwarf mice.

It should be indicated that abnormalities of the endocrine system in hereditary dwarf mice are not limited to primary deficiency of GH. These animals are also hypothyroid,[6,24] probably due to a primary deficiency of adenohypophyseal TSH,[11] combined with the apparent failure of the thyroid to differentiate normally in the absence of

GH.[25,26] The evidence for primary PRL deficiency in hereditary dwarf mice will be reviewed in some detail in the section dealing with the use of *dw/dw* and *df/df* mice in the study of the effects of PRL on the testis and the pituitary. The gonadal status of hereditary dwarf mice will be discussed in the same section.

Dwarf mice have been used in demonstrating the involvement of the anterior pituitary and, specifically, GH in the control of diverse physiological processes. These include:

1. Regulation of cell size in various organs[27–30]
2. Control of the appearance of multiple DNA classes (ploidy) in some tissues[31]
3. Control of RNA polymerase levels in liver[137]
4. Stimulation of protein synthesis in the diaphragm[32]
5. Control of the postnatal maturation of the skeleton[29] and the peripheral nerves[30]
6. Determination of the nerve fiber to muscle fiber ratio within the motor units[33]
7. Regulation of serum somatomedin levels[34]
8. Morphological differentiation of the interscapulary brown fat[35] and the submaxillary glands[36]
9. Metabolic responses to reduced environmental temperatures[37,38]
10. Control of the diurnal activity rhythm[39]
11. Development of the immune system[40–45]

It is of interest that the severity of immunodeficiency in homozygous *dw/dw* mice is modified by the genetic background and apparently can be further influenced by husbandry practices. In some colonies, dwarf mice have numerous symptoms of abnormal immune function,[40-45] are extremely susceptible to disease, and, consequently, have reduced life spans.[46] In contrast, in dwarf mice from other colonies the morphological development of the immune system and the ability to develop delayed hypersensitivity are not affected,[47] and homozygous dwarfs live as long as their normal littermates.[32,47-49] Studies in hereditary dwarf mice have also demonstrated a role of pituitary hormones in the control of spontaneous tumor development,[50] growth of transplanted tumors,[51] expression of endogenous tumor viruses,[50] and susceptibility to various chemical carcinogens.[52-54]

In two studies of the hormonal control of excessive fat deposition, *dw* genes were combined in the same individual with genes causing hereditary obesity. This work will be described in a separate section of this chapter, together with other information on anterior pituitary function in obese-hyperglycemic syndromes.

In the discussion of hereditary hormone deficiencies leading to growth retardation, at least two mouse mutants other than *dw* deserve to be mentioned. Ames dwarf *(df/df)* mice were described by Schaible and Gowen[55] among the descendants of a stock used in an irradiation experiment and are phenotypically indistinguishable from *dw/dw* animals. The endocrine status of Ames dwarf mice has not been studied very extensively, but the results of histological and hormone-replacement studies strongly suggest that these animals are GH and PRL-deficient and hypothyroid, much like the *dw/dw* dwarfs.[21,25,56] Thus, two mutations which have arisen independently at two different loci appear to produce identical, or at least very similar, endocrine syndromes.

Little *(lit/lit)* mice are smaller than their normal littermates, but differ from *dw* and *df* dwarfs in having adult rather than immature body proportions and by the ability of females to reproduce.[57] These animals have reduced stores of pituitary GH and PRL and grow when treated with GH or pituitary grafts.[57]

In contrast to *dw/dw*, *df/df*, and *lit/lit* animals, the proportional dwarfism of pigmy *(pg/pg)* mice is due to the unresponsiveness of peripheral tissues to GH, rather than to a deificiency of GH production.[58] These animals have biologically detectable amounts of GH in their pituitaries and fail to grow when treated with daily implants of pituitaries from normal animals or with a purified GH preparation.[58]

Strain differences in serum and pituitary GH levels in laboratory mice will be discussed in the section dealing with the hormonal correlates of genetic differences in mammary tumor incidence. Schindler et al.[59] described significant strain differences in serum GH levels in the rabbit. Strain differences in responsiveness to GH have also been described in mice.[60]

III. ENDOCRINE STUDIES IN ANIMALS WITH HEREDITARY PROLACTIN DEFICIENCY

Investigations of the effects of PRL on the gonadal and pituitary function and on the hepatic RNA metabolism in *dw/dw* and *df/df* mice provide an example of advantages of using genetic models in basic endocrine studies.

A chance observation in 1963 by the author that some female dwarf mice caged together with normal adult males were mating at regular 4- to 5-day intervals, but never became pregnant, led Yochim[140] to suggest that homozygous *dw/dw* and *df/df* animals are PRL deficient. This suggestion was consistent with the previously demonstrated absence of acidophilic cells in their pituitaries[6,25] and was soon confirmed by results of replacement therapy with purified ovine PRL or with PRL-producing ectopic transplants of pituitaries from normal mice.[61] Subsequently, PRL deficiency in the pituitaries of dwarf mice was confirmed using disc electrophoresis,[62] immunohistochemistry,[63] and radioimmunoassay.[15] Presence of reduced but detectable amounts of immunoreactive PRL in the peripheral circulation of *dw/dw* mice[15] can probably be explained by a nonspecific interaction of some substance(s) present in the serum of dwarf mice with the antibody used in the assay. The same assay detected only minimal amounts of PRL in the pituitaries of dwarf animals,[15] and the rat PRL radioimmunoassay usually detects measurable quantities of "PRL" in the peripheral circulation of hypophysectomized animals.[64,65]

Untreated female dwarf mice are invariably sterile, even though they can cycle, mate, and produce fertilizable ova.[56,61] Treatment with PRL or PRL-producing pituitary grafts allows these animals to become pregnant, carry to term, deliver live young, and raise them to weaning.[56,61] The demonstration that exogenous PRL is not required during the second half of pregnancy[66] is consistent with the known ability of murine placenta to produce a lactogenic hormone.[66] These observations have suggested that the secretion of adenohypophyseal gonadotropins (LH and FSH) can be adequate in these animals and that dwarf mice provide a unique model for studying the role of PRL in the regulation of reproductive processes. The advantages of using dwarf mice in the study of PRL physiology are further underlined by difficulties in producing immunodeficiency of PRL, particularly in chronic experiments,[67,68] and by the unsettled question of whether chronic suppression of pituitary PRL release with ergot alkaloids can be both complete and specific in terms of preserving normal release of LH and FSH.[69,70]

Male dwarf mice were used to determine whether PRL plays a role in the pituitary control of testicular function. At the time these studies were initiated, no effects of PRL on the testis were established, even though experiments of Woods and Simpson[71] in hypophysectomized rats suggested that PRL may potentiate the action of gonadotropins on spermatogenesis. Moreover, it was still open to question whether the pituitary of an adult male releases any PRL into the general circulation. Treatment of male dwarf mice with PRL increased the weight of the testes and the accessory reproductive glands,[72] stimulated spermatogenesis,[72,73] increased testicular stores of esterified cholesterol,[74] enhanced the activities of testicular 3β-hydroxysteroid dehydrogenase[75] and

17β-hydroxysteroid dehydrogenase,[76] and induced fertility.[56,61] It is interesting to note that the fertility of male dwarf mice treated with daily implants of nondwarf pituitaries had already been reported in 1932.[77] However, the inhibitory effect of the hypothalamus on PRL release and the active secretion of PRL by pituitaries transplanted to ectopic sites were not discovered until some 20 years later, and therefore this early observation was not interpreted as an indication that PRL may influence testicular function. Recent studies indicate that treatment of male dwarf mice with PRL increases the ability of their testes to bind LH[78] and to produce testosterone in response to human chorionic gonadotropin (a hormone with LH activity) in vitro.[79] Studies on the effects of PRL in hereditary dwarf mice indicate that this hormone can increase testicular responsiveness to the steroidogenic action of LH and suggest several mechanisms by which PRL may exert this effect. It is of particular significance that this previously unsuspected action of PRL on testicular function has since been described in genetically "normal" mice[80] and in other species,[81,82] possibly including man.[83]

The advantages of using hereditary dwarf mice as a model for studying the action of PRL are by no means limited to the physiology of the reproductive system. Chen et al.[84] have demonstrated that treatment of *dw/dw* mice with PRL stimulates hepatic synthesis of RNA and that a single injection of PRL is sufficient to cause a demonstrable assembly of liver ribosomes into polyribosomes. These observations are of great interest since the mammalian liver contains high levels of PRL receptors[85] and thus appears to be an important target tissue for PRL, but the physiological role of PRL in the regulation of liver function is not understood. Because of the structural similarities between GH and PRL and known overlaps between the biological activities of these hormones, it is difficult to relate these findings to the demonstration that GH can normalize the depressed levels of RNA polymerase in the liver of dwarf mice.[137,138]

The effects of PRL on the release of pituitary gonadotropins are presently being examined using dwarf and Ames dwarf mice. Contrary to expectations,[61] plasma FSH levels are significantly lower in dwarf males than in their normal littermates. In both *dw/dw* and *df/df* males, the concentration of FSH in the plasma increases after treatment with PRL (Table 1) or pituitary grafts.[79] These results extend earlier observations that intrahypothalamic implants of PRL can increase FSH release and advance puberty in immature female rats.[86] It appears that PRL may have a function in stimulating the release of pituitary gonadotropins before sexual maturation.

Nude mice, which have no thymus, have reduced levels of PRL and elevated levels of LH.[139] Thymus grafts normalize the levels of both hormones, suggesting that the endocrine and immune systems interact during development.

IV. SEARCH FOR HORMONAL BASIS OF GENETIC DIFFERENCES IN THE INCIDENCE OF MAMMARY TUMORS

The high incidence of breast cancer in women continues to stimulate great interest in the study of factors controlling the development and growth of mammary tumors. The importance of genetic factors is evident from the comparison of tumor incidence in different inbred strains of laboratory mice.[87] Epidemiological studies suggest that familial, possibly genetic, factors influence the risk of breast cancer in women.[88]

In mice and rats, PRL exerts major effects on the occurrence and growth of mammary tumors. Chronic elevation of peripheral PRL levels by ectopic pituitary grafts greatly increases tumor incidence,[89-92] while suppression of PRL release with ergot alkaloids prevents the development of mammary cancers[93,94] and causes regression of spontaneous[95] and carcinogen-induced[96,97] tumors. Several lines of evidence suggest that GH may also influence the development of mammary neoplasms.[98]

Against the background of this information, it is of considerable interest to deter-

TABLE 1

Effects of Hereditary Prolactin (PRL) Deficiency and Treatment with PRL on Plasma FSH Levels in Mice (Results Expressed as ng NIAMDD Rat FSH-RP-1 per mℓ ± SE)

	dwarf, *dw*		Ames dwarf, *df*	
Genotype and treatment	n	FSH (ng/mℓ)	n	FSH (ng/mℓ)
Adult nondwarf (?/+) males of the same strain	58	948±65	55	746±30
Dwarf males	66	132±22[a]	57	171±14[a]
Dwarf males treated with PRL (125μg/day for 2 weeks)	23	202±27	9	255±13

[a] In both dwarf and Ames dwarf strains, plasma FSH levels in control (untreated or saline-injected) dwarf males were significantly lower than in adult normal (nondwarf) males or in dwarfs treated with PRL.

mine whether the genetic differences in the susceptibility to mammary tumors can be traced to hereditary variations in PRL and GH levels. A series of studies by Sinha and his colleagues[99-102] were addressed to this problem. These investigations were based on comparisons of inbred mouse strains that were known to differ in the incidence of spontaneous mammary tumors with particular emphasis on the C3H mice, most of which develop these lesions, and C57BL animals that rarely develop tumors. The concentration of PRL and GH in the pituitary is significantly greater in C3H than in C57BL females.[99] However, serum levels of GH do not differ in these two strains, while serum PRL levels are lower in C3H mice between the ages of 30 and 80 days and do not differ in older animals.[99] Comparison of the effects of nursing on pituitary and peripheral PRL levels in C3H and C57BL mice revealed an interesting difference between these strains, namely, in the tumor-susceptible C3H animals, nursing produced a proportionally greater depletion of pituitary PRL, but a smaller elevation in serum PRL levels.[100] These observations and the demonstration that urinary PRL levels are higher in C3H than in C57BL animals[101] led the authors to postulate that the rate of PRL metabolism is greater in females of the tumor-susceptible C3H strain than in those of the tumor-resistant C57BL strain.[100] Increased metabolism of a hormone without a change in its concentration in the serum implies a greater production rate of this hormone. The dynamics of production, secretion, transport, and clearance of polypeptide hormones are poorly understood, but these observations suggest that the biological effects of PRL may correlate with the rate of its production, rather than with its concentration in peripheral serum, much as has been shown for the gonadal and adrenal steroids.

The same investigators have later extended their studies to include other inbred strains of mice.[102] The results indicate that strains with higher incidence of mammary tumors generally have higher levels of PRL and GH in the pituitary, and GH in the serum, than the strains with low tumor incidence. Resting serum levels of PRL do not correlate with tumor incidence, while perphenazine stimulation causes proportionally greater elevation in serum PRL levels of tumor-resistant strains, even though pituitary stores of PRL are depleted in tumor-resistant and tumor-susceptible animals to a similar extent. These results were interpreted as lending further support to the conclusion that tumor susceptibility is associated with increased ability to metabolize PRL.

However, the relationship between the production of pituitary PRL and the development of mammary tumors is very complex and far from being completely elucidated. Responsiveness of the mammary glands to PRL is greater in C3H than in

C57BL/6 mice.[103] In addition, development of the tumors is related to the milk-transmitted mammary tumor virus, to the levels of ovarian steroids, and to reproductive history.[98] Complex interrelationships between the reproductive cycle, PRL levels, ovarian steroidogenesis, pregnancy, and lactation make the relative contributions of these factors very difficult to define.

Importantly, PRL may mediate some of the hereditary differences in the occurrence of breast cancer in women. Kwa et al.[104] have shown that serum PRL levels were higher in women from families with high risk of mammary cancer than in women from the general population.

V. ANTERIOR PITUITARY HORMONES AND HEREDITARY OBESITY-HYPERGLYCEMIA SYNDROMES

Both diabetes and obesity are common in human populations, difficult to control, and associated with reduced life expectancy. It is, therefore, not surprising that mutants causing excessive fat deposition and hyperglycemia in laboratory animals attracted considerable attention. Studies on the regulation of carbohydrate metabolism in these animals, including measurements of food intake, metabolic rate, fat deposition, blood glucose and insulin levels, tissue responsiveness to insulin, and levels of insulin receptors, are outside the scope of this chapter. A reader interested in this field is referred to the chapter 5 by Woodrow in volume 2 and to reviews on hereditary obesity and diabetes in men[105] and in experimental animals.[106]

The involvement of the anterior pituitary in the development of hereditary obesity and hyperglycemia in mice was suspected from the well-documented function of GH in the regulation of carbohydrate metabolism, the weight loss observed in genetically obese animals after hypophysectomy,[107] and the reproductive disorders associated with hereditary obesity.

The results of Desjardins[108] indicate that genetically diabetic *(db/db)* mice have elevated levels of GH and GH-releasing factor (GH-RF) during the early stages of the appearance of the diabetic syndrome and reduced GH and GH-RF levels after the development of severe hyperglycemia. In the obese-hyperglycemic *(obese, ob/ob)* mice, Roos et al.[109] found normal levels of GH, while Sinha et al.[110] reported reduced levels of PRL and GH in pituitary and serum. The latter investigators also demonstrated that the ability to release PRL in response to perphenazine stimulation is impaired in *ob/ob* animals.[110] A subsequent study of obese mice and their normal (lean) littermates between the ages of 2 and 26 weeks confirmed the observation that serum levels of both PRL and GH are reduced in *ob/ob* animals of both sexes.[111] These results suggest abnormalities in hypothalamic-pituitary function of genetically obese and diabetic animals, but do not necessarily imply that the alterations in release of anterior pituitary hormones contribute to the development of excessive fat deposition or hyperglycemia. Ingenious experiments in which the genes causing hereditary obesity were combined in the same individual with genes causing GH and PRL deficiency suggest that these hormones are not required for the excessive fat deposition. Wolff[112] produced mice which were homozygous for the *dw* gene (and therefore GH and PRL deficient) and heterozygous for the A^y gene, which causes a variety of phenotypic alterations including obesity, and observed that these animals weighed considerably more than the nonyellow dwarfs and that this weight difference was due almost entirely to increased fat deposition in the *dw/dw* A^y/a individuals. Joosten et al.[113] reported that genetically obese dwarf mice *(ob/ob dw/dw)* developed obesity and hyperinsulinemia in spite of electrophoretically confirmed GH deficiency.

Abnormal hypothalamic-pituitary function in genetically obese *(ob/ob)* mice appears to account for, or at least contribute to, their sterility. Swerdloff et al.[114] have demonstrated that plasma LH and FSH levels are lower in obese males than in lean animals of the same strain. In addition, the magnitude of the postcastration increase in peripheral gonadotropin levels was reduced in *ob/ob* mice, and plasma LH levels in castrated obese males could be suppressed with a much lower dose of testosterone than was required in the lean controls.[114]

VI. HEREDITARY VARIATIONS IN GONADOTROPIN LEVELS

Strain and breed differences in fertility in both experimental and farm animals have been studied in considerable detail (see chapter 5 by Land and Carr in this volume), but information on the genetic control of the levels of LH and FSH is relatively scarce. In laboratory mice, Karande et al.[115] reported strain differences in the pituitary content of FSH, in the proportional increase in pituitary FSH stores after gonadectomy, and in the time-course of this response. Differences in plasma FSH levels were found in males from strains selected for different ages of sexual maturation.[116] Peripheral gonadotropin levels are reduced in obese *(ob/ob)*, dwarf *(dw/dw)*, and Ames dwarf *(df/df)* males,[79,114] as discussed in the preceding sections of this chapter. Pituitary and peripheral gonadotropin levels are elevated in mice carrying the gene substitutions pink-eyed dilution (*p*) and p-unstable (p^{un}).[117] In p-sterile mutants (p^{6}, p^{bs}, and p^{25}) at the same locus, Melvold[118] found fewer gonadotropin-staining cells in sections of pituitaries. Johnson and Hunt[119] found degenerative changes in the *pars nervosa* and decreased estrogen binding to the hypothalamus of mice homozygous for p^{25}.

In male rats and mice hemizygous for testicular feminization *(tfm)*, peripheral tissues are unresponsive to androgens.[120] This insensitivity interferes with the normal negative-feedback control of gonadotropin secretion by testicular steroids and, as a result, plasma LH levels are significantly elevated.[120] In pseudohermaphroditic *vestigial testes* ("vet") rats, Leydig cells fail to differentiate normally and androgen synthesis is defective.[120] In the absence of an inhibitory influence of testicular androgens, both LH and FSH levels in peripheral circulation are elevated.[120] In restricted (H^{re}/H^{re}) rats, which are characterized by germinal cell aplasia and deficiency of testicular-androgen-binding protein, plasma testosterone levels are somewhat reduced, while LH and FSH levels are significantly elevated.[121] In sterile steel (Sl/Sl^{d}) mice, congenital absence of germinal cells in the testis is associated with significantly elevated serum LH and FSH levels, even though there are no apparent changes in testicular testosterone production.[122] Thus, alteration in gonadotropin levels can be a secondary effect of the genetically determined failure of gonadal function or reflect a hereditary defect in the pituitary-gonadal feedback regulation. However, a hereditary difference in gonadotropin levels can also be a cause for altered gonadal activity. In both dwarf and obese mice, reproductive failure appears to be secondary to the abnormal function of the hypothalamic-pituitary axis. Male mice of C57BL/10 and DBA/2 strains differ with respect to testicular weight, sperm production, plasma testosterone levels, copulatory behavior, and ability to produce pheromones.[123-125] These differences are due to a difference in serum LH levels after sexual maturation.[126,141]

Selection for improved reproductive performance is a standard practice in animal husbandry, and numerous studies have been directed at determining the heritability of various traits related to female and male fertility. The levels of gonadotropins were examined in some of the selection experiments in an attempt to elucidate the possible hormonal basis of the response of reproductive characteristics to selection. In the ewe, plasma LH levels measured at 30 days, or at 5 months of age, were found to be significantly elevated in stocks selected for high incidence of multiple births.[127,128] Land[129] reported that selection based solely on litter size (ovulation rate) in mice and sheep results in parallel changes in testicular weight in males of the selected lines. He suggested that this correlation of responses in both sexes can be explained by assuming that selection acted by way of affecting endocrine function, e.g., gonadotropin levels. In further support of this hypothesis, selection for testis weight in mice resulted in correlated responses in the ovulation rate of selected lines.[130]

Land and Falconer[131] selected mice for different rates of natural and induced ovulation. Their findings indicate that the response to selection could generally be explained by changes in the ovarian sensitivity, except for the animals selected for high natural ovulation, which had an increased "FSH activity" as defined from their dose-response experiments.[131] Murr et al.[132] examined plasma LH and FSH levels at different stages of the estrous cycle in mice from lines selected for differences in ovulation rate, embryo survival and litter size and in a control unselected line. There were no differences in plasma gonadotropin levels between these lines, suggesting that selection must have altered the responsiveness of the ovaries to gonadotropins, rather than the rate of gonadotropin release. Differences in ovarian responsiveness to exogenous gonadotropins in animals from lines used by Murr et al.[132] were subsequently demonstrated by Bindon and Pennycuik.[133] Explanation of the response to selection in terms of differences in the gonadal sensitivity to gonadotropins may also apply to other similar experiments. Parks and Wolfe[134] have shown that the ability of the ovaries to bind FSH in vitro was significantly greater in mice selected for high ovulatory response to exogenous gonadotropins than in those from a line selected for low response. Other observations on the same lines suggest that selection for difference in ovulatory response to the pregnant mare serum-human chorionic gonadotropin regimen may have altered gonadal responsiveness to gonadotropins in both sexes. The ability of the testes to produce testosterone in response to pregnant mare serum gonadotropin in vitro is greater in animals from the line selected for high ovulatory response than in animals from the line selected for low ovulation rate.[135] The differences in the testicular sensitivity to gonadotropins cannot be readily explained by differences in endogenous LH or FSH levels in these animals.[135]

A new dimension to the study of the genetic control of plasma gonadotropin levels was added by the recent demonstration of strain differences in the in vitro response of the pituitary to hypothalamic luteinizing hormone-releasing hormone (LH-RH).[4,136] In these studies, anterior pituitaries of adult male mice were incubated in the presence of LH-RH and the accumulation of LH in the medium was measured by radioimmunoassay. Comparison of four inbred strains, C57BL/6, C3H/He, 129/Re, and NAW, revealed significant strain differences in the amount and rate of LH release, and this work is being extended to include pituitary response in F_1 hybrids in a diallel design.

ACKNOWLEDGMENTS

The writing of this chapter and the previously unpublished studies from this laboratory were supported by N.I.H. through a Research Career Development Award HD70369 and Grants HD06867 and HD09584. I thank Drs. H. G. Wolfe and D. Sustarsic for access to their unpublished results.

REFERENCES

1. **Nicoll, C. S.**, Physiological actions of prolactin, in *Handbook of Physiology — Endocrinology* Vol. 4 (Part 2), Knobil, E. and Sawyer, W. H., Eds., American Physiological Society, Washington, D. C., 1974, 253.
2. **Shire, J. G. M.**, The forms, uses and significance of genetic variation in endocrine systems, *Biol. Rev.*, 51, 105, 1976.
3. **Seavey, B. K., Singh, R. N. P., Lewis, U. J., and Geschwind, I. I.**, Bovine growth hormone: evidence for two allelic forms, *Biochem. Biophys. Res. Commun.*, 43, 189, 1971.
4. **Sustarsic, D. L. and Wolfe, H. G.**, Differences in male reproductive physiology between C3H/HeWe and C57BL/6We inbred strains of mice, *Genetics*, 83, s74, 1976.
5. **Snell, G. D.**, Dwarf, a new mendelian recessive character of the house mouse, *Proc. Natl. Acad. Sci. U.S.A.*, 15, 733, 1929.
6. **Grüneberg, H.**, *The Genetics of the Mouse*, Martinus Nijhoff, The Hague, 1952, 122.
7. **deBeer, G. R. and Grüneberg, H.**, A note on the pituitary dwarfism in the mouse, *J. Genet.*, 39, 297, 1940.
8. **Francis, T.**, *The Development of the Pituitary and Hereditary Anterior Pituitary Dwarfism in Mice*, Munksgaard, Copenhagen, 1944.
9. **Ortman, R.**, A study of some cytochemical reactions and the hormone content of the adenohypophysis in normal and in genetic dwarf mouse, *J. Morphol.*, 99, 417, 1956.
10. **Rennels, E. G. and McNutt, W.**, The fine structure of the anterior pituitary of the dwarf mouse, *Anat. Rec.*, 131, 591, 1958.
11. **Elftman, H. and Wegelius, O.**, Anterior pituitary cytology of the dwarf mouse, *Anat. Rec.*, 135, 43, 1959.
12. **Peterson, R. R.**, Electron microscope observations on the pituitary gland of the dwarf mouse, *Anat. Rec.*, 133, 322, 1959.
13. **Smith, P. E. and Mac Dowell, E. C.**, The differential effect of hereditary mouse dwarfism on the anterior pituitary hormones. *Anat. Rec.*, 50, 85, 1931.
14. **Lewis, U. J., Cheever, E. V., and VanderLaan, W. P.**, Studies on the growth hormone of normal and dwarf mice, *Endocrinology*, 76, 210, 1965.
15. **Sinha, Y. N., Salocks, C. B., and VanderLaan, W. P.**, Pituitary and serum concentrations of prolactin and GH in Snell dwarf mice, *Proc. Soc. Exp. Biol. Med.*, 150, 207, 1975.
16. **Weitze, M.**, The action of the anterior pituitary gland on the growth of mice shown by parabiosis. *Acta Pathol. Microbiol. Scand.*, 22, 151, 1945.
17. **Snell, G. D.**, Effect of injection of anterior pituitary extract on the thyroids of mice with hereditary dwarfism, *Anat. Rec.*, 47, 316, 1930.
18. **Bates, R. W., Laanes, T., Mac Dowell, E. C., and Riddle, O.**, Growth in silver dwarf mice with and without injections of anterior pituitary extracts, *Endocrinology*, 31, 53, 1942.
19. **Rouse, C. A. and Osborn, C. M.**, Early growth hormone therapy in hereditary dwarf mice. *Anat. Rec.*, 101, 717, 1948.
20. **Nielsen, E. L.**, Studies on hereditary dwarfism in mice. XIII. Effect of the growth hormone and thyroxin on the growth of bones in mice with hereditary pituitary dwarfism, *Acta Pathol. Microbiol. Scand.*, 30, 10, 1951.
21. **Bartke, A.**, The response of two types of dwarf mice to growth hormone, thyrotropin and thyroxine, *Gen. Comp. Endocrinol.*, 5, 418, 1965.
22. **Wallis, M. and Dew, J. A.**, The bioassay of growth hormone in Snell's dwarf mice: effects of thyroxine and prolactin on the dose-response curve, *J. Endocrinol.*, 56, 235, 1973.
23. **Carsner, R. L. and Rennels, E. G.**, Primary site of gene action in anterior pituitary dwarf mice, *Science*, 131, 829, 1960.
24. **Chai, C. K. and Dickie, M. M.**, Endocrine variations, in *Biology of the Laboratory Mouse*, 2nd ed., Green, E. L., Ed., Dover, New York, 1975, 387.
25. **Bartke, A.**, Histology of the anterior hypophysis, thyroid and gonads of two types of dwarf mice, *Anat. Rec.*, 149, 225, 1964.
26. **Bartke, A.**, The response of dwarf mice to murine thyroid-stimulating hormone, *Gen. Comp. Endocrinol.*, 11, 246, 1968.
27. **Cheek, D. B., Powell, G. K., and Scott, R. E.**, Growth of muscle cells (size and number) and liver DNA in rats and Snell Smith mice with insufficient pituitary, thyroid, or testicular function, *Bull. Johns Hopkins Hosp.*, 117, 306, 1965.
28. **Winick, M. and Grant, P.**, Cellular growth in the organs of the hypopituitary dwarf mouse, *Endocrinology*, 83, 544, 1968.
29. **Dawson, A. B.**, The influence of hereditary dwarfism on the differentiation of the skeleton of the mouse, *Anat. Rec.*, 61, 485, 1935.

30. **Reier, P. J., Froelich, J. S., Sawchak, J. A., and Hughes, A. F. W.,** Maturation of nonmyelinated fiber bundles in a strain of dwarf (Snell's) mice, *Anat. Rec.,* 178, 103, 1974.
31. **Leuchtenberger, C., Helweg-Larsen, H. F., and Murmanis, L.,** Relationship between hereditary pituitary dwarfism and the formation of multiple deoxyribose nucleic acid (DNA) classes in mice, *Lab. Invest.,* 3, 245, 1954.
32. **Nutting, D. F.,** Effects of growth hormone, thyroxine, and age on diaphragm muscle from dwarf mice, *Endocrinology,* 99, 1423, 1976.
33. **Viola-Magni, M.,** Cell number deficiencies in the nervous system of dwarf mice, *Anat. Rec.,* 153, 325, 1965.
34. **Holder, A. T. and Wallis, W.,** Regulation of serum somatomedin levels and growth in dwarf mice by growth hormone, prolactin and thyroxine, *J. Endocrinol.,* 71, 82p, 1976.
35. **Mazza, L., Martinazzi, M., and Magrini, U.,** Morfologia del grasso bruno nel topo con nanismo ipofisario: effetto degli ormoni preipofisari, *Boll. Soc. Ital. Biol. Sper.,* 39, 247, 1963.
36. **Martinazzi, M. and Baroni, C.,** Controllo ormonico della ghiandola sottomascellare del topo con nanismo ereditario preipofisario, *Boll. Soc. Ital. Biol Sper.,* 39, 648, 1963.
37. **Boettiger, E. G.,** The relation of oxygen consumption and environmental temperature to the growth of dwarf mice, *Am. J. Physiol.,* 129, 312, 1940.
38. **Mollenbach, C. J.,** Studies on hereditary dwarfism in mice. IV. On the function of metabolic active hormones on the anterior pituitary dwarf mouse, *Acta Pathol. Microbiol. Scand.,* 18, 169, 1941.
39. **Osborn, C. M.,** Spontaneous diurnal activity in a genetically hypopituitary animal, the dwarf mouse, *Anat. Rec.,* 78, 137, 1940.
40. **Pierpaoli, W., Baroni, C., Fabris, N., and Sorkin, E.,** Hormones and immunological capacity. II. Reconstitution of antibody production in hormonally deficient mice by somatotropic hormone, thyrotropic hormone and thyroxin, *Immunology,* 16, 217, 1969.
41. **Baroni, C. D., Fabris, N., and Bertoli, G.,** Effects of hormones on development and function of lymphoid tissues. Synergistic action of thyroxin and somatotropic hormones in pituitary dwarf mice, *Immunology,* 17, 303, 1969.
42. **Arezzini, C., De Gori, V., Tarli, P., and Neri, P.,** Weight increase of body and lymphatic tissues in dwarf mice treated with human chorionic somatomammotropin, *Proc. Soc. Exp. Biol. Med.,* 141, 98, 1972.
43. **Baroni, C. D., Scelsi, R., Mingazzini, P. L., Cavallero, A., and Uccini, S.,** Delayed hypersensitivity in the hereditary pituitary dwarf Snell/Bagg mouse, *Nature (London), New Biol.,* 237, 219, 1972.
44. **Duquesnoy, R. J., Kalpaktsoglou, P. K., and Good, R. A.,** Immunological studies of the Snell-Bagg dwarf mouse, *Proc. Soc. Exp. Biol. Med.,* 133, 201, 1970.
45. **Duquesnoy, R. J.,** Studies of the mechanism of prevention of immunologic deficiency in suckling dwarf mice, *Adv. Exp. Med. Biol.,* 12, 387, 1971.
46. **Fabris, N., Pierpaoli, W., and Sorkin, E.,** Lymphocytes, hormones, and ageing, *Nature (London),* 240, 557, 1972.
47. **Schneider, G. B.,** Immunological competence in Snell-Bagg pituitary dwarf mice: response to the contact-sensitizing agent oxazolone, *Am. J. Anat.,* 145, 371, 1976.
48. **Shire, J. G. M.,** Growth hormone and premature ageing, *Nature (London),* 245, 215, 1973.
49. **Bartke, A.,** Low mortality and long survival of dwarf mice (dw/dw), *Mouse News Lett.,* 56, 63, 1977.
50. **Chen, H. W., Meier, H., Heiniger, H.-J., and Huebner, R. J.,** Tumorigenesis in strain DW/J mice and induction by prolactin of the group-specific antigen of endogenous C-type RNA tumor virus, *J. Natl. Cancer Inst.,* 49, 1145, 1972.
51. **Rennels, E. G., Anigstein, D. M., and Anigstein, L.,** A cumulative study of the growth of sarcoma 180 in anterior pituitary dwarf mice, *Tex. Rep. Biol. Med.,* 23, 776, 1965.
52. **Bielschowksy, F. and Bielschowsky, M.,** Carcinogenesis in the pituitary dwarf mouse. The response to methylcholanthrene injected subcutaneously, *Br. J. Cancer,* 13, 302, 1959.
53. **Bielschowsky, F. and Bielschowsky, M.,** Carcinogenesis in the pituitary dwarf mouse. The response to 2-aminofluorene, *Br. J. Cancer,* 14, 195, 1960.
54. **Bielschowsky, F. and Bielschowsky, M.,** Carcinogenesis in the pituitary dwarf mouse. The response to dimethylbenzanthracene applied to the skin, *Br. J. Cancer,* 15, 257, 1961.
55. **Schaible, R. and Gowen, J. W.,** A new dwarf mouse, *Genetics,* 46, 896, 1961.
56. **Bartke, A.,** Influence of luteotropin on fertility of dwarf mice, *J. Reprod. Fertil.,* 10, 93, 1965.
57. **Beamer, W. G. and Eicher, E. M.,** Stimulation of growth in the little mouse, *J. Endocrinol.,* 71, 37, 1976.
58. **Rimoin, D. L. and Richmond, L.,** The pygmy (pg) mutant of the mouse — a model of the human pygmy, *J. Clin. Endocrinol. Metab.,* 35, 467, 1972.
59. **Schindler, W. J., Hutchins, M. O., Laird, C. W., and Fox, R. R.,** Effect of strain and sex variation of growth hormone in rabbit serum, *Proc. Soc. Exp. Biol. Med.,* 147, 820, 1974.

60. **Moon, H. D., Simpson, M. E., Li, C. H., and Evans, H. M.,** Effect of pituitary growth hormone in mice, *Cancer Res.,* 12, 448, 1952.
61. **Bartke, A.,** Prolactin deficiency in genetically sterile dwarf mice, *Mem. Soc. Endocrinol.,* 15, 193, 1967.
62. **Cheever, E. V., Seavey, B. K., and Lewis, U. J.,** Prolactin of normal and dwarf mice, *Endocrinology,* 85, 698, 1969.
63. **Dubois, M. and Bartke, A.,** unpublished observations.
64. **Neill, J. D. and Reichert, L. E., Jr.,** Development of a raioimmunoassay for rat prolactin and evalutation of the NIAMD rat prolactin radioimmunoassay, *Endocrinology,* 88, 548, 1971.
65. **Lu, K. H., Grandison, L., Huang, H. H., Marshall, S., and Meites, J.,** Relation of gonadotropin secretion by pituitary grafts to spermatogenesis in hypophysectomized male rats, *Endocrinology,* 100, 380, 1977.
66. **Bartke, A.,** Differential requirement for prolactin during pregnancy in the mouse, *Biol. Reprod.,* 9, 379, 1973.
67. **Morishige, W. K., Billiar, R. B., and Rothchild, I.,** Radioimmunologic assessment of the level of circulating LH antibodies after passive immunization in the rat: relation to the level of LH secretion, *Endocrinology,* 96, 1437, 1975.
68. **Bartke, A., Scaramuzzi, R., and Stylos, W.,** unpublished observations.
69. **Wuttke, W., Cassell, E., and Meites, J.,** Effects of ergocornine on serum prolactin and LH and on hypothalamic content of PIF and LRF, *Endocrinology,* 88, 737, 1971.
70. **Seki, M., Seki, K., Yoshihara, T., Watanabe, N., Okumura, T., Tajima, C., Huang, S.-Y., and Kuo, C.-C.,** Direct inhibition of pituitary LH secretion in rats by CB-154 (2-Br-α-ergocryptine), *Endocrinology,* 94, 911, 1974.
71. **Woods, M. C. and Simpson, M. E.,** Pituitary control of the testis of the hypophysectomized rat, *Endocrinology,* 69, 91, 1961.
72. **Bartke, A. and Lloyd, C. W.,** Influence of prolactin and pituitary isografts on spermatogenesis in dwarf mice and hypophysectomized rats, *J. Endocrinol.,* 46, 321, 1970.
73. **Cavallero, C., Martinazzi, M., Baroni, C., and Magrini, U.,** Pituitary control of mouse testis in hereditary dwarfism; histological and cytochemical observations, *Gen. Comp. Endocrinol.,* 3, 636, 1963.
74. **Bartke, A.,** Prolactin changes cholesterol stores in the mouse testis, *Nature (London),* 224, 700, 1969.
75. **Hafiez, A. A., Philpott, J. E., and Bartke, A.,** The role of prolactin in the regulation of testicular functions: the effect of prolactin and luteinizing hormone on 3β-hydroxysteroid dehydrogenase activity in the testes of mice and rats, *J. Endocrinol.,* 50, 619, 1971.
76. **Musto, N., Hafiez, A. A., and Bartke, A.,** Prolactin increases 17β-hydroxysteroid dehydrogenase activity in the testis, *Endocrinology,* 91, 1106, 1972.
77. **Laanes, T.,** The role of the endocrines in development; mice, *Carnegie Inst. Washington Yearb.,* 31, 47, 1932.
78. **Bohnet, H. G. and Friesen, H. G.,** Effect of prolactin and growth hormone on prolactin and LH receptors in the dwarf mouse, *J. Reprod. Fertil.,* 48, 307, 1976.
79. **Bartke, A., Goldman, B. D., Bex F., and Dalterio, S.,** Effects of prolactin (PRL) on pituitary and testicular function in mice with hereditary PRL deficiency, *Endocrinology,* 101, 1760, 1977.
80. **Bartke, A.,** Effects of prolactin on spermatogenesis in hypophysectomized mice, *J. Endocrinol.,* 49, 311, 1971.
81. **Hafiez, A. A., Lloyd, C. W., and Bartke, A.,** The role of prolactin in the regulation of testes function: the effects of prolactin and luteinizing hormone on the plasma levels of testosterone and androstenedione in hypophysectomized rats, *J. Endocrinol.,* 52, 327, 1972.
82. **Bex, F. J. and Bartke, A.,** Testicular LH binding in the hamster: modification by photoperiod and prolactin, *Endocrinology,* 100, 1223, 1977.
83. **Rubin, R. T., Poland, R. E., and Tower, B. B.,** Prolactin-related testosterone secretion in normal adult men, *J. Clin. Endocrinol. Metab.,* 42, 112, 1976.
84. **Chen, H. W., Hamer, D. H., Heiniger, H.-J., and Meier, H.,** Stimulation of hepatic RNA synthesis in dwarf mice by ovine prolactin, *Biochim. Biophys. Acta,* 287, 90, 1972.
85. **Posner, B. I.,** Regulation of lactogen specific binding sites in rat liver: studies on the role of lactogens and estrogens, *Endocrinology,* 99, 1168, 1976.
86. **Voogt, J. L., Clemens, J. A., and Meites, J.,** Stimulation of pituitary FSH release in immature female rats by prolactin implant in median eminence, *Neuroendocrinology,* 4, 157, 1969.
87. **Murphy, E. D.,** Characteristic tumors, in *Biology of the Laboratory Mouse,* 2nd ed., Green E. L., Ed., Dover, New York, 1975, 521.
88. **MacMahon, B., Cole, P., and Brown, J.,** Etiology of human breast cancer: a review, *J. Natl. Cancer Inst.,* 50, 21, 1973.
89. **Mühlbock, O. and Boot, L. M.,** Induction of mammary cancer without the mammary tumor agent by isografts of the hypophyses, *Cancer Res.,* 19, 402, 1959.

90. **Heston, W. E.**, Induction of mammary gland tumors in strain C_{57}BL/He mice by isografts of hypophyses, *J. Natl. Cancer Inst.*, 32, 947, 1964.
91. **Hagen, E. O. and Rowlinson, H. E.**, The induction of mammary cancer in male mice by isologous pituitary implants, *Cancer Res.*, 24, 59, 1964.
92. **Boot, L. M.**, *Induction by Prolactin of Mammary Tumors in Mice,* North-Holland, Amsterdam, 1969.
93. **Yanai, R. and Nagasawa, H.**, Inhibition by ergocornine and 2-Br-α-ergocryptin of spontaneous mammary tumor appearance in mice, *Experientia,* 27, 934, 1971.
94. **Welsch, C. W. and Gribler, C.**, Prophylaxis of spontaneously developing mammary carcinoma in C3H/HeJ female mice by suppression of prolactin, *Cancer Res.*, 33, 2939, 1973.
95. **Quadri, S. K. and Meites, J.**, Regression of spontaneous mammary tumors in rats by ergot drugs, *Proc. Soc. Exp. Biol. Med.*, 138, 999, 1971.
96. **Nagasawa, H. and Meites, J.**, Suppression by ergocornine and iproniazid of carcinogen-induced mammary tumors in rats; effects on serum and pituitary prolactin levels, *Proc. Soc. Exp. Biol. Med.*, 135, 469, 1970.
97. **Cassell, E. E., Meites, J., and Welsch, C. W.**, Effects of ergocornine and ergocryptine on growth of 7,12-dimethyl-benzanthracene-induced mammary tumors in rats, *Cancer Res.*, 31, 1051, 1971.
98. **Sinha, Y. N., Salocks, C. B., and VanderLaan, W. P.**, Circulating levels of prolactin and growth hormone and natural incidence of mammary tumors in mice, *J. Toxicol. Environ. Health Suppl.*, 1, 131, 1976.
99. **Sinha, Y. N., Selby, F. W., and VanderLaan, W. P.**, The natural history of prolactin and GH secretion in mice with high and low incidence of mammary tumors, *Endocrinology,* 94, 757, 1974.
100. **Sinha, Y. N., Salocks, C. B., Lewis, U. J., and VanderLaan, W. P.**, Influence of nursing on the release of prolactin and GH in mice with high and low incidence of mammary tumors, *Endocrinology,* 95, 947, 1974.
101. **Sinha, Y. N., Selby, F. W., and VanderLaan, W. P.**, Radioimmunoassay of prolactin in the urine of mouse and man, *J. Clin. Endocrinol. Metab.*, 36, 1039, 1973.
102. **Sinha, Y. N., Salocks, C. B., and VanderLaan, W. P.**, Prolactin and growth hormone levels in different inbred strains of mice: patterns in association with estrous cycle, time of day, and perphenazine stimulation, *Endocrinology,* 97, 1112, 1975.
103. **Nagasawa, H., Yanai, R., Iwahashi, H., Fujimoto, M., and Kuretani, K.**, Difference in mammary gland susceptibility to prolactin between a high and a low mammary tumor strains of mice, *Endocrinol. Jpn.*, 14, 351, 1967.
104. **Kwa, H. G., Engelsman, E., De Jong-Bakker, M., and Cleton, F. J.**, Plasma-prolactin in human breast cancer, *Lancet,* 1, 433, 1974.
105. **Bennett, P. H., Rushforth, N. B., Miller, M., and LeCompte, P. M.**, Epidemiologic studies of diabetes in the Pima Indians, *Recent. Prog. Horm. Res.*, 32, 333, 1976.
106. **Stauffacher, W., Orci, L., Cameron, D. P., Burr, I. M., and Renold, A. E.**, Spontaneous hyperglycemia and/or obesity in laboratory rodents: an example of the possible usefulness of animal disease models with both genetic and environmental components, *Recent. Prog. Horm. Res.*, 27, 41, 1971.
107. **Herbai, G.**, Weight loss in obese-hyperglycaemic and normal mice following transauricular hypophysectomy by a modified technique, *Acta Endocrinol., (Copenhagen),* 65, 712, 1970.
108. **Desjardins, C.**, Pituitary growth hormone and its hypothalamic releasing factor in normal and genetically diabetic mice, *Proc. Soc. Exp. Biol. Med.*, 130, 1, 1969.
109. **Roos, P., Martin, J. M., Westman-Naeser, S., and Hellerström, C.**, Immunoreactive growth hormone levels in mice with the obese-hyperglycemic syndrome (Genotype obob), *Horm. Metab. Res.*, 6, 125, 1974.
110. **Sinha, Y. N., Salocks, C. B., and VanderLaan, W. P.**, Prolactin and growth hormone secretion in chemically induced and genetically obese mice, *Endocrinology,* 97, 1386, 1975.
111. **Larson, B. A., Sinha, Y. N., and VanderLaan, W. P.**, Serum growth hormone and prolactin during and after the development of the obese-hyperglycemic syndrome in mice, *Endocrinology,* 98, 139, 1976.
112. **Wolff, G. L.**, Hereditary obesity and hormone deficiencies in yellow dwarf mice, *Am. J. Physiol.*, 209, 632, 1965.
113. **Joosten, H. F. P., van der Kroon, P. H. W., and Buis, A. J. M.**, Development of the obese-hyperglycemic syndrome in mice with a growth hormone deficiency, *Metab. Clin. Exp.*, 24, 573, 1975.
114. **Swerdloff, R. S., Batt, R. A., and Bray, G. A.**, Reproductive hormonal function in the genetically obese (ob/ob) mouse, *Endocrinology,* 98, 1359, 1976.
115. **Karande, K. A., Sheth, N. A., and Ranadive, K. J.**, Follicle-stimulating hormone content of the pituitary gland of intact and ovariectomized mice of different strains, *J. Endocrinol.*, 48, 457, 1970.
116. **Bartke, A., Weir, J. A., Mathison, P., Roberson, C., and Dalterio, S.**, Testicular function in mouse strains with different age of sexual maturation, *J. Hered.*, 65, 204, 1974.

117. **Wolfe, H. G.,** Genetic influence on gonadotropic activity in mice, *Biol. Reprod.,* 4, 161, 1971.
118. **Melvold, R. W.,** The effects of mutant *p*-alleles on the reproductive system in mice, *Genet. Res.,* 23, 319, 1974.
119. **Johnson, D. R. and Hunt, D. M.,** Endocrinological findings in sterile pink-eyed mice, *J. Reprod. Fertil.,* 42, 51, 1975.
120. **Bardin, C. W., Bullock, L. P., Sherins, R. J., Mowszowicz, I., and Blackburn, W. R.,** Androgen metabolism and mechanism of action in male pseudohermaphroditism: a study of testicular feminization, *Recent Prog. Horm. Res.,* 29, 65, 1973.
121. **Musto, N. and Bardin, C. W.,** unpublished observations.
122. **Younglai, E. V. and Chui, D. H. K.,** Testicular function in sterile steel mice, *Biol. Reprod.,* 9, 317, 1973.
123. **Shire, J. G. M. and Bartke, A.,** Strain differences in testicular weight and spermatogenesis with special reference to C57BL/10J and DBA/2J mice, *J. Endocrinol.,* 55, 163, 1972.
124. **Bartke, A. and Shire, J. G. M.,** Differences between mouse strains in testicular cholesterol levels and androgen target organs, *J. Endocrinol.,* 55, 173, 1972.
125. **Bartke, A.,** Increased sensitivity of seminal vesicles to testosterone in a mouse strain with low plasma testosterone levels, *J. Endocrinol.,* 60, 145, 1974.
126. **Selmanoff, M. K., Goldman, B. D., and Ginsburg, B. E.,** Developmental changes in serum luteinizing hormone, follicle stimulating hormone and androgen levels in males of two inbred mouse strains, *Endocrinology,* 100, 122, 1977.
127. **Bindon, B. M.,** Genetic differences in plasma luteinizing hormone of the prepubertal lamb, *J. Reprod. Fertil.,* 32, 347, 1973.
128. **Trounson, A. O., Chamley, W. A., Kennedy, J. P., and Tassell R.,** Primordial follicles numbers in ovaries and levels of LH and FSH in pituitaries and plasma of lambs selected for and against multiple births, *Aust. J. Biol. Sci.,* 27, 293, 1974.
129. **Land, R. B.,** The expression of female sex-limited characters in the male, *Nature (London),* 241, 208, 1973.
130. **Mafizul Islam, A. B. M., Hill, W. G., and Land, R. B.,** Ovulation rate of lines of mice selected for testis weight, *Genet. Res.,* 27, 23, 1976.
131. **Land, R. B. and Falconer, D. S.,** Genetic studies of ovulation rate in the mouse, *Genet. Res.,* 13, 25, 1969.
132. **Murr, S. M., Geschwind, I. I., and Bradford, G. E.,** Plasma LH and FSH during different oestrous cycle conditions in mice, *J. Reprod. Fertil.,* 32, 221, 1973.
133. **Bindon, B. M. and Pennycuik, P. R.,** Differences in ovarian sensitivity of mice selected for fecundity, *J. Reprod. Fertil.,* 36, 221, 1974.
134. **Parks, R. and Wolfe, H. G.,** Genetic differences in ovarian FSH binding in mice, *Genetics,* 86 (Suppl. 2), s47, 1977.
135. **Wolfe, H. G., Bartke, A., Dalterio, S., and Bex, F.,** Genetic differences in the production of testosterone by mouse testes *in vitro, Genetics,* 86(Suppl. 2), s70, 1977.
136. **Sustarsic, D. L. and Wolfe, H. G.,** unpublished observations.
137. **Bouhnik, J., Michel, O., Gaundry, M., and Michel, R.,** Spécificité des hormones thyroïdiennes et de l'hormone de croissance sur les propriétés et la proténogenèse des particules sub-cellulaires. II. Souris génétiquement naines "dwarf", *Biochimie,* 54, 493, 1972.
138. **Priestley, G. C. and Robertson, M.,** Nucleic acids and polyribosomes in organs from mice with genetically different growth capacities, *J. Cell Biol.,* 55, 208a, 1972.
139. **Pierpaoli, W., Kopp, H. G., and Bianchi, E.,** Interdependence of thymic and neuroendocrine functions in ontogeny, *Clin. Exp. Immunol.,* 24, 501, 1976.
140. **Yochim, J. M.,** personal communication.
141. **Bartke, A., Roberson, C., and Dalterio, S.,** Concentration of gonadotrophins in the plasma and testicular responsiveness to gonadotrophic stimulation in androgen-deficient, *J. Endocrinol.,* 75, 441, 1977.

Chapter 7

HUMAN GROWTH HORMONE

Z. Laron

TABLE OF CONTENTS

I. PHYSIOLOGICAL ASPECTS

Human growth hormone (hGH), together with adrenocorticotropin (ACTH), thyrotropin (TSH), prolactin (Pr), and the gonadotropins (LH and FSH), is synthesized in the anterior pituitary. The human pituitary gland already has the capacity to synthesize and store the pituitary hormones early in fetal life. Histochemical, immunofluorescent, and electromicroscopic examination of fetal pituitary cells, bioassay and immunochemical measurement of the hormonal content of fetal pituitary glands, and radioimmunoassay of pituitary hGH in the fetal circulation have demonstrated synthesis, storage, and secretion of fetal pituitary growth hormone between the 7th and 10th week of gestation,[1] with a marked increase during the 16th and 21st weeks.[2] The progressive increase in pituitary weight during gestation is paralleled by an increase in the hGH content of the fetal pituitary gland,[3] which rises from 0.4 μg at 10 to 14 weeks of gestation to 578 μg at 30 to 34 weeks and to 675 μg at 35 to 40 weeks.

The ontogeny of growth hormone secretion by the human fetus and the quantitative relationship between pituitary content and serum concentration are shown in Figure 1.

There is no transfer of GH through the placenta[5,6] and thus, in the newborn the level of GH is higher in the arterial cord blood than in the venous cord blood. After birth there is a rapid rise in plasma hGH concentration that usually peaks between 24 and 48 hr.[7] During the first 3 days of life, plasma hGH ranges between 20 to 50 ng/mℓ, although it may also be as high as 200 ng/mℓ (Figure 2). In prematures the level can be even higher,[9,10] while large babies and babies born to diabetic mothers are liable to have lower concentrations of hGH in the plasma.[11] At 4 to 6 weeks of life, serum hGH decreases to levels of 1 to 4 ng/mℓ, although in prematures this decrease is slower. During later infancy, childhood, and adulthood, the levels of fasting hGH are

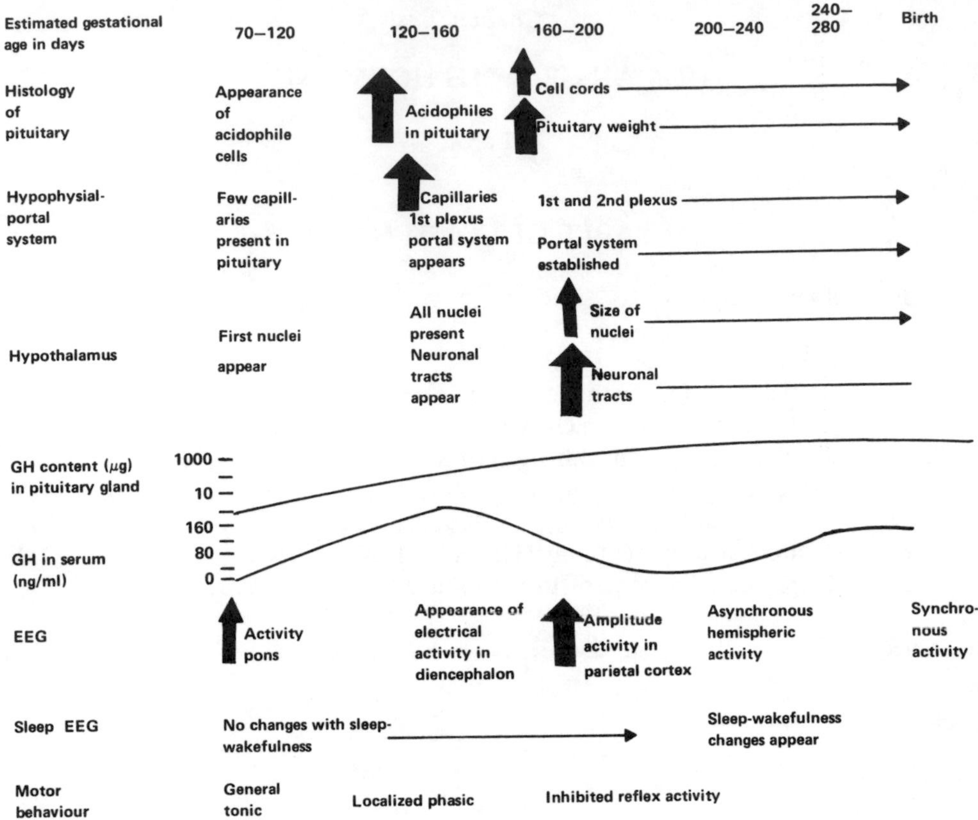

FIGURE 1. The ontogeny of growth hormone secretion by the human fetus. (From Grumbach, M. M. and Kaplan, S. L., *Foetal and Neonatal Physiology*, 1973, 464. With permission.)

usually very low and may even be undetectable. In adolescent girls and young adult women, however, the fasting plasma hGH may be elevated, possibly due to an estrogen-potentiating effect[12] or to nonspecific stress more apt to be present in females. In old age, growth hormone is still being secreted[13] but there is evidence that the pituitary reserve is slightly less than that present in children and young adults.[8]

Human growth hormone is a polypeptide. The amino acid sequence proposed by Li et al.[14] in 1969 proved to be not entirely correct and a revised version was reported by this same group of workers in 1971,[15] as well as by Niall.[16] On the basis of their findings, hGH consists of 191 amino acids with two S-S bonds and has a molecular weight of 21,500 and an isoelectric point at pH 4.9. The amino acid sequence is shown in Figure 3.

For years it has been evident from the different electrophoretic patterns obtained that hGH preparations made from the pituitary lack uniformity.[17-19] More recent methods of gel filtration on Sephadex® (G-75 or G-100) and radioimmunoassay have demonstrated that the hGH circulating in the serum is also heterogeneous.[20,21] The major component, which corresponds approximately to a molecular weight of 22,000, is termed "little" growth hormone, whereas a second component that is double in molecular weight is a "big" growth hormone. Frohman and Stachmura[22] observed a third peak of intermediate size. Gel chromatography of hGH obtained from tissue cultures of fetal pituitary glands aged 15 to 16 weeks revealed only components of high molecular weight and no monomeric hGH.[23] Fetal pituitaries obtained at the end of gestation or soon after birth were found to contain a "big-big" component.[24] Plasma samples of premature newborns had a smaller proportion of the "big" IR-

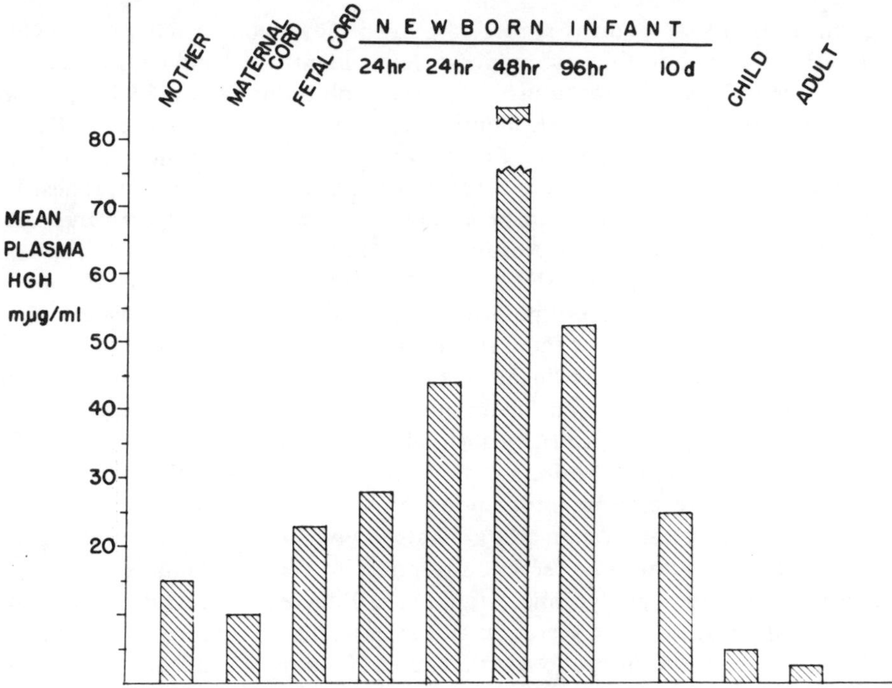

FIGURE 2. Mean plasma hGH concentrations in the mother, at birth, in the newborn, infant, child, and adult. (From Laron, Z., *Paediatric Endocrinology,* Hubble, S. W., Ed., 1969, 35. With permission.)

NH_2-Phe-Pro–Thr-Ile—Pro-Leu-Ser-Arg-Leu-Phe-Asp-Asn-Ala–Met-Leu-Arg-Ala–His–Arg-Leu-
1 5 10 15 20

His–Gln–Leu-Ala–Phe-Asp-Thr–Tyr–Gln–Glu–Phe-Glu–Glu–Ala–Tyr–Ile—Pro–Lys-Glu-Gln–
25 30 35 40

Lyc–Tyr–Ser–Phe-Leu-Gln–Asn-Pro–Gln–Thr–Ser–Leu–Cys-Phe-Ser–Glu–Ser–Ile—Pro–Thr–
45 50 55 60

Pro–Ser–Asn-Arg-Glu–Glu–Thr–Gln–Lys–Ser–Asn–Leu–Gln–Leu-Leu-Arg-Ile—Ser-Leu-Leu-
65 70 75 80

Leu-Ile—Gln–Ser–Trp–Leu–Glu–Pro–Val—Gln–Phe–Leu–Arg–Ser–Val–Phe-Ala–Asn-Ser–Leu-
85 90 95 100

Val–Tyr–Gly–Ala–Ser–Asn-Ser–Asp-Val–Tyr–Asp-Leu-Leu-Lys-Asp-Leu-Glu-Glu-Gly-Ile—
105 110 115 120

Gln-Thr-Leu-Met-Gly–Arg-Leu-Glu-Asp-Gly–Ser–Pro–Arg-Thr-Gly–Gln–Ile—Phe-Lys-Gln-
125 130 135 140

Thr–Tyr–Ser–Lys–Phe-Asp-Thr–Asn-Ser–His–Asn-Asp-Asp-Ala–Leu-Leu-Lys-Asn-Tyr-Gly-
145 150 155 160

Leu-Leu-Tyr–Cys-Phe-Arg-Lys-Asp-Met-Asp-Lys–Val–Glu–Thr–Phe-Leu-Arg-lie—Val–Gln–
165 170 175 180

Cys–Arg–Ser–Val–Glu–Gly–Ser–Cys-Gly–Phe-COOH
185 190

FIGURE 3. Amino acid sequence of hGH. (From Li, C. H. and Dixon, J. S., *Arch. Biochem. Biophys.,* 146, 233, 1971. With permission.)

hGH components than did those of full-term newborns and older children. It would appear that with maturation there is a gradual decrease in the percentage of the bigger components of hGH in favor of the monomer. The main question still to be resolved is whether the bigger components are aggregates or represent hormone precursors.[25]

Growth hormone secretion is regulated by central nervous mechanisms, which include a GH-releasing hormone as yet incompletely identified[26] and a GH-release-inhibiting hormone (GH-RIH or somatotropin-release-inhibiting factor, SRIF, or somatostatin),[27,28] which has been isolated, identified, and synthesized (Figure 4). There have been recent advances in establishing the main pathways of brain monoaminergic neurotransmitters[29] and their role in the control of hypothalamic neurohormones.[30] It has been demonstrated that alpha- and beta-adrenergic receptors, respectively, stimulate and inhibit the secretion of GH.[31] Results concerning the role of specific monoamines, dopamine (DA), norepinephrine (NE), and Serotonin (5-HT) in the hGH control system are contradictory, and recent pathologic studies in acromegaly have cast doubt as to the site at which monoamines act in the regulation of GH secretion.[32]

Synthetic somatostatin in its linear or cyclized form has been shown to suppress growth hormone secretion in man[33] in animals,[34] and in isolated pituitary tissue,[35] confirming the lack of species specificity seen with hGH. Somatostatin has a very short biological half-life, less than 4 min, and to demonstrate a measurable effect on plasma GH it must be administered by intravenous infusion. Somatostatin not only suppress growth hormone secretion in man and animals in vivo and in vitro, but also abolishes or reduces the growth hormone secretion response to various stimuli such as exercise, sleep, insulin-induced hypoglycemia, arginine, L-dopa, etc. It acts directly on the somatotroph cells to inhibit GH secretion and release. These findings imply that its site of action is distal to that of cyclic AMP. The immunohistochemical finding of somatostatin in nerve terminals[28] suggests that somatostatin may be a neurotransmitter. This hormone has also been found to be a potent inhibitor of insulin and glucagon[36] and, interestingly, has been shown to be secreted by cells in the pancreatic islets as well.[37] There is direct and indirect evidence, obtained in man under normal conditions, which supports the existence of a stimulatory role of dopamine receptor activation in the release of GH while, conversely, activation of the serotonin system inhibits GH release.[38] In acromegaly, dopaminergic drugs suppress GH release, denoting an abnormality in the hypothalamic-pituitary regulation of GH release.[38]

Basal (resting or nonstress) levels of IR-hGH in the plasma of children and adults are usually low although determinations made at frequent intervals during the day and night show fluctuations of various intensity. These are often related to meals, i.e., there may be a rise after ingestion of amino acids or during a fall in the blood glucose level,[39] but the most consistent and largest bursts occur during the first part of nocturnal sleep.[40] The number and magnitude of the spontaneous bursts of GH occuring during sleep are in part age dependent; Finkelstein et al.[41] showed that during the transition period from early to late puberty they increase in number and intensity.

Since basal GH levels are usually low and measurements of the release taking place during sleep are inconvenient to both subject and technician, stimulation tests are generally employed for standardization of the secretory capacity of GH by the pituitary.[8] These include exercise, insulin hypoglycemia, arginine infusion, propranolol, L-dopa, ingestion of an amino acid mixture, and others. A lack of response of plasma GH to these stimuli is considered to constitute evidence for an insufficiency of hypothalamic-pituitary secretion of GH. An exception is obesity, a condition in which IR-hGH secretion is blunted;[42] these children, however, grow normally or even beyond the normal rate.[43]

All three of the major classes of metabolic substrate — carbohydrates, proteins, and fats — affect GH secretion and are in turn affected by the activity of GH. Thus, GH

H—Ala—Gly—Cys—Lys—Asn—Phe—Trp—Lys—Thr—Phe—Thr—Ser—Cys—OH

FIGURE 4. Structure of somatostatin.

exhibits a diabetogenic effect. In healthy individuals it interferes with glucose tolerance;[44] acromegalic patients often suffer from diabetes mellitus. This effect is probably due to a decrease in the peripheral uptake of glucose. Administration of hGH results in mobilization of fat, as evidenced by a rise in plasma NEFA and reduction of the skinfold thickness.[45] Growth hormone stimulates protein synthesis, possibly by increased synthesis of ribonucleic acid.[46] Intracellular transport of amino acids and their incorporation into protein are increased[47] and clinically nitrogen retention is observed.[48] hGH also has an effect on Na, K, PO_4, Ca, and other minerals.[49,50] The large retention of K and PO_4 is due to the increase in protoplasm which accompanies growth. Growth hormone does not have just a single target organ, as is true of some of the other pituitary hormones, but acts on many different tissues of varied origin. It affects cellular growth and proliferation, whether of the muscle or of the cartilage cells,[51] and ultimately influences skeletal and linear body growth.[52,53]

In recent years evidence has accumulated, indicating that growth hormone does not act directly but induces the formation of a mediating substance, actually a hormone, which is the true stimulator of growth. This factor, which is probably synthesized in the liver,[54] was originally termed a "sulfation factor" because it stimulates the incorporation of radioactive sulfate into glucosaminoglycans of cartilage[55] and is now known as somatomedin.[56] Investigation has shown that the plasma contains more than one growth-promoting substance controlled by growth hormone and it is probable that there is a family of somatomedins.[57,58] Some of the properties of these growth factors are shown in Table 1. Somatomedin A, C, and NSILA, as defined by various investigators, are very closely related and may even be variants of the same molecule, of which the active form mediates the effects of growth hormone. The feedback mechanism between growth hormone and somatomedin secretion has not yet been fully elucidated but clear evidence of the relationship between them in various clinical entities is being obtained.

II. CLINICAL ASPECTS

The known clinical entities of hypo- and hypersecretion of growth hormone, with special emphasis on the genetic forms, are described in this section.

A. Deficiency of Growth Hormone Secretion

The term "pituitary dwarfism" is used for those forms of marked short stature that are secondary to a deficiency of hGH. An isolated lack of TSH is extremely rare and, with the easily recognized signs of hypothyroidism that develop, will not remain undi-

TABLE 1

Some Characteristics of the Somatomedins (SM) and of the Nonsuppressible Insulin-like Activity (NSILA)

	SM-A	SM-B	SM-C	NSILA
Dependent on GH activity	+	+	+	+
Molecular weight	7600	5000	7600	7600
SO_4 incorporation in cartilage	+	−	+	+
Growth promoting activity in cells in vitro		+	+	+
Insulin like activity in fat cells	+	−	+	+
Competes with insulin for its receptor	+		+	+

agnosed for long. Furthermore, a deficiency of ACTH, prolactin, or the gonadotrophins does not lead to dwarfism.

Growth hormone deficiency may be isolated (IGHD) or associated with other pituitary hormone deficiencies, i.e., multiple pituitary hormone deficiencies (MPHD; panhypopituitarism). The deficiency or deficiencies may be progressive, partial or total, and transitory or permanent. The site of the lesion may be in the pituitary or hypothalamus or in both. The cause of the lesion may be found in congenital abnormalities, trauma (including perinatal damage), tumors (including congenital tumors) such as craniopharyngioma, infections, systemic disease, malignancy, or irradiation or it may be idiopathic.[8] Many of these disease entities are hereditary. Recently it has been found that pituitary dwarfism may constitute the clinical expression of a lack in somatomedin generation and possibly a receptor defect.[59]

B. Isolated (Monotropic) Growth Hormone Deficiency

Isolated growth hormone deficiency exists in both hereditary and sporadic form.[8,60] In most cases it appears to be inherited as an autosomal recessive trait (Figure 5).[61] There are, however, reports of nonconsanguineous families in which the father and some of the offspring are affected, a finding which also suggests the possibility of an autosomal dominant inheritance.[62,63]

The clinical characteristics of these patients include dwarfism, acromicria, frontal bossing, relative obesity, sparse hair, small genitalia, slowness of motor development, dental maturation and nail growth, and a high-pitched voice.[64] Skeletal age is retarded. Puberty is delayed but normal and there is normal reproductive function. The facial skin wrinkles much earlier than is normal and is thin, making these patients appear older than they actually are.

These patients have a hypersensitivity to insulin and a tendency to hypoglycemia. It has been found that serum somatomedin A and C activity is low in these cases.[65,66] The endogenous insulin secretion in patients with growth hormone deficiency is reduced and rises upon administration of hGH, thus proving that hGH has a definite insulinotropic effect.[67]

While most patients with isolated growth hormone deficiency show insulinopenia, there exists a subgroup that displays neither insulin sensitivity nor hypoinsulinism and may even have hyperinsulinism.[68] There also appears to be yet another subgroup in

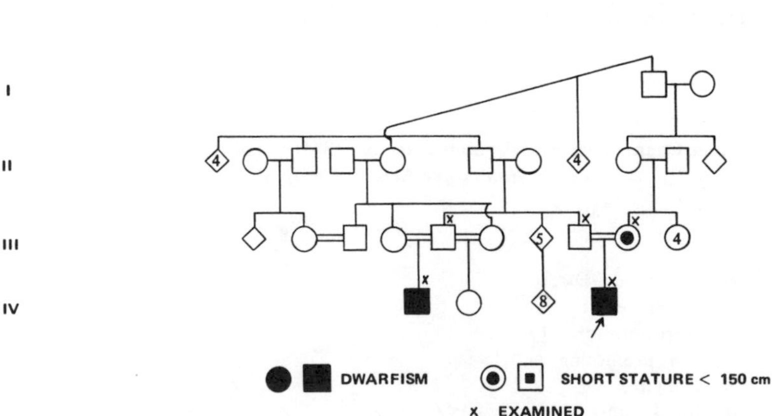

FIGURE 5. Pedigree of two related families with isolated GH deficiency — illustrating recessive heredity in consanguinous parents. (From Pertzelan, A., Adam, A., and Laron, Z., *Isr. J. Med. Sci.*, 9, 1599, 1973. With permission.)

this category of isolated GH deficiency. Some patients have an hereditary total lack of growth hormone and a consequent lack of immunotolerance for hGH.[69] These patients are characterized by a short birth length and early onset of growth retardation. The initial response to hGH therapy is marked, but this is followed by a progressive development of a high titer of antibodies to hGH and arrest of growth. It is the only group classified as isolated growth hormone deficiency in which treatment with exogenous hGH is unsuccessful.[70,71,72]

From the theoretical point of view, hereditary, congenital, or acquired isolated growth hormone deficiency can be caused by a lack of releasing hormone (GH-RH) or a lack of GH synthesis by the pituitary cells. Less probable is a permanent oversecretion of somatostatin.

C. Pituitary Dwarfism with High Plasma IR-hGH (Laron-type Dwarfism)

In 1966 a syndrome of familial dwarfism was described which was indistinguishable both clinically (compare Figures 6 and 7), and in many of the laboratory findings from pituitary dwarfism,[73] but in which there were abnormally high plasma concentrations of immunoreactive human growth hormone (IR-hGH). In recent years additional clinical and laboratory findings have been reported in these and more recently discovered

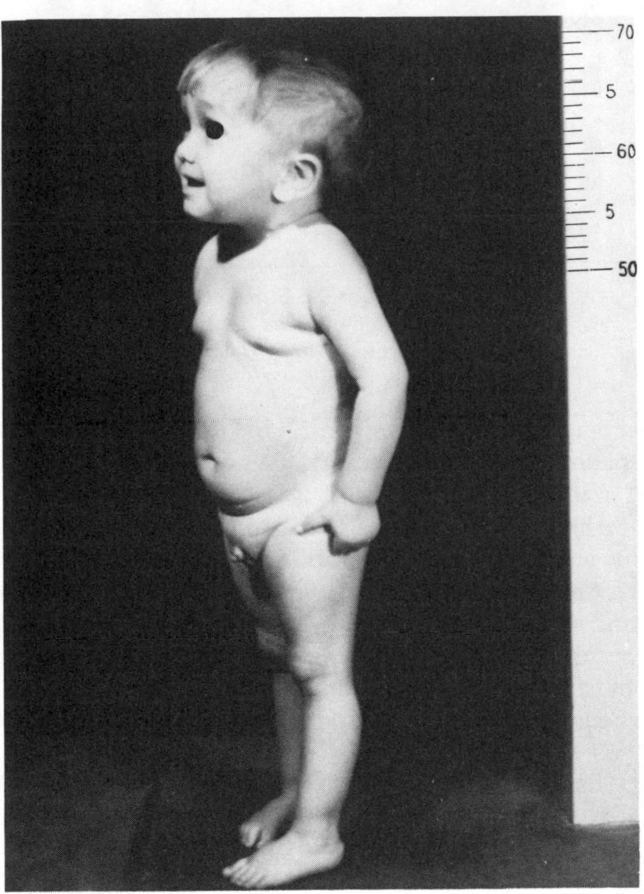

FIGURE 6. Typical appearance of isolated growth hormone deficiency. Patient E.I., male aged 4 years.

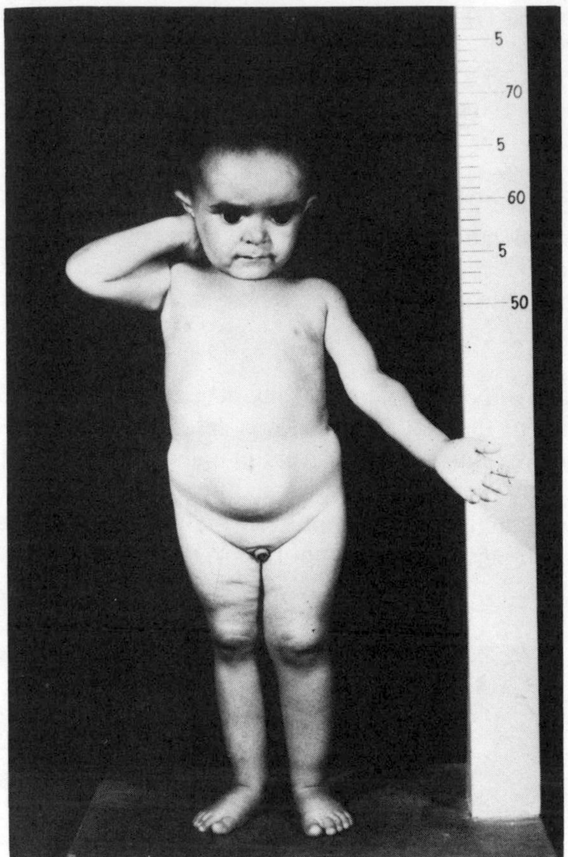

FIGURE 7. Typical appearance of pituitary dwarfism with high plasma IR-hGH (Laron-type dwarfism). Patients Y.I. age 7 years. Note resemblance to isolated GH deficiency.

patients, all of whom were of Jewish origin,[74,75] the total number studied by the author so far being 30 patients. Genetic studies of our population[61] and the distribution of affected patients in their respective families indicated an autosomal recessive mode of inheritance (Figure 8), although the occurrence of this disorder in a father and two of his children, a boy and a girl, raises the possibility that it is inherited as an autosomal dominant as well. An increasing awareness that this syndrome may also occur in non-Jewish populations led to the discovery of such patients in other countries,[61,76-82] with clear evidence for hereditary foci among the Arab population in Lebanon and Saudi Arabia, in Holland and in Dutch emigrants to Canada, in Spain, and in France. Sporadic cases have been observed in Denmark, Holland, Italy, and recently in Japan and New Zealand.

At the present time the basic defect in this syndrome is unknown. It may be assumed, however, that there is at least one basic inherited defect which leads to specific clinical and metabolic changes indistinguishable from those present in isolated hereditary hGH deficiency. A plausible explanation is the primary inability of the liver to generate somatomedin A.[59,65,66] There are still two other possibilities to be ruled out: an end-organ receptor defect and the synthesis of a slightly abnormal molecule which is immunologically identical to that of normal hGH but is biologically inactive. Several recent studies[20,83-86] provide evidence which speaks against the latter possibility. Another explanation would be end-organ refractoriness due to an intracellular enzymatic

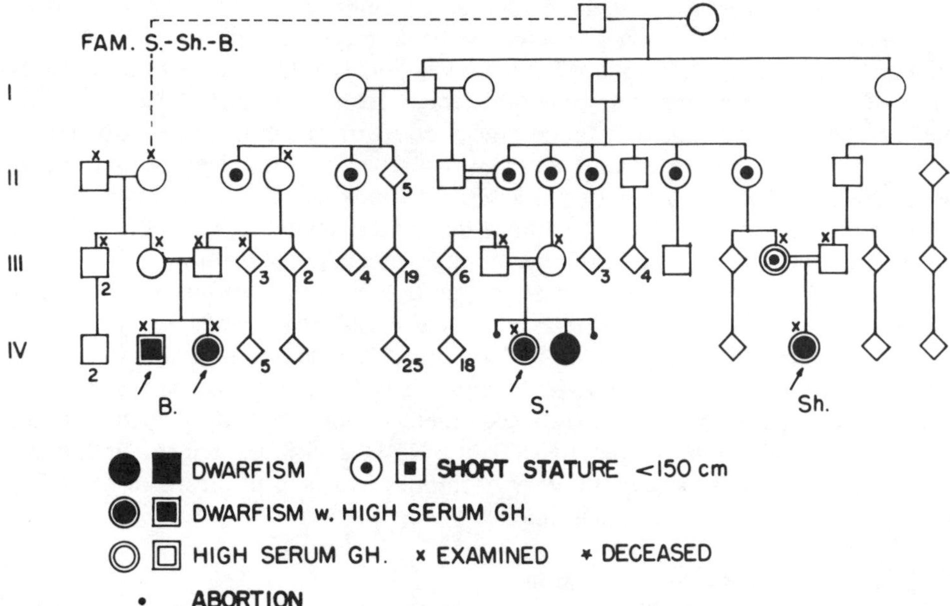

FIGURE 8. Pedigree of three related children with pituitary dwarfism and high IR-hGH Laron-type dwarfism. (From Pertzelan, A., Adam, A., and Laron, Z., *Isr. J. Med. Sci.*, 9, 1599, 1973. With permission.)

defect, but this would not explain the lack of somatomedin generation, implying a feedback mechanism between target cells and hypothalamic GH-RH.[87] At least part of the resistance to exogenous hGH of these patients would seem to be due to competitive saturation of peripheral tissue receptors of hGH by the endogenous hormone. Such a mechanism has been found to be present in active acromegaly and healthy newborns, both conditions in which there are high concentrations of circulating serum hGH.[59]

It is to be hoped that in the not too distant future, purified or synthetic somatomedin will be available in amounts sufficient for clinical trials so that the etiopathology of this syndrome can be clarified.

D. The African Pygmies

The members of this interesting population residing in the tropical rain forests of Africa are dwarfed and have been found to have insulinopenia and insulin hypersensitivity similar to that seen in isolated hGH deficiency.[88,89] Levels of IR-hGH and somatomedin activity are normal,[90] however, and clinically they do not exhibit the truncal obesity and wrinkled skin typical of pituitary dwarfs. They are completely unresponsive to the free-fatty-acid-mobilizing, insulinotropic, and nitrogen-retaining properties of hGH, and it may be assumed that their small size is due to a partial peripheral nonresponsiveness to circulating growth hormone at the receptor or intracellular level or to a factor generated by hGH. Up to now, no peripheral unresponsiveness to hGH and/or somatomedin has been described in any other ethnic group.

E. Familial Mulitple Pituitary Hormone Deficiencies

The familial occurrence of a deficiency of several pituitary hormones including growth hormone is rare.[91] The hormone deficiency most frequently associated with that of growth hormone is gonadotropin deficiency, followed in order by TSH deficiency, and then by partial ACTH deficiency. There is, however, inter- and intrafamilial variability in these associated hormone deficiencies: in some families one individual may lack most of the hormones secreted by the anterior pituitary while other members may lack only a single hormone.[92] Evidence suggests that there is an X-linked recessive form of multiple pituitary hormone deficiency. Schimke et al.[93] have described two half brothers with this disease who are the product of one mother and two fathers. In another family,[94] three male children from two separate sibships and a maternal uncle were affected. Recently a family was described[98] in which 8 of 12 siblings were found to have multiple deficiencies of pituitary hormones, including GH, TSH, and gonadotrophins. The parents and four other siblings were in good health.

It should be stressed that most cases of multiple pituitary hormone deficiencies are sporadic, many of them being due to organic disease.[8] The site of the lesion may be in the hypothalamus, the pituitary, or both. As yet, there are no laboratory methods for the direct measurement of the hypothalamic releasing hormones that would make a more precise diagnosis possible. Until such methods have been developed, administration of the available hormones LH-RH and TRH and measurement of the change taking place in the respective pituitary hormones is a helpful means of assessing the pituitary function for individual hormones.[95]

F. Hypersecretion of Growth Hormone

Hypersecretion of growth hormone in childhood results in gigantism. In adults it leads to acromegaly, a syndrome characterized by the typical enlargment of the acrae and the tongue and by visceromegaly.[96] The diagnosis is made on the basis of the very high plasma levels of hGH. Although the majority of cases of acromegaly are sporadic, many families have been reported in which multiple members are affected.[91,97] Some descriptions suggest autosomal-dominant inheritance, but the finding of acromegaly in two cousins in a highly inbred family also indicates that it may be autosomal recessive.

REFERENCES

1. **Kaplan, S. L., Grumbach, M. M., and Aubert, M. L.,** The ontogenesis of pituitary hormones and hypothalamic factors in the human fetus: maturation of central nervous system regulation of anterior pituitary function, *Recent Prog. Horm. Res.*, 32, 161, 1976.
2. **Baker, B. L. and Jaffe, R. B.,** The genesis of cell types in the adenohypophysis of the human fetus as observed with immunocytochemistry, *Am. J. Anat.*, 143, 137, 1975.
3. **Kaplan, S. L., Grumbach, M. M., and Shepard, T. H.,** The ontogenesis of human fetal hormones. I. Growth hormon and insulin, *J. Clin. Invest.*, 51, 3080, 1972.
4. **Grumbach, M. M. and Kaplan, S. L.,** The ontogeny of GH secretion, in *Foetal and Neonatal Physiology,* Comline, R. S., Ed., Cambridge University Press, London 1973, 464.
5. **Laron, Z., Mannheimer, S., and Guttman, S.,** Lack of transplacental passage of growth hormone in rabbits, *Experientia,* 22, 831, 1966.
6. **Laron, Z., Mannheimer, S., Pertzelan, A., Goldman, J., and Guttman, S.,** Lack of placental transfer of human growth hormone, *Acta Endocrinol. (Copenhagen),* 53, 687, 1966.
7. **Laron, Z., Mannheimer, S., Pertzelan, A., and Nitzan, M,.** Serum growth hormone concentration in full term infants, *Isr. J. Med. Sci.*, 6, 770, 1966.
8. **Laron, Z.,** The hypothalamus and the pituitary gland (hypophysis), in *Paediatric Endocrinology,* Hubble, S. W., Ed., Blackwell Scientific, Oxford, 1969, 35.
9. **Cornblath, M., Parker, M. L., Reisner, S. H., Forbes, A. E., and Daughaday, W. H.,** Secretion and metabolism of growth hormone in premature and full term infants, *J. Clin. Endocrinol. Metab.*, 25, 209, 1965.

10. **Keret, R., Mathiash, S., Brown, M., Pertzelan, A., Levy, I., and Laron, Z,.** Correlation between plasma growth hormone and insulin and blood glucose concentrations in premature infants, *Horm. Res.*, 7, 313, 1976.
11. **Laron, Z., Mannheimer, S., Nitzan, M., and Goldman, J.**, Growth hormone, glucose and free fatty acid levels in mother and infant in normal, diabetic and toxaemic pregnancies, *Arch. Dis. Child.*, 42, 24, 1967.
12. **Frantz, A. G. and Rabkin, M. T.**, Effects of estrogen and sex difference on secretion of human growth hormone, *J. Clin. Endocrinol. Metab.*, 25, 1470, 1965.
13. **Laron, Z., Doron, M., and Amikam, B.**, Plasma growth hormone in men and women over 70 years of age, in *Physical Activity and Aging, Medicine and Sport,* Vol. 4, Brunner, D., Ed., S. Karger, Basel, 1970, 126.
14. **Li, C. H., Dixon, J. S., and Liu, W. K.**, Human pituitary growth hormone. XIX. The primary structure of the hormone, *Arch. Biochem. Biophys.*, 133, 70, 1969.
15. **Li, C. H. and Dixon, J. S.**, Human pituitary growth hormone. XXXII. The structure of the hormone: revision, *Arch. Biochem. Biophys.*, 146, 233, 1971.
16. **Niall, H. D.**, Revised primary structure for human growth hormone, *Nature (London),* 23, 90, 1971.
17. **Laron, Z. and Assa, S.**, Immunochemical studies of human pituitary growth hormone, *Acta Endocrinol. (Copenhagen),* 40, 311, 1962.
18. **Laron, Z., Yed-Lekach, A., Assa, S., and Kowadlo-Silbergeld, A.**, Immunochemical properties of bovine and human pituitary growth hormone after pepsin digestion, *Endocrinology,* 74, 632, 1964.
19. **Lewis, N. J., Singh, R. N. P., Peterson, S. M., and Vanderlaan, W. P.**, Human growth hormone: a family of proteins, in *Growth Hormone and Related Peptides,* Pecile, A. and Müller, E. E., Eds., Excerpta Medica, Amsterdam, 1976, 64.
20. **Goodman, A. D., Tanenbaum, R., and Rabinowitz, D.**, Existence of two forms of immunoreactive growth hormone in human plasma, *J. Clin. Endocrinol. Metab.*, 35, 868, 1972.
21. **Gorden, P., Hendriks, C. M., and Roth, J.**, Evidence for "big" and "little" components of human plasma and pituitary growth hormone, *J. Clin. Endocrinol Metabo.*, 36, 178, 1973.
22. **Frohman, L. A. and Stachmura, M. E.**, Evidence for possible precursors in the synthesis of growth hormone by rat and human fetal anterior pituitary in vitro, *Mt. Sinai J. Med., (N.Y.),* 40, 414, 1973.
23. **Assa, S., Laron, Z., Sheridan, R., and Pasteels, J. L.**, Heterogenity of IR-hGH in media of cultured foetal pituitaries (Abstract), *Ricerca Scientifica ed Educazione Permanente,* 2 (Suppl. 1, Abstr.), 16, 1975.
24. **Eshet, R., Assa, S., and Laron, Z.**, Heterogeneity of pituitary and endogenous plasma human growth hormone from fetuses, premature, and full-term newborns, *Biol. Neonat.*, 29, 354, 1976.
25. **Soman, V. and Goodman, A. D.**, Studies of the composition and radioreceptor activity of "big" and "little" human growth hormone, *J. Clin. Endocrinol Metab.*, 44, 569, 1977.
26. **Müller, E. E.**, The nervous control of human growth hormone, in *Advances in Human Growth Hormone Reserach,* Raiti, S., Ed., No. 74—612, Department of Health, Education, and Welfare, Washington, D.C., 1973, 192.
27. **Brazeau, P., Vale, W., Burgus, R., Ling, N., Butcher, M., Rivier, J., and Guillemin, R.**, Hypothalamic polypeptide that inhibits the secretion of immunoreactive pituitary growth hormone, *Science,* 179, 77, 1973.
28. **Pimstone, B. L., Berelowitz, M., and Kronheim, S.**, Somatostatin, 1976, *S. Afr. Med. J.*, 50, 1471, 1976.
29. **Fuxe, K.**, Evidence for the existence of monomine neurons in the central nervous system. IV. Distribution of monoamine nerve terminals in the central nervous system., *Acta. Physiol. Scand. Suppl.*, 247, 39, 1965.
30. **McCann, S. M., Fawcett, C. P., and Krulich, I.**, Hypothalamic hypophyseal releasing and inhibiting hormones, in *Endocrine Physiology,* McCann, S. M., Ed., University Park Press, Baltimore, 1974, 31.
31. **Martin, J. B.**, Neural regulation of growth hormone secretion, *N. Engl. J. Med.*, 288, 1384, 1973.
32. **Liuzzi, A., Chiodim, P. G., Botalla, L., Silvestrini, F., and Müller, E. E.**, Growth hormone (GH) — releasing activity of TRH and GH — lowering effect of dopamine drugs in acromegaly: homogeneity in the two responses, *J. Clin. Endocrinol. Metab.*, 39, 871, 1974.
33. **Hall, R., Besser, R. M., Schally, A. V., Coy, D. H., Evered, D., Goldie, D. J., Kastin, A. J., McNeilly, A. S., Mortimer, C. H., Phenekos, C., Tunbridge, W. M. G., and Weightman, D.**, Action of growth hormone-release inhibitory hormone in healthy men and in acromegaly, *Lancet,* 2, 581, 1973.
34. **Brazeau, P., Rivier, J., Vale, M,. and Guillemin, R.**, Inhibition of growth hormone secretion in the rat by synthetic somatostatin., *Endocrinology,* 94, 184, 1974.
35. **Borgeat, P., Labrie, F., Drouin, J., Belanger, A., Immer, H., Sestani, K., Nelson V., Gotz, M., Schally, A. V., Coy, D. H., and Coy, E. J.**, Inhibition of adenosine 3′,5,-monophosphate accumulation in anterior pituitary gland in vitro by growth-hormone-release inhibiting hormone, *Biochem. Biophys. Res. Commun.*, 56, 1052, 1974.

36. **Mortimer, C. H., Can, D., Lund., T., Bloom, S. R., Mallinson, C. W., Schally, A. C., Tunbridge, W. M. G., Yeomans, L., Coy, D., Kastin, A., Besser, G. M., and Hall, R.**, Effects of growth hormone release inhibiting hormone on circulating glucagon, insulin and growth hormone in normal, diabetic and acromegalic and hypopituitary patients, *Lancet,* 1, 697, 1974.
37. **Luft, R., Efendic, S., Hükfelt, T., Johansson, O., and Arimura, A.**, Immunohistochemical evidence for the localization of somatostatin-like immunoreactivity in a cell population of the pancreatic islets, *Med. Biol.*, 52, 428, 1974.
38. **Liuzzi, A., Panerai, A. E., Chiodini, P. G., Secchi, C., Cocchi, D., Botalla, L., Silverstrini, F., and Müller, E. E.**, Neuroendocrine control of growth hormone secretion: experimental and clinical studies in *Growth Hormone and Related Peptides,* Pecile, A. and Müller, E. E., Eds., Excerpta Medica, Amsterdam, 1976, 236.
39. **Rabinowitz, D. and Zierler, K. L.**, A metabolic regulating device based on the actions of human growth hormone and of insulin, singly and together on the human forearm, *Nature (London),* 199, 913, 1963.
40. **Takahashi, Y., Kipnis, D. M., and Daughaday, W. H.**, Growth hormone secretion during sleep, *J. Clin. Invest.*, 47, 2079, 1968.
41. **Finkelstein, J. W., Roffwarg, H. P., Boyer, R. M., Kream, J., and Hellman, L.**, Age-related change in the twenty-four hour spontaneous secretion of growth hormone, *J. Clin. Endocrinol. Metab.*, 35, 665, 1972.
42. **Carnelutti, M., Del Guercio, M. J., and Chimello, G.**, Influence of growth hormone on the pathogenesis of obesity in childhood, *J. Pediatr.*, 77, 285, 1970.
43. **Laron, Z., Ben-Dan, I., Shrem, M., Dickerman, Z., and Lilos, P.**, Puberty in simple obese boys and girls, *Symp. on Obesity in Childhood,* Academic Press, New York, in press.
44. **Mitchell, M. L., Raben, M. S., and Ernesti, M.**, Use of growth hormone as a diabetic stimulus in man, *Diabetes,* 19, 196, 1970.
45. **Laron Z., Karp. M., Dudek, M., Kowadlo-Silbergeld, A., and Harel, D.**, A contribution to the fat mobilizing activity of human growth hormone, *Helv. Paediatr. Acta,* 23, 37, 1968.
46. **Korner, A.**, Growth hormone control of messenger RNA synthesis, *Biochem. Biophys. Res. Commun.*, 13, 386, 1963.
47. **Kostyo, J. L.**, Rapid effects of growth hormone on amino acid transport and protein synthesis, *Ann. N. Y. Acad. Sci.*, 148, 389, 1968.
48. **Knorr, D. and Butenandt, O.**, Erfahrunger mit dem Stickstoff-Retentionstest mit humanem, hypophysärem Wachstrumshormon, *Monatsschr. Kinderheilkd.*, 115, 308, 1967.
49. **Henneman, P. H., Forbes, A. P., Moldawer, M., Dempsey, E. F., and Carroll, E. L.**, Effects of human growth hormone in man, *J. Clin. Invest.*, 39, 1223, 1960.
50. **Prader, A., Zackmann, M., Polen, J. R., and Illig, R.**, The metabolic effect of a small uniform dose of human growth hormone in hypopituitary dwarfs and in control children. I. Nitrogen, α-amino N, creatine-creatinine and calcium excretion and serum urea N, α-amino-N, inorganic phosphorus and alkaline phosphatase, *Acta Endocrinol. (Copenhagen),* 57, 115, 1968.
51. **Cheek, D. B.**, Cellular growth hormones, nutrition and time, *Pediatrics,* 41, 30, 1968.
52. **Raben, M. S.**, Treatment of a pituitary dwarf with human growth hormone. *J. Clin. Endocrinol. Metab.*, 18, 901, 1958.
53. **Pertzelan, A., Kauli, R., Assa, S., Greenberg, D., and Laron, Z.**, Intermittent treatment with hGH in isolated growth hormone deficiency and in multiple pituitary hormone deficiencies, *Clin. Endocrinol.*, 5, 15, 1976.
54. **Daughaday, W. H., Phillips, L. S., and Herington, A. C.**, Regulation of somatomedin generation, in *Growth Hormone and Related Peptides,* Pecile, A. and Müller, E. E., Eds. Excerpta Medica, Amsterdam, 1976, 169.
55. **Salmon, W. D. Jr. and Daughaday, W. H.**, A hormonally controlled serum factor which stimulates sulfate incorporation by cartilage in vitro, *J. Lab. Clin. Med.*, 49, 825, 1957.
56. **Daughaday, W. H., Hall, K., Raben, M. S., Salmon, W. D., Jr., Van den Brande, J. L., and Van Wyk, J. J.**, Somatomedin: a proposed designation for the "sulfation factor", *Nature (London),* 235, 107, 1972.
57. **Van Wyk, J. J., Underwood, L. E., Lister, R. C., and Marshall, R. N.**, The somatomedins — a new class of growth regulating hormones, *Am. J. Dis. Child.*, 126, 705, 1973.
58. **Shields, R.**, Growth hormones and serum factors, *Nature (London),* 267, 308, 1977.
59. **Laron, Z., Pertzelan, A., Karp, M., Kowadlo-Silbergeld, A., and Daughaday, W. H.**, Administration of growth hormone to patients with familiar dwarfism with high plasma immunoreactive growth hormone: measurements of sulfation factor, metabolic and linear growth responses, *J. Clin. Endocrinol. Metab.*, 33, 332, 1971.
60. **Rabinowitz, D. and Merimee, T. J.**, Isolated human growth hormone deficiency and related disorders, *Isr. J. Med. Sci.*, 9, 1599, 1973.
61. **Pertzelan, A., Adam, A., and Laron, Z.**, Genetic aspects of pituitary dwarfism due to absence or biological inactivity of growth hormone, *Isr. J. Med. Sci.*, 4, 895, 1968.

62. **Rayner, P. H. W., Hubble, D. V., and Brown, G. A.,** Hereditary isolated growth hormone (GH) deficiency, *Exerpta Med. Int. Congr. Ser.,* 142, 42, 1967.
63. **Sheikholislam, B. M. and Stempfel, R. S.,** Familial growth hormone (GH) deficiency, *Pediatr. Res.,* 1, 205, 1967.
64. **Laron, Z. and Sarel, R.,** Penis and testicular size in patients with growth hormone insufficiency, *Acta Endocrinol. (Copenhagen),* 63, 625, 1970.
65. **Takano, K., Hall, K., Ratzen, M., Iselius, L., and Sievertsson, H.,** Somatomedian — a in human serum determined by radioreceptor assay, *Acta Endocrinol. (Copenhagen),* 82, 449, 1976.
66. **D'Ercole, A. J., Underwood, L. E., and Van Wyk, J. J.,** Serum somatomedin-C in hypopituitarism and in other disorders of growth, *J. Pediatr.,* 90, 375, 1977.
67. **Laron, Z., Mimouni, M., Josefsberg, Z., Zadik, Z., and Doron, M.,** The effect of hGH deficiency on the insulin response to glucagon after oral glucose loading, *Diabetologia,* 13, 447, 1977.
68. **Merimee, T. J., Burgess, J. A., and Rabinowitz, D.,** An influence of growth hormone on insulin secretion: studies of growth hormone deficient dwarfs, *Diabetes,* 15, 478, 1967.
69. **Illig, R.,** Growth hormone antibodies in patients treated with different preparations of human growth hormone (HGH), *J. Clin. Endocrinol. Metab.,* 31, 679, 1970.
70. **Tanner, J. M., Whitehouse, R. H., Hughes, P. C. R., and Vince, F. P.,** Effect of human growth hormone treatment for 1 to 7 years on growth of 100 children with growth hormone deficiency, low birthweight, inherited smallness, Turner's syndrome and other compliants, *Arch. Dis. Child.,* 46, 745, 1971.
71. **Prader, A., Ferrandez, A., Zachmann, M., and Illig, R.,** Effect of HGH treatment on growth, bone age and skinfold thickness in 44 children with growth hormone deficiency in *Growth and Growth Hormone,* Pecile, A. and Müller, E. E., Eds., Excerpta Medica, Amsterdam, 1972, 452.
72. **Laron, Z. and Pertzelan, A.,** Intermittent versus continuous HGH treatment of hypopituitary dwarfism in *Growth Hormone and Related Peptides,* Pecile, A., and Müller, E. E., Eds., Excerpta Medica, Amsterdam, 1976, 297.
73. **Laron, Z., Pertzelan, A., and Mannheimer, S.,** Genetic pituitary dwarfism with high serum concentration of growth hormone. A new inborn error of metabolism?, *Isr. J. Med. Sci.,* 2, 152, 1966.
74. **Laron Z., Karp, M., Pertzelan, A., Kauli, R., Keret, R., and Doron, M.,** The syndrome of familial dwarfism and high plasma immunoreactive human growth hormone (IR-hGH), in *Growth and Growth Hormone,* Pecile, A. and Müller, E. E., Eds., Excerpta Medica, Amsterdam, 1972, 459.
75. **Laron, Z.,** Syndrome of familial dwarfism and high plasma immunoreactive growth hormone, *Isr. J. Med. Sci.,* 10, 1247, 1974.
76. **Merimee, T. J., Hall, J., Rabinowitz, D., McKusick, V. A., and Rimoin, D. L.,** An unusual variety of endocrine dwarfism. Subresponsiveness to growth hormone in a sexually mature dwarf, *Lancet,* 2, 919, 1968.
77. **Van Gemund, J. J., Laurent De Angelo, M. S., and Van Gelderen, V. V.,** Familial prenatal dwarfism with elevated serum immunoreactive growth hormone levels and endorgan unresponsiveness, *Maandschr. Kindergeneeskd.,* 37, 372, 1969.
78. **Najjar, S. S., Khachadurian, A. K., Ilbawi, M. N., and Blizzard, R. M.,** Dwarfism with elevated levels of plasms growth hormone, *N. Engl. J. Med.,* 284, 809, 1971.
79. **Elders, M. J., Garland, J. T., Daughaday, W. H., Fisher, D. A., Whitney, J. E., and Highes, E. F.,** Laron's Dwarfism. Studies on the nature of the defect, *J. Pediatr.,* 83, 253, 1973.
80. **Kastrup, K. W., Andersen, H., and Hanssen, K. F.,** Increased immunoreactive plasma and urinary growth hormone in growth retardation with defective generation of somatomedin A (Laron's syndrome), *Acta Paediat. (Stockholm),* 64, 613, 1975.
81. **Rappaport, R., Czernichow, P., Prevost, C., and Jullien, M.,** Retard de croissance avec somathormone circulante élevée et incapacité à générer la somatomedine (Nanisme de type Laron), *Ann. Pediat. (Paris),* 24, 63, 1977.
82. **Takano, K., Toledo, S. P. A., Gluckman, P. D., Ferrandez, A., Bailey J., and Pierson, M.,** personal communications.
83. **Eshet, R., Laron, Z., Brown, M., and Arnon, R.,** Immunoreactive properties of the plastma HGH from patients with the syndrome of familial dwarfism and high plasma IR-HGH, *J. Clin. Endocrinol. Metab.,* 37, 919, 1973.
84. **Eshet, R., Laron, Z., Brown, M., and Arnon, R.,** Immunological behavior of HGH from plasma of patients with familial dwarfism and high IR-HGH in radioimmunoassay system, *Horm. Metab. Res.,* 6, 80, 1974.
85. **Jacobs, L. S., Sneid, S. D., Garland, J. T., Laron, Z., and Daughaday, W. H.,** Receptor-active growth hormone in Laron-dwarfism, *J. Clin. Endocrinol. Metab.,* 42, 403, 1976.
86. **Nevo, Z., Nof, D., Bier-Adler, M., Mimouni, M., Pertzelan, A., and Laron, Z.,** Serum sulfate levels and plasma hGH in patients with low and excessive hGH secretion, *Pediatr. Res.,* 10 (Abstr.). 876, 1976.

87. **Laron, Z.**, Syndrome of familial dwarfism and high plasma immunoreactive growth hormone (IR-hGH) — Laron-type dwarfism, *Paediatrician*, 6, 106, 1977.
88. **Rimoin, D. L., Merimee, T. J., Rabinowitz, D., McKusick, V. A., and Cavalli-Sforza, L. L.**, Growth hormone in African Pygmies, *Lancet*, 2, 523, 1967.
89. **Merimee, T. J., Rimoin, D. L., Rabinowitz, D., Cavalli-Sforza, L. L., and McKusick, V. A.**, Metabolic studies in the African Pygmy, *Trans. Assoc. Am. Physicians*, 81, 221, 1968.
90. **Rimoin, D. L., Merimee, T. J., Rabinowitz, D., Cavalli-Sforza, L. L., and McKusick, V. A.**, Peripheral subresponsiveness to human growth hormone in the African pygmies, *N. Engl. J. Med.*, 281, 1383, 1969.
91. **Rimoin, D. L. and Schimke, R. N.**, *Genetic Disorders of the Endocrine Glands*, C. V. Mosby, St. Louis, 1971, 32.
92. **Rimoin, D. L., Merimee, T. J., Rabinowitz, D., and McKusick, V. A.**, Genetic aspects of clinical endocrinology., *Recent Prog. Hormon. Res.*, 24, 365, 1968.
93. **Schimke, R. N., Spaulding, J. J., and Hollowell, J. F.**, X-linked congenital panhypopituitarism, *Birth Defects Orig. Artic. Ser.*, 7, 21, 1971.
94. **Phalan, P. D., Connelley, J., Martin, F. I. R., and Weltenhall, H. N. B.**, X-linked recessive hypopituitarism, *Birth Defects Orig. Artic. Ser.*, 7, 24, 1971.
95. **Dickerman, Z., Prager-Lewin, R., and Laron, Z.**, The effect of repeated injections of synthetic LH-RH on the response of plasma LH and FSH in young hypogonadotrophic-hypogonadal patients, *Fertil. Steril.*, 27, 162, 1976.
96. **Lawrence, J. H., Tobias, C. A., Linfoot, J. A., Born, J. L., Lyman, J. T., Chang, C. Y., Manonginn, E., and Wei, W. C.**, Successful treatment of acromegaly: metabolic and clinical studies in 145 patients, *J. Clin. Endocrinol. Metab.*, 31, 180, 1970.
97. **Leva, J.**, Über familiäre Akromegalie, *Med. Klin. (Munich)*, 11, 1266, 1915.
98. **Adler-Bier, M., Pertzelan, A., Laron, Z., Lieberman, E., and Moses, S.**, Multiple pituitary hormone deficiencies in eight siblings of one Jewish Moroccan family, *Acta Paediatr. Scand.*, in press.

Chapter 8

GENETIC VARIATION IN THE ENDOCRINE SYSTEMS OF THE NEUROHYPOPHYSIS

A. D. Stewart

TABLE OF CONTENTS

I. INTRODUCTION

This chapter outlines areas where there is significant knowledge of genetic variation affecting the neurohypophysial octapeptide hormones of vetebrates, analyzes some of the experimental uses of this variation, and discusses the more general biological significance (especially in evolutionary terms) of such variation.[1,2]

Genetic variation in an endocrine system is generally observed in the first place because of some effect which is secondary to (or, in genetic terminology, a pleiotropic effect[3] of) the primary effect of the genetic locus or loci concerned. The primary effect is very often not known. For example, considerable genetic variation has been demonstrated in the kinetics of the response of mice to a gastric water load.[4-6] This could clearly result from variant genetic loci having their primary actions at any point from the synthesis of vasopressin in the hypothalamus, its transport down the axons of the biosynthetic neurones, its storage in and release from the posterior pituitary, its interaction with the kidney, and its ultimate breakdown by the liver or kidney.[7] Each of these processes is itself complex. The observed phenotypic variation might even have nothing to do with the neurohypophysial endocrine system; it might arise if some mice are more susceptible to stress than others and reduce the glomerular filtration rate by some other mechanism entirely. For these reasons, it is always important to try and define the primary effects of genes as closely as possible; by the same token, it is impossible to organize this discussion in a completely rational way when this objective has inevitably not been attained in many cases. Genetic variation affecting the biosynthesis and storage of hormones will be described first and then that which affects the action and breakdown of these hormones at their target organs.

Extremely good and comprehensive reviews of the biochemistry, physiology, and pharmacology of the neurohypophysial and related octapeptide hormones are available.[7,8] The review of some genetic aspects of the biosynthesis, storage, and secretion of the hormones by Valtin and his colleagues[9] is especially relevant.

II. SYNTHESIS AND STORAGE OF NEUROHYPOPHYSIAL HORMONES

A. The Mole-Ratio

The amounts of the octapeptide hormones stored in the adult neurohypophysis vary widely in different species.[10-12] Clearly, as variation between species implies variation within a species at some time, there could be genetic variation in these stores. It is worth considering the different methods available to establish this conclusion.

Restricting the discussion to mammals, where the hormones (vasopressin and oxytocin) are sufficiently well characterized for one to have confidence in the figures, much of this variation between species is, not surprisingly, correlated with body weight. However, even closely related species may still differ considerably in the quantities of hormones stored, whether or not correction is made for body weight or neural lobe weight. On the other hand, the mole-ratio of vasopressin to oxytocin is similar in closely related species, but differs significantly between taxonomic groups. The degree of variation between groups increases as higher taxons are considered (for a statistical analysis, see Valtin and colleagues).[9] It has been argued from this one fact that the mole-ratio is "an inherited characteristic"[10] (or "under genetic control"[11]) and that it is of adaptive significance. These arguments seem to lack rigor. First, comparison between species is an inappropriate technique for demonstrating genetic variation. Second, selection (or the lack of it) can result in either similarities or differences between different animal populations, depending on the circumstances.[13,14]

The two arguments must proceed separately. There are two studies which demonstrate genetic variation in the storage of vasopressin and oxytocin. The hormones stored in the pituitaries of five inbred strains of mice have been bioassayed.[15,16] The strain differences paralleled the species differences, in that considerable variation was found between strains whether or not body-weight was taken into consideration; however, with the exception of the Peru strain, there was no significant variation in the mole-ratio of vasopressin to oxytocin. In the Peru strain, taking account of the fact that the [8-lysine]-vasopressin elaborated by the mice at that time[17] has a lower activity than [8-arginine]-vasopressin (produced by the other strains) in the rat-pressor bioassay, it was found that the mole-ratio was higher than in the other strains. Since all the mice were maintained under identical conditions and standardized for age and sex, it is highly probable that these differences are genetic in origin. Valtin[9] calculated the variation in the mole-ratio that might arise by free genetic recombination in crosses between the five strains of mice referred to above. It must be emphasized that this is very much a maximum figure, depending as it does on the completely unverified assumption that the strain differences in the two stores are independently determined (i.e., by mutually exclusive sets of genetic loci).

However, Waring and Landgrebe,[18] in the second valid study, reported that the mole-ratio was significantly more variable in a genetically heterogeneous (i.e., segregating) stock of guniea pigs than in pure lines. Although experimental details seem to be lacking, this is one of the classic techniques for demonstrating genetic control of a quantitative character.[13]

The character studied here (quantity of hormone stored) is clearly not very specific and variation in it could be attributed to several causes. Other interesting parameters, such as the increase in the rate of biosynthesis following the stimulation of hormone release,[9] the distribution of the hormone in a heterogeneous store,[19-21] and the sensitivity of the hypothalamic-neurophypophysial system to standard stimuli[22-26] have yet to be studied. However, the very specific character of the structure of the hormones has been given considerable attention.

TABLE 1

Chemical Structure of Known, Naturally Occurring, Octapeptide Hormones

General Structure of Octapeptide Hormones

1 2 3 4 5 6 7 8 9
CyS-Tyr-A-B-Asn-CyS-Pro-C-Gly-NH_2

Common name of hormone	Amino acids present A	B	C
Arginine vasopressin	Phe	Gln	Arg
Lysine vasopressin	Phe	Gln	Lys
Arginine vasotocin	Ile	Gln	Arg
Lysine vasotocin	Ile	Gln	Lys
Oxytocin	Ile	Gln	Leu
Valitocin	Ile	Gln	Val
Mesotocin	Ile	Gln	Ile
Isotocin	Ile	Ser	Ile
Glumitocin	Ile	Ser	Gln
Aspartocin	Ile	Asn	Leu

B. Hormone Structure

1. Naturally Occurring Hormones

The structures of the octapeptide hormones that have been identified in extracts of posterior pituitary glands and pineal glands[9] are shown in Table 1. This list is probably incomplete, as peptides that are inactive in the current bioassay systems (few of them based on lower vertebrates) will not have been detected. The phylogenetic distribution of these hormones has often been reviewed.[9,12,27-32]

Population geneticists estimate that a fairly high proportion — perhaps 25% or more — of all structural genetic loci are polymorphic among the members of natural populations of a particular species, at the level of the amino acid sequence of the polypeptide chain specified by that locus. Opinions are however divided as to the functional and evolutionary significance of this variation.[14] There is, therefore, a strong theoretical interest in attempting to ascertain the extent of genetic variation in the structure of the neurohypophysial hormones. The small size of the molecules and the specificity of the methods available mean that it is relatively easy to identify these hormones, and the extent of our knowledge of their function, at least in higher vertebrates, means that the functional significance of variation in structure is open to investigation.

Unfortunately, there has not yet been any systematic attempt to investigate the extent of genetic variation within species of octapeptide hormones, apart perhaps from the report of Ferguson and Heller.[11] This is partly because of the difficulty of analyzing material from single animals. In the future, wider use of sensitive and specific methods, such as radioimmunoassay (utilizing antibodies with a known spectrum of cross-reactions with analogues) combined with preliminary chromatographic separations, may overcome these difficulties. In the meantime, there are a number of reports indicative or suggestive of genetic variation.

2. Basic Octapeptides

Arginine vasotocin (AVT) is found throughout the vertebrates. This probably includes the mammals, which, although elaborating vasopressin in the neurohypophysis when adult, probably possess AVT in the fetal neurohypophysis[33,34] and adult pineal gland[35-40] and subcommissural organ.[41] The only exception to this may be the domestic pig, where lysine vasotocin (LVT) has been reported in the pineal.[42]

Nearly all mammals produce arginine vasopressin (AVP) in the adult neurohypophysis. In the Suiformes, there are well-authenticated reports of polymorphism.[11,43,44] The domestic pig apparently possess only lysine vasopressin (LVP), but all the feral species so far investigated (warthog, collared peccary, white-lipped peccary, giant forest hog, European wild boar, and the hippopotamus) may be polymorphic. The polymorphism is particularly well documented in the warthog and collared peccary.[44] In the hippopotamus, there are conflicting claims. LVP alone was first reported[11] and AVP was found in addition in a later study,[45] yet a further study of animals from the same population by Uttenthal and Hope[46] revealed only AVP. Some of the methodological problems have been discussed,[46] but the situation still remains confused especially in view of the relatively small numbers of animals examined.

LVP has also been reported in the Peru strain of the house mouse, following chromatographic and pharmacological studies and amino acid analysis, whereas several other strains of the mouse elaborated AVP.[17] This was confirmed in an Edinburgh subline by specific radioimmunoassay as late as 1972.[47] Recent studies indicate that the present sublines of the Peru strain no longer elaborate LVP, but instead have the more usual AVP.[48] Unless doubt is cast on the original report, the most likely explanations are either that the line has been contaminated at some point or that the original Peru stock was itself polymorphic and different sublines diverged. Such divergence is very common and it should be remembered that the Peru strain was not very highly inbred at the time of the first studies.

There does not seem to be any particular reason why polymorphism in the vasopressins should be restricted to the mouse and the Suiformes. The selective pressures for or against LVP may depend to a large extent on the sensitivity of the target organs to it when it appears in a particular population for the first time (see Section IV).

3. Neutral Octapeptides

The literature on the neutral octapeptides, especially in the lower vertebrates, is large and confusing. The confusion results partly because of the variety of octapeptides elaborated, partly because of methodological problems in distinguishing between the octapeptides, and partly because conflicting reports have often been interpreted, not as indicating the *possibility* of natural polymorphic variation which should be directly investigated, but as a result of poor methodology by one or another group.

To start on solid ground, Pickering[49] demonstrated by pharmacological criteria and by amino acid analysis that both oxytocin (OT) and mesotocin (MT) were present in pooled pituitaries of the cobra. The presence of both octapeptides in reptiles was confirmed, using pharmacology and chromatography only, by Follett, who examined pooled extracts from a few glands of the grass snake and the green turtle and also a single gland from a loggerhead turtle.[50]

Turning to the amphibia, there are some conflicting reports. In the American leopard frog, Munsick found, by pharmacological and chromatographic methods, a peptide that was significantly different from MT but identical in its properties with OT. He obtained his frogs from Wisconsin.[51] Acher and his colleagues, apparently perturbed by the claimed presence of OT rather than MT (which is certainly more common in amphibians), demonstrated fairly conclusively by pharmacology, chromatography, and amino acid analysis that these animals elaborated MT and no detectable OT. He obtained his animals from a dealer in California.[52]

Similarly, the frog *Rana esculenta* was found by Acher and his colleagues to possess AVT and MT, whereas Morel and co-workers found AVT and some other compound with higher natriferic activity than either MT or OT.[53] This peptide, if it exists, has yet to be identified.

A similar situation seems to exist in the African lungfish. Fish from Lake George, Uganda apparently possessed MT,[54] whereas those from Lake Victoria, Uganda elaborated OT.[55,56] A later batch of pituitaries from Lake George apparently did contain some MT as well as OT[57] (see Sawyer for an account of some of the methodological problems of this work).[58]

What conclusion should be drawn? The pharmacological methods used (notably the relative uterotonic activity of the peptides in the presence and absence of Mg^{++}) are admittedly subject to unexplained variation,[58] but they can still provide useful information if adequate control experiments with known MT and OT are carried out simultaneously. This area definitely needs further systematic study, preferably with more reliable methods. So far, only a small number of species has been examined; for many of these, there is only a single report of a single population. It will be some time before it is clear how commonly both MT and OT are to be found within a species. Meanwhile in view of the fairly definitive work of Pickering on the cobra, the accounts of both hormones in the lungfish, reptiles, and amphibia, seem plausible.

A variety of neutral octapeptides other than OT and MT have been found in lower vetebrates (Table 1). Knowledge of the phylogenetic distribution of these, especially the recently reported valitocin (VT) and aspartocin (AT), is rather deficient. Progress may be aided if the possibility of natural genetic variation is remembered.

4. Genetic Determination

a. Potential Primary Sites of Action

It is generally assumed, especially in discussions of the evolution of hormone structure, that the complete structure of any octapeptide hormone is determined by a single genetic locus (i.e., that a hormone is an unmodified template protein, or an unmodified part of a template protein, specified by a particular mRNA species).[12,28-32] It would then follow that any variation in the structure of the hormone would be entirely genetically determined by variation at that one structural locus. The evidence that an octapeptide is part of a precursor template protein rather than a product of sequential enzymatic synthesis derives almost entirely from the elegant series of experiments on the biosynthesis of vasopressin by Sachs and his colleagues, especially his kinetic studies on the effect of puromycin[9,59] (see also Section II.C.2.c on the theory that neurophysin A and vasopressin are derived from a common precursor in the rat). However, this does not rule out the possibility that different octapeptides could be produced from separate structural loci at different seasons or (as with AVT and AVP in mammals) at different developmental stages; or even that structure of the octapeptide could be enzymatically modified (in addition to its cleavage from the precursor molecule) after its ribosomal synthesis. Genetic variation at a regulatory or enzymatic locus could then give rise to structural variation in the hormones. The fact that many of the amino acid changes which have taken place during the evolution of the octapeptide hormones can be explained with single base changes[9] does *not* constitute evidence that they are due to template changes. Acceptable amino acid substitutions, by whatever method they occur, will involve amino acids with similar properties.

b. The AVP/LVP Polymorphism

The evidence does seem to be contrary to the possibility of environmental or developmental effects for the AVP-LVP polymorphism. In the case of the Peru mice, the animals were maintained under the same conditions and were the same age as the other strains that elaborated AVP rather than LVP.[17] In the case of the feral Suiformes, these factors were not controlled, but Ferguson has studied the relative frequencies of animals possessing either AVP, LVP or both in the warthog, and the collared peccary.[44] These were found to be in accordance with the Hardy-Weinberg equilibrium.[13] This fact can be interpreted in various ways, depending on the particular assumption underlying the theoretical distribution which it is desired to test. As there is only one degree of freedom, a prior choice has to be made as to which this should be. The distribution has been used by Ferguson to test the assumption that there is no selection between the three putative genotypes, but this is an unprofitable way to use the data as the sample was too small to be of significant help in this respect,[17] and deviation from Hardy-Weinberg is in any case an extremely inefficient method for detecting selection.[60-62] It seems better to use the data to support the assumption that the population polymorphism is due to the segregation of the three genotypes (corresponding to the two homozygotes and the heterozygote) which segregate with two alleles at a single genetic locus in the population. Thus, developmental and epigenetic environmental effects are again ruled out.

The simplest explanation of the polymorphisms would be that they are due to mutation by a single base change in a codon for arginine to a codon for lysine in the structural gene for vasopressin.[12,29] This is certainly the most likely explanation, but the possibility of subsequent enzymatic modification of structure after ribosomal synthesis arises from two rather unexpected observations. These are both cases of a parallel change in two octapeptides, vasopressin and vasotocin. In Brattleboro rats, with hypothalamic diabetes insipidus and absence of detectable AVP, AVT is apparently also absent from the pineal[39] (see Section II.C.2). Similarly, in domestic pigs, which possess LVP rather than AVT, the pineal elaborates LVT rather than AVT.[42] These observations could both be due to coincidence (for a possible explanation of the Brattleboro situation, see Section II.C.2.e) or to a change in the specificity of a modifying enzyme system.

An interesting genetic experiment that would provide important population information and would also discriminate between these possibilities would be to examine the structure of the octapeptides in the pineal and pituitary of feral suina polymorphic for LVP and AVP. If AVP were found in the absence of AVT, or LVP in the absence of AVT (or vice versa), this would demonstrate that the structures of vasotocin and vasopressin are independently determined and not affected by a common system (or, in genetic terms, that there are two separate loci). This test is similar in concept to the use of a segregating hybrid generation (see Chapter 1), but is in fact still more powerful. This is because in a natural population, even if the two loci are very closely linked, all the possible chromosomal types (AVP-AVT, AVP-LVT, LVP-AVT, LVP-LVT) will be present at frequencies governed (except in the case of strong linkage disequilibrium) only by the allele frequencies at the two loci.[14] Besides resolving the point at issue, this experiment would provide interesting evidence about the time at which the change from AVT to LVT occurred in the ancestry of the pig and might produce further evidence of genetic polymorphism.

c. The MT/OT Polymorphism

The case of polymorphism at a single locus in those species where both MT and OT may have been found is not so clear, apart from the methodological problems, because it has not been possible to examine individual animals. Thus, the situation in the cobra could be explained either as the result of gene duplication, followed by mutation at one of the two loci, or as a result of polymorphism following mutation at a single locus. The latter alternative is simpler, especially as most reptiles only elaborate two octapeptide hormones; cases (such as may exist in the American leopard frog and in the African lungfish) of geographical variation in the hormone produced could then be interpreted in terms of the two different alleles becoming more frequent or fixed in different populations.

C. Major Defects in the Production and Secretion of Octapeptides

1. The Variety of Defects

As with the natural quantitative variation discussed in Section II.A, a major defect in hormone synthesis and release could occur owing to a large variety of different causes, from the detection of the releasing-stimulus by the nervous system, through the different stages of synthesis in the hypothalamus, to the storage and release of the hormone at the neurohypophysis. In genetic defects, the modes of inheritance may vary accordingly. These principles are illustrated very clearly by hypothalamic diabetes insipidus.[63] Reported examples of defects in the brain include some sort of general hypothalamic disturbance, leading to a syndrome that also includes optic atrophy, diabetes mellitus, and neurosensory hearing loss in man[64] (probably autosomal recessive),[65] and defective thirst mechanism in mice (autosomal recessive).[66] Presumptive failure in the production of vasotocin has been reported in the chick (autosomal recessive)[63] and of vasopressin in man (both autosomal dominant and X-linked forms),[65,68,79] and the rat (recessive).[70]

In man, there has been some dispute as to whether the condition is due to incomplete synthesis of variable severity or to defective release (perhaps involving the osmoreceptors). There is evidence for neuronal atrophy in some cases, but it is quite possible that each of the reported forms is itself heterogeneous, with defects occurring at different stages.[71-73] The conditions in laboratory animals are more amenable to experimentation and are therefore better understood. In the chick, bioassays revealed a deficiency of antidiuretic, vasopressor, and frog-bladder activities in neurohypophyses of affected White Leghorn birds compared with normal animals.[74] There may be some vasotocin (or even a relatively inactive structural variant) present in affected animals, as there was more frog bladder activity than could be attributed to the measured oxytocin. A defect in the regulation of hormone synthesis, or neuronal atrophy as in man, of variable severity could account for this and the fact that the water consumption by affected animals is rather variable. Clearly, this situation now has potential for an intensive research effort of the kind that has been expended on the Brattleboro rat (which is so great that it is considered separately in Section II.C.2 below).

Genetic variation could also be involved in excessive secretion of vasopressin of unexplained origin in children and adults,[75] and in determining whether or not ectopic secretion of vasopressin occurs in association with certain pathological states.[76] There is no evidence on these points.

There is a striking lack of reports of major defects in the production and release of oxytocin. Except in the case of ectopic secretion, where there is some evidence that oxytocin is rarely involved,[76] this is likely to be a result of an inherent bias between the systems, rather than because mutations causing such defects do not occur. In the case of domestic and laboratory animals, a defect in oxytocin production or release would probably lead to increased perinatal mortality, resulting in strong selection against such mutations. In man, difficulties of the sort that would presumably be caused by a hypothalamic deficiency during childbirth and breast feeding are common,[77,78] but a wide variety of different causes may be involved,[79] which are usually not investigated in detail. Rather, they are commonly overcome, where medical facilities are available, by means such as the use of uterotonic drugs[80] and artificial feeding. It would, however, be very interesting if such an abnormality were found.

2. The Brattleboro Rat

a. Initial Observations

The Brattleboro rat with hypothalamic diabetes insipidus was first described by Valtin in 1961.[70,71] Early studies naturally concentrated on defining the nature of the defect, but the potential for investigations of vasopressin biosynthesis soon became obvious. It has also been widely used in the study of the physiological actions of vasopressin, both on the kidney and other organs. This is similar in concept to the traditional use of hypophysectomized animals but with the advantage that there is much more specific alteration to the system.

This section does not aim to deal with all this work in detail, but to give examples of the ways in which the Brattleboro rat has been used by endocrinologists and found an important and accepted place in the literature. Brattleboro rats are derived from the Long-Evans strain, and a single autosomal locus is involved. Homozygous affected animals drink three quarters of their body weight per day and excrete up to 20 times as much urine as a normal animal. They elaborate oxytocin, but no detectable vasopressin or vasopressin-associated neurophysin. The high fluid turnover can be corrected by chronic administration of vasopressin. The secretory neurones show evidence of increased metabolic activity, being hypertrophied with enlarged nuclei and nucleoli (unlike the condition in man). Heterozygous animals are intermediate for most parameters, but may resemble one or another homozygote more closely depending on the particular character considered.[9,70,71]

b. One Cell-One Hormone Hypothesis

The Brattleboro rat has been used to provide evidence for two types of neurones, producing *either* oxytocin *or* vasopressin. Recent work has used a variety of techniques. Vandesande and Dierickx,[81] using immunoenzyme cytochemical techniques on normal rats (of undefined strain!), demonstrated separate vasopressin- and oxytocin-containing neurones in both the supraoptic and paraventricular nuclei of the hypothalamus and neurohypophysis; vasopressin-containing neurones were also found in the suprachiasmatic nuclei. Similar, but more weakly staining, oxytocin-containing neurones were found in the Brattleboro rat, but many neurones did not contain oxytocin. No vasopressin-containing neurones were identified at any location.[81] Similar results were obtained by Swaab et al.[82] using an immunofluroescence technique; they too stained alternate sections for oxytocin and vasopressin and found no neurones containing both hormones. Heterozygous Brattleboro animals were similar to the normal animals; they constitute an important control experiment, often neglected. Both reports used antisera with little cross-reactivity between oxytocin and vasopressin. Earlier findings of some material reactive with vasopressin antisera[83] are thus likely to be due to cross-reactivity, probably with oxytocin-containing neurons. This interpretation is strengthened by the consistent failure, not just by bioassay but even with sensitive and specific radioimmunoassay techniques,[39] to detect any vasopressin in extracts from homozygous Brattleboro rats. Thus, these results afford very good evidence in favor of the one neurone-one hormone hypothesis, which has also found support on other grounds (see Livett[84]).

In addition, Rosenbloom and Fisher[39] found that the pineal gland, which contains vasotocin in the secretory ependymal cells in normal animals, did not contain any vasotocin in homozygous Brattleboro animals. This finding should be reinvestigated, together with the presence or absence of vasotocin in the subcommissural organ where it has been reported in normal animals,[41] since it is critical for the efforts to determine the primary site of the biochemical defect (see Section II.C.2.e below, and Section II.B.4.g above).

c. The Hypothesis of a Common Precursor Molecule of Vasopressin and Neurophysin A

In view of the idea that octapeptide hormones and neurophysins were derived from a common precursor, it is natural to inquire whether the different neurones, synthesizing vasopressin or oxytocin, also elaborate specific neurophysins. The interpretation of many results is confused by the fact that specific methods for distinguishing between the rat neurophysins have only recently been developed. Quantitative studies using nonspecific radioimmunoassay methods should be disregarded entirely[85] (see discussion after Pickering et al).[86]

The clearest demonstration of three specific neurophysins in the rat is given by various biochemical techniques. The polyacrylamide gel electrophoretic (PAGE) method of Burford and Pickering has been particularly useful, either in combination with isotopic techniques[86] or with densitometric quantification.[87] The initial use of Brattleboro homozygotes with both methods was to show that the neurophysin A of Pickering's group,[86] corresponding to the neurophysin I of Sunde and Sokol,[87] is not detectable in the neural lobe. Taken together with the absence of neurosecretory granules and neurophysin from many hypothalamic and neurohypophysial neurones in these animals, this would readily be explained if neurophysin A and vasopressin are both absent in the same cells in the hypothalamus and neurohypophysis. This interpretation was strengthened by the fact that the greater neurohypophysial stores of oxytocin resulting from correction of water balance with exogenous vasopressin are accompanied by an increased density of neurosecretory granules[9] and was recently confirmed by the finding of Vandesande and Dierickx that it is the same neurones in Brattleboro homozygotes which contain both oxytocin and neurophysin.[81]

These findings do not in themselves rule out the possibility that when it does occur, neurophysin A could be associated with oxytocin or that when vasopressin is elaborated, it is also associated with neurophysins B and C. Here in the absence of integrated studies using immunocytochemical methods specific for vasopressin, oxytocin, and neurophysins A, B, and C, we have to rely on the quantitative studies of the behavior of the various neurophysins compared with that of vasopressin and oxytocin under different physiological conditions and using the three different genotypes[86,87] (see below).

The results of other studies of the homozygous Brattleboro animal, most usually using heterologous antisera that do not discriminate between neurophysins A, B, and C, can now be examined. Leclerc and Pelletier,[88] using electron-microscopic techniques with an antihuman-neurophysin that cross-reacts with all rat neurophysins, obtained consistent observations, but interpreted the absence of staining in some neurones as due to a very high turnover of the secretory granules in them in accordance with a previous ultramicroscopical study by Kalimo and Rinne.[89] Similarly, Watkins[83] attributed the large number of cells not stained for neurophysin in the hypothalamus to the chronically dehydrated condition of the animals. On the other hand, Zimmerman et al.[90] and Vandesande and Dierickx[81] with the light microscope and the sensitive immunoperoxidase technique interpret their results in terms of a synthetic defect leading to complete absence of neurophysin, while admitting that it is possible (from the swollen nature of the terminal processes of the neurones and their large Herring bodies in the neural lobe) that some secretory substances are being produced. Thus, although there is disagreement concerning the mechanisms involved, all these observations are consistent with the hypothesis that separate neurones contain separate neurophysins and that neurophysin A is associated with vasopressin. The Brattleboro rat has thus been of considerable value in confirming this conclusion in the rat, in line with observations of the association of vasopressin and oxytocin with specific neurophysins in other species.[84]

A simple explanation of this association of neurophysin A with vasopressin in specific neurones would be to postulate that they are both formed from the common precursor of Sachs and his colleagues[59] (see above). The simultaneous absence of both in Brattleboro rats has sometimes been taken as conclusive evidence for this hypothesis, but Valtin's group has clearly shown that there are possible alternative explanations for this phenomenon, notably coordinate regulation of vasopressin and neurophysin production.[9] Sunde and Sokol tested the hypothesis further by estimating the mole-ratio of neurophysin A to vasopressin in the neural lobe under various physiological conditions and found it to be nearly one in homozygous normal and heterozygous Brattleboro animals.[87] Pickering described a similar correspondence for the rate of synthesis, which is a more critical parameter as differential release could subsequently occur.[86]

Although these experiments could be done with increased accuracy and in a wider variety of physiological states, it seems reasonable to accept the hypothesis provisionally. The relationship between oxytocin and neurophysins B and C is less clear, although it has been suggested that neurophysin C may merely be a breakdown product of neurophysin B.[86] Brattleboro and normal rats have been used to identify proteins which may represent the precursors of vasopressin and neurophysin A, oxytocin and neurophysin B, and intermediate breakdown products.[218] The octapeptide and neurophysin sequences are not necessarily adjacent in the precursor molecule.[219]

Valtin proposed a critical test for the hypothesis on the supposition that structural genetic variants of a specific neurophysin and its corresponding octapeptide might be found in some species; under the hypothesis, the same genetic locus would be responsible for both effects and this could be ascertained in a suitable breeding experiment with a segregating generation.[9] Attempts to find structural variants in different strains of mice have, however, failed.[91] This is not too surprising in view of the high degree of similarity in the amino acid sequences of neurophysins A and B and their binding properties for vasopressin and oxytocin, and the evolutionary conservation of neurophysin structure which this seems to imply.[86] However, the possibility should be borne in mind, and further investigation of the neurophysins of feral Suina in relation to the type of vasopressin elaborated in single glands[46] would be worthwhile.

d. The Roles of the Supraoptic and Paraventricular Nuclei in the Rat

There is a considerable amount of evidence from traditional types of experimentation in a variety of species that oxytocin-containing neurones predominate in the paraventricular nucleus and vasopressin-containing neurones in the supraoptic nucleus.[84]. The Brattleboro animal has been used to throw light on the problem in the rat. The fundamental assumption is made that the diabetes insipidus gene does not affect the distribution of oxytocin- and vasopressin-containing neurones, but only the synthetic activity of the vasopressin-type neurone; however, there is some evidence to support this.[82] Several studies of homozygous Brattleboro animals indicate that about half or more of the neurones in both the supraoptic and paraventricular nuclei do not secrete neurophysin.[83,88] Further, Swaab and colleagues, in one of the few papers to contain good quantitative data, likewise found no difference between the nuclei in the proportions of vasopressin- and oxytocin-containing neurones in the normal animal.[82] Vandesande and Dierickx give a similar impression in their studies of the distribution of vasopressin, oxytocin, and neurophysin in normal and Brattleboro animals.[81] (However, both these groups did comment on a differential distribution of neurones within each of these nuclei, with more oxytocin-containing cells in the rostral part and more vasopressin-containing cells in the caudal part of each nucleus.[81,82]) Since the supraoptic nucleus has two (or more) times as many cells as the paraventricular nucleus, it might also elaborate more oxytocin.[81,82] This conclusion is in contradiction to the evidence from traditional experiments in the rat. Bilateral destruction of the paraventricular nucleus in the rat resulted in a loss of neurohyphysial oxytocin, and destruction of the supraoptic nucleus resulted in a loss of neurohypophysial vasopressin and the induction of diabetes insipidus.[84] Burford et al. showed similar effects on the rates of specific neurophysin synthesis.[92] The discrepancy could be due either to methodological problems (for example, in the incomplete destruction of the hypothalamic nuclei or in the histochemical techniques), to differential activity of neurones that look similar (for example, Watkins[83] observed more intense vasopressin staining in the supraoptic nucleus than the paraventricular nucleus), or to the control pathways for the release of the hormones operating predominantly through one or another nucleus.

e. The Nature of the Primary Defect

It is now possible to consider what the nature of the defect in Brattleboro rats might be. Many different observations have to be taken into account. First, there is the considerable hypertrophy of the neurosecretory neurones, their nuclei, and their nucleoli in both heterozygous and homozygous animals; this affects the oxytocin-containing neurones as well.[9] In addition, ultramicroscopic observations characteristic of active protein synthesis have been made in neurones devoid of neurosecretory granules.[89] Some authors also report the presence of extragranular neurophysin and octapeptides in all heterozygous neurosecretory cells and in the oxytocin-containing cells of homozygotes.[88] Although it is by no means clear whether or not this extragranular material represents an artifact of fixation or biochemical extraction procedures, this is apparently also characteristic of normal animals subject to chronic osmotic stimulation when parallel studies are performed.[21] It seems quite likely that all these observations describe secondary consequences of the deficiency in vasopressin and neurophysin in Brattleboro animals, which would lead to increased chronic stimulation of both types of neurosecretory cells (whether through the hypothalamic osmoreceptors or by an intraneuronal feedback mechanism).[71]

Second, Moses and Miller[93] and Sunde and Sokol[87] have claimed that heterozygous animals are defective in their ability to release vasopressin and neurophysin A, respectively, into the circulation during dehydration. The initial observations were that the rate of neural lobe vasopressin depletion[93] and neurophysin depletion[87] were low relative to the stores, as was the vasopressin-repletion rate during rehydration.[93] However, I have already remarked above that the heterozygous animal displays symptoms of chronic stimulation of the neurosecretory system. Plasma levels of vasopressin in the heterozygote are probably about 75% as high as in the normal animal, when allowed water *ad libitum.*[94] They rise considerably on dehydration in both genotypes, with heterozygotes having a plasma level of 50% of normal animals.[94] Assuming that the rate of breakdown of hormone in plasma is proportional to its concentration,[95] this implies that the rate of release of hormone in these animals is also about 50% of normal. Taken together, these results are entirely consistent with the view that the synthetic capacity of heterozygotes for vasopressin is 50% of normal, the higher osmotic stimulation of heterozygotes even when hydrated resulting in a secretion rate of 75% of normal and a pituitary repletion rate of less than 50% during rehydration. The results for neurophysin cannot be adequately evaluated in the absence of accurate data permitting estimation of synthesis and secretion rates during dehydration, preferably parallel with observations on vasopressin. In general though, the synthetic rate of neurophysin A parallels that of vasopressin.[86,87] Thus, the *release* of vasopressin and neurophysin does not seem to be defective in relation to the synthetic capability of the animals. The observations on the percentage changes during depletion of the stores could be explained by the existence of the "readily releasable" pools of both hormone and neurophysin in the neural lobe of unstressed animals;[19-21] the already-stressed heterozygote would not be expected to release the same proportion of its store as the normal animal when dehydrated. Therefore, I do not find the evidence for a defect in the release of either vasopressin or neurophysin A at all compelling.

Where, then, does the primary defect lie? Present information only permits speculation; the possibilities have been clearly outlined by Valtin.[9] The complete absence of detectable vasopressin or neurophysin in affected neurones, even in the hypothalamus and even with very sensitive techniques, argues against the suggestion of a defect either in packaging within the neurosecretory granules and consequent rapid enzymatic breakdown or in the enzymatic cleavage of precursor to yield neurophysin A and vasopressin.[96] In either case, the same defect would have to affect vasotocin synthesis in the pineal,[39] but not the synthesis of oxytocin in the same nuclei of the hypothalamus.

The absence of neurosecretory granules is perhaps more likely to be a secondary consequence of the absence of neurophysin.[71] Accepting the common precursor theory, and considering that there is no evidence for any effect on cell differentiation apart from that on precursor synthesis, it seems that the primary effect is in the synthesis of the precursor.[71] Thus, the Brattleboro gene could be a regulatory or structural mutant of the precursor-determining genetic locus.[9] It is unlikely to be a regulatory mutant unlinked to the structural gene acting through a diffusible product and affecting transcription, translation, or incorporation into neurosecretory granules, if it is accepted that 50% of normal levels of the primary polypeptide products are found in the heterozygote with comparable osmotic stimulation. This would not be expected with such a mutant except by chance. This is unfortunate, as such a regulatory mutant might also have explained the absence of vasotocin from the pineal. If the absence of vasotocin from the pineal is taken as definite (a crucial point), then this also rules out otherwise feasible ideas that the mutation might be in an initiator, operator, promoter,[97] or other closely linked regulatory mutant of the kind claimed in other eukaryotic systems;[98-101] or that it might cause premature chain termination of precursor synthesis. Not only is there little evidence in mammalian systems for such regulatory loci controlling more than one structural locus, but in the present case there is no evidence for coordinate snythesis within any one cell of vasopressin and vasotocin. However, if the vasotocin- and vasopressin-precursor loci have evolved from a more primitive vasotocin locus by tandem gene duplication during the evolution of the early mammals, these loci may well be closely linked.[9] I, therefore, retreat to the mammalian geneticist's last resort and suggest that the primary defect is a very small deletion covering both structural loci — a last resort, because it is unsatisfactory to have to explain a single syndrome in terms of two primary effects.[3]

f. Other Uses of Brattleboro Rats

Many studies have made use of Brattleboro rats as experimental tools, in elucidating the role of vasopressin in various physiological systems. It is particularly useful to have animals with a specific defect in vasopressin synthesis, which is not affected in other ways (unlike, for example, a hypophysectomized animal); although it must always be borne in mind that a primary defect may result in secondary, and unexpectedly far-reaching, consequences, and also, as discussed above, that the primary defect is not completely understood.

One example, of potential practical utility relevant to the preceding sections, will be discussed first to illustrate an important methodological point. Tasso's group,[102] using cytochemical methods that are believed to detect glycoproteins at the ultrastructural level, demonstrated two distinct types of secretory neurones within the neural lobe and within the hypothalamic magnocellular nuclei of Sprague-Dawley rats. In homozygous Brattleboro rats, there were, however, no neurones containing reactive granules, and it was, therefore, proposed that the reactivity was associated with vasopressin- (and presumably neurophysin A) containing granules, oxytocin being stored in nonreactive granules. This is a plausible idea, and when more is known about the specificity of the cytochemical stains, it may be of considerable importance. Unfortunately, there is an alternative explanation; rats of the Brattleboro strain might differ from Sprague-Dawley animals in their biochemical properties, quite apart from the diabetes insipidus gene. This may seem fairly improbable, but the point is that a much more unequivocal result could easily have been obtained by the simple expedient of comparison with homozygous normal and heterozygous animals from the same strain (Long-Evans) instead of the Sprague-Dawley strain.

An illustrative list of some of the uses of Brattleboro animals follows. The question of whether chlorpropamide has a direct renal effect in potentiating the action of vasopressin or acts by stimulating vasopressin-release (even from patients with hypothalamic diabetes insipidus, who often have only a partial deficiency of vasopressin) was investigated with contrasting interpretations.[104-106] The role of vasopressin in sodium balance, during sodium depletion, or more normal circumstances has been examined, and it is suggested that vasopressin might have some action in the loop of Henle, such as increasing sodium transport in the ascending limb.[106-108] The independence of lanthanum-tight junctions of the renal collecting duct from vasopressin has been studied.[109] The Brattleboro homozygous animal has been examined in studies of the renal handling of lithium[110,111] and has also been used as a bioassay subject for vasopressin as an antidiuretic hormone.[112-115] Homozygotes appear to suffer from a renal defect in concentrating ability, which is probably a developmental consequence of the lack of vasopressin, perhaps mediated by K^+ deficiency in affected animals.[116-118] The possibility of such secondary damage complicates the interpretation of results[106] and is a drawback of the use of severely affected genetic variants, rather than variation within normality.

The relationships between the adrenal gland, pituitary, and kidney with respect to water and electrolyte metabolism have been examined,[119-121] as has the plasma renin response to vasopressin.[122] Significant evidence for a physiological role for vasopressin in the mitotic response of bone marrow cells to hemorrhage has been produced.[123] This would represent an interesting complementary effect to that on blood pressure in response to the same stimulus, which may also be of physiological significance.[124,125]

A variety of studies on the nervous system have been reported. Wooten and colleagues[126] describe an inhibitory effect of vasopressin on the release of dopamine-β-hydroxylase from sympathetic nerves in the adrenal medulla, but believe that this may be an indirect effect mediated by the influence of intravascular volume on sympathetic nerve activity. This case highlights the need for genetic studies to be combined with a range of physiological and pharmacological techniques. De Wied and his coworkers[127-129] report a wide range of behavioral differences between Brattleboro homozygotes, heterozygotes, and normal animals, including sleep, memory, passive avoidance, open-field activity, and threshold to electric shock. These are attributed to vasopressin, but the possibility that these effects may be due to either a deficiency in the secretion of vasotocin into the cerebrospinal fluid[130-133] or to indirect effects such as the influence of plasma electrolytes[116] on nerves must also be considered.

This gives an indication of the extraordinarily wide range of experiments in which Brattleboro animals have been used.

III. ACTIONS AND BREAKDOWN OF NEUROHYPOPHYSIAL HORMONES

A. Sites of Variation in the Actions Octapeptide Hormones

1. The Actions of Octapeptide Hormones

The octapeptide hormones have a wide variety of actions. In mammals, oxytocin seems to be involved in the control of uterine contractions during parturition[77,78,134] and in the neuroendocrine reflex of milk ejection (by action on the myoepithelium of the mammary gland) during lactation.[135] The principal role of vasopressin in mammals and vasotocin in birds seems to be as an antidiuretic hormone,[136,138] but it may also be important as a vasoconstrictor in some circumstances.[24,124,139] Other actions, such as effects on lipid and carbohydrate metabolism, may also be significant.[140] In the lower vertebrates, the actions of the octapeptides are not as well understood,[138,141] However, in the amphibians vasotocin is the effective water balance principle, acting on skin and bladder to affect sodium transport and water permeability. Vasotocin may also be active on the oviduct of lower vetebrates.[142] Clearly, the well-known actions in mammals are the more amenable to genetical investigations; the antidiuretic action of vasopressin is discussed separately in Section III.B.

2. Possible Sites of Genetic Variation

Variation in the response of a target organ to endogenous or exogenous hormone can be due to an alteration in a wide range of parameters. Thus, apparent strain differences in the sensitivity of mice[4] and rats[143] to intraperitoneal and intravenous injections of vasopressin as an antidiuretic agent could be attributable to variation in the absorption of the hormone into the circulation, binding to plasma proteins, interaction with the renal receptors, the structure of the kidney, or the rate of inactivation of the vasopressin by kidney and liver. To add to the complexity of the situation, some of these factors could be assessed by a variety of methods at different organizational levels. Thus, the hormone-receptor affinity of different octapeptides could in principle be investigated by direct measurements of binding with isolated receptors[144,145] or with tubule fragments in vitro.[146,147] by the degree of adenyl cyclase activation,[148] by measurement of the tubular antidiuresis in vitro,[149] or by the relative antidiuretic potencies of the octapeptide hormones in the whole animal. This situation is analyzed in more detail below. Individual difference in the antidiuretic response are known in man, could be genetically determined, and are medically important in hypothalamic diabetes insipidus (whether of genetic or environmental origin.)[150]

In comparison with the effort expended on the antidiuretic action of mammals, knowledge in other areas is scanty. Resistance to hepatic actions of vasopressin in inhibiting fatty acid and cholesterol synthesis has been claimed in obese *(ob/ob)* mice and may throw some light on the primary defect in these animals.[140] Oxytocin could be involved in parameters of importance in the breeding of dairy cattle, such as the completeness of milking, and further studies in this area are indicated.[151]

3. Receptor Studies with Oxytocin

The characterization of oxytocin receptors seems to be an area where genetics could make a contribution. Oxytocin receptors can be characterized (in the traditional pharmacological way) by the relative responsiveness of the target organ to a variety of different analogues[152] or by the extent to which such analogues are bound. Variation in the spectrum of responses might be found if strains differ in the molecular structure of the receptor-sites or in the proportion of two types of receptor with different affinities, but variation in the morphological structure of the organ could not itself cause such variation. Evidence that the strains differed at a single genetic locus affecting the receptors might then be obtained from a segregating generation. Such variation could be useful in two ways. First, attempts to isolate receptors[153] would be authenticated if the isolated receptors were controlled by the same gene. Second, it is difficult to know whether the oxytocin receptors in different target organs (uterus and mammary myoepithelium) are identical or not, as the different milieus could well affect their pharmacological characterization.[154] However, a demonstration that they were controlled by the same gene would again overcome this problem. In principle, these concepts could also be applied to vasopressin but the problems of characterizing the receptors of such an anatomically and functionally complex organ as the mammalian kidney are greater than for smooth muscle.

B. Vasopressin as the Antidiuretic Hormone

1. Antidiuretic Assays, Adenyl Cyclase, and the Renal Inactivation of Vasopressin

a. Preliminary Observations

Much work on the effects of vasopressin in the intact animal has been done using the whole-animal antidiuretic assay.[155] The experimental subject is water-loaded, and the degree of hydration is usually then kept constant: once water diuresis is established, the effects of intravenous injections of hormones on urine flow, conductivity, inulin clearance, or related parameters are monitored. Animals of the same genotype often vary considerably in their sensitivity to vasopressin for unknown reasons (perhaps such variables as the osmotic gradient into the renal medulla are important), so that this parameter may not always be very useful. The more specific character of relative potencies of different analogues — especially AVP and LVP — which is not affected by such variables is, therefore, often used.[156] The potency of a hormone can empirically be measured in a number of ways, including the maximum percentage decrease in the rate of urine flow (equivalent to the conductivity increase for a tubular antidiuresis) or by the percentage fall in the total urine flow over a set period following the injection. This latter parameter depends on the duration of the antidiuretic response, as well as its intensity. The choice of parameter does not much matter if a hormone is being standardized against another sample of the same chemical form (except with regard to statistical efficiency). However, different analogues vary in both these parameters, so that their relative potencies even in defined animals may vary considerably according to the criteria which are chosen. Log-dose/response curves for AVP and LVP are often nonparallel. Clearly, if relative potency is to be of critical use as a character, the situation requires further analysis.[156]

An alternative approach is to look at major defects in the antidiuretic response, so that the variation between individuals of the same genotype in their antidiuretic responses is smaller than the variation between genotypes. Such variation is discussed in section III.B.2 below.

b. A Model for the Hormone-Receptor Interaction in Antidiuretic Assays

As noted above, vasopressin analogues (notably AVP and LVP) differ not just in the intensity of the antidiureses induced by equimolar doses, but in the duration of the response to doses which induce an antidiuresis of the same initial intensity. However, this is not related to the half-life of the vasopressin in the plasma; it has repeatedly been observed that AVP promotes an antidiuresis of longer duration than LVP in the rat, despite the fact that it is cleared more rapidly from the circulation.[156] In addition, the half-life of the antidiuretic response is longer than the half-life of the hormone in plasma.[26,95,156] If one accepts that cyclic AMP acts as a second messenger to mediate the effects of the hormone, and the action of the hormone is confined to its interaction with the membrane receptor, which in turn activates adenyl cyclase on the serosal surface of the cell,[157] neither can the difference in duration of antidiuresis be due to an effect on the breakdown of cAMP within the cell. Again, because the antidiuretic effect commences rapidly and persists after the hormone levels have dropped, the magnitude of the response in the system is not likely to depend on the *rate* of formation or breakdown of the hormone-receptor complex. Thus, the difference in the duration of antidiuresis probably results from differences in the hormone-receptor interaction and in particular the stability of the hormone-receptor complex.[156] The relevant factors may be represented in a crude model of the hormone-receptor interactions in an antidiuretic assay, which contains many simplifying assumptions[48] (see DeHaven and Shapiro).[158]

The number of hormone-receptor complexes, [HR], will be governed by reaction parameters such as k_1 and k_2:

$$[H] + [R] \xrightarrow{k_1} [HR] \xrightarrow{k_2} [H^*] + [R]$$

where [H] is the plasma hormone concentration entering the kidney, [R] the number of unoccupied receptors, and [H*] represents the form in which the hormone leaves the receptor (whether active or inactive). Ignoring possible cooperative or interfering effects and taking k_1 and k_2 to be constant, the net rate of formation of hormone-receptor complexes will be given by:

$$\frac{d[HR]}{dt} = [H]\ [R]\ k_1 - [HR]\ k_2 \qquad (1)$$

It may also be assumed that, after the initial hormone dose has been given, the plasma hormone concentration will decline exponentially:

$$[H] = H_1 e^{-k_3 t} \qquad (2)$$

where H_1 is the initial hormone concentration. Further, if the total number of hormone-receptors is $[R_T]$, and this remains constant for the duration of the assay, then:

$$[R_T] = [R] + [HR] \qquad (3)$$

Substituting for [R] and [H] in Equation 1 yields:

$$\frac{d[HR]}{dt} = [H]\ k_1([R_T] - [HR]) - [HR]\ k_2 \qquad (4)$$

$$= k_1 H_1{}^{-k_3 t}([R_T] - [HR]) - [HR]\ k_2$$

This rather cumbersome equation can be solved analytically in the form of a convergent infinite series by the substitution $t_1 = e^{-kt}$, when it is related to Bernoulli's equation. Of more practical interest, it can also be solved by numerical methods on the computer. Various approaches can now be taken. It is now becoming technically feasible to measure k_1 and k_2, at least in vitro on isolated tubules and perhaps on isolated receptor preparations.[144-147] Further, methods for measuring k_3 are also available.[95] The relation between the number of hormone-receptor complexes formed and the degree of adenyl cyclase activation for different analogues is also amenable to study.[146] The intrinsic activities of AVP and LVP as judged by adenyl cyclase activition do not appear to differ.[148] The relationship between adenyl cyclase activation and antidiuretic activity may be complex, at any rate for larger doses of vasopressin (especially if the increased permeability of the tubules and consequent water flow results in significant diminution of the osmotic gradient), even if the relation between cAMP concentrations and tubule permeability is simple. However, even this relationship will probably yield to study eventually.[152]

For the time being, a simplistic approach ignoring these complexities can be taken to arrive at some qualitative conclusions. Approximate values for k_2 and k_3 are known directly[95,146,147] and support the suggestion in the initial discussion of this problem that k_2 must be small, relative to k_3. (Note that this conclusion will not necessarily apply to all analogues, e.g., carba-vasopressin analogues which apparently have a high degree of metabolic stability.[159]) For the naturally occurring hormones under these conditions, the following simplified generalizations may be made: (1) the half-life of the decay in the number of receptors occupied is effectively determined by k_2 and (2) the maximum number of receptors occupied is determined primarily by the ratio k_1/k_2 (the hormone-receptor affinity), but is also affected by k_3 insofar as this determines the hormone concentration at the time of this maximum.[48] Hence, it can be concluded that the antidiuretic potency of hormones, as conventionally tested by the antidiuretic response over a period of time, is influenced as much by k_2 as by the hormone-receptor affinity.

It is interesting to compare this with the situation where the hormone is infused continuously into the circulation. In this equilibrium situation, the hormone concentration will depend strongly on k_3 (with the proviso that since the hormone cannot diffuse out of the circulation into other fluid compartments, k_3 may be smaller in this situation than in a conventional antidiuretic assay). The number of hormone-receptor sites occupied will again depend on the hormone-receptor affinity, k_1/k_2, but k_2 will have no independent effect. Thus, this situation, especially if the plasma hormone concentration could be monitored, would be much more directly comparable to the dose-response curves obtained for in vitro adenyl-cyclase activation. Such antidiuretic assays, though difficult, are feasible.[160] It is hard to say which situation will more accurately reflect the situation with respect to the endogenous secretion of vasopressin under natural conditions, as there is some evidence that the secretion of vasopressin may, like that of oxytocin, be episodic.

c. Quantitative Genetic Variation in the Antidiuretic Response

Stewart, using the crude technique of intraperitoneal injections of very large doses of LVP, observed strain differences in the effect on the kinetics of water and electrolyte excretion after water-loading in mice.[4] Kar et al. reported differences in the sensitivity of rats of vasopressin as an antidiuretic agent.[143] Such variation could be due to factors such as the rates of absorption and breakdown of vasopressin, or to differences in kidney structure, which are known to exist between strains. This situation has not been adequately analyzed, and, indeed, there has been no systematic genetic study of the clearance rates of octapeptides in normal animals. However, an attempt has been made to ascertain the relative sensitivities of both CBA/FaCam and Peru mice to AVP and LVP by intravenous injection. The use of relative sensitivity at once eliminates the effect of variation in kidney structure, for example, as this would affect the action of both hormones equally. It was reported that Peru mice were relatively more responsive to LVP than CAB/FaCam mice, but that the LVP was nevertheless slightly less active than AVP in Peru animals. There was no difference in these assays in the duration of antidiureses of equal intensity induced by AVP and LVP and log-dose/response curves were parallel.[161] However, the experiments on the Peru animals were technically difficult because of the inhibition of diuresis in them by any form of stress. Only a small proportion of the experimental animals gave satisfactory results, so it is believed the results must be treated with considerable caution. Nevertheless, this approach should be extended in the future and a wider range of animals and analogues could profitably be used in the genetical and pharmacological characterization of the renal hormone-receptor system.

A lack of correlation has been observed between the antidiuretic and natriuretic effects of vasopressin in different strains of mice.[4] The natriuretic effect of vasopressin is often claimed to be a secondary consequence of the water retention that results from its antidiuretic effect. However, Morel observed that different analogues differed in their effects on electrolyte excretion even when the degree of water-loading was controlled, suggesting that different sets of renal receptors may mediate the two responses.[160] Either explanation would be compatible with the genetic differences in the reltionship between the antidiuretic and natriuretic effects: in the one case if the strains differ in their response to changes in extracellular fluid volume, in the other if they differ in the proportions of the two types of receptor. The genetic variation should provide good material for further investigation of this problem.

d. The Significance of Renal Inactivation of Vasopressin

Vasopressin is inactivated largely by the liver and the kidney.[95] The topic is raised here because the hypothesis that the hormone is inactivated in the kidney as a result of its interaction with the receptor molecule, rather than by a separate enzymatic system, has been suggested. Smith, working in the rat, found a positive correlation between the rates of inactivation of various octapeptide analogues by kidney slices in vitro and their in vivo antidiuretic potencies.[162] On the other hand, incubation of hormone with an adenyl cyclase membrane fraction resulted in enzyme activation, but not in hormone breakdown.[163] This may be because of the relatively small amount of tissue present the usual ionic environment, or the rather short period of incubation compared with that used in inactivation experiments. The question is an important one, because if this theory is correct, analysis of the breakdown products of vasopressin could provide information about the way in which the hormone interacts with the receptor.

Stewart[16] incubated mouse-kidney slices from different strains with AVP and LVP according to the method of Smith[162] and measured their rates of inactivation. Inactivation was approximately log-linear; AVP was inactivated about twice as quickly as LVP by kidneys from CBA/FaCam and A/Cam mice, but Peru kidney slices inactivated both hormones at the same rate. As with the results of other workers described above, there is a correlation (in this case, genetic) between the potency of a hormone and its rate of inactivation. This provides the material for a test of whether this genetic correlation is a causal one by examining individual animals of a genetically segregating generation such as a backcross (or recombinant inbred strains) for their antidiuretic sensitivities to, and their rates of inactivation of, the two hormones. If both variables are affected by the same gene (presumably determining the hormone receptor), then the correlation will be maintained, but if there are different physiological (and hence genetic) systems, the correlations will disappear. However, before this is attempted, a more critical look at the theoretical factors must be taken. It has generally been assumed, on the basis of the hypothesis, that a positive correlation between the in vivo antidiuretic assays and in vitro rates of inactivation is to be expected. Leaving aside factors that might affect the in vitro system requiring further investigation, such as the influence of the ionic composition of the incubation medium, this is not necessarily reasonable. Under the conditions of an inactivation experiment, using the previous notation:

the rate of [HR] formation, and A = rate of [HR] breakdown,

$$\therefore A = k_1\,[H]\,[R] = k_2\,[HR]$$

Hence,

$$\frac{1}{A} = \frac{1}{[R_T]}\left(\frac{1}{k_2} + \frac{1}{k_1\,[H]}\right) \qquad (5)$$

This equation is very different in form from Equation 4. In particular, the affinity (k_1/k_2) is not important in itself, whereas the magnitudes of k_1 and k_2 are, and a smaller value of k_2, which would lead to a *more intense and prolonged* antidiuresis in vivo, should also result in a *lower* rate of inactivation in vitro, if the same receptors are involved. However, larger values of k_1 would increase both in vivo potency and in vitro inactivation and would provide the basis of a positive correlation between them. Thus, the type of correlation to be expected depends on which of the two parameters is varying between strains and between analogues. Thorn and Willumsen[164] did not find AVP to be inactivated more rapidly than LVP in rats. However, it is clear that this result does not disprove the hypothesis as k_2 probably varies between AVP and LVP in this system.[156] Some methodological problems raised by them, such as possible interference by impurities, are of little importance in a geneticstudy, as they are unlikely to be the cause of a genetic difference, but measurements of k_1, k_2, and k_3 are necessary in any critical genetic test of the hypothesis. There are several reports which lend some support to the hypothesis. Dicker and Eggleton[165] found that a larger proportion of exogenous vasopressin is excreted in the urine of patients with inherited nephrogenic diabetes insipidus than by normal subjects. If the binding and action of antidiuretic hormone is blocked, either by low pH or by SH blockers, then the inactivation of vasopressin is also inhibited.[166-168] It is also relevant to note that there is considerable inactivation of oxytocin by the mammary glands of lactating rats, but not in nonlactating animals.[169,170] The hypothesis deserves further investigation, using more sophisticated genetic and experimental methods.[164,171]

e. The Role of Adenyl Cyclase

It is widely held that the antidiuretic action of vasopressin on mammalian kidney is mediated by adenosine 3′,5′-cyclic phosphate (cAMP), acting as a second messenger (in a manner yet to be determined)[172,173] as a result of the activation of membrane-bound adenyl cyclase by the hormone-receptor complex in the distal convoluted tubular and collecting ducts.[157,174-178] The evidence for this has often been reviewed (but see Thorn for a critical view),[179] and consists basically of the observations that:

1. Vasopressin-responsive adenyl cyclase can be found in appropriate regions of the kidney, notably the medullary collecting ducts.
2. Vasopressin administration increases the levels of intracellular cAMP.
3. cAMP and its analogues, as well as theophylline and similar substances which inhibit the breakdown of cAMP, mimic the effect of vasopressin.

It must be admitted that evidence of this sort is much more compelling for the action of vasotocin (or, more often, vasopressin!) on an isolated toad bladder than it is in such an anatomically and physiologically complex organ as the mammalian kidney. In recent years, however, techniques for studying isolated tubules have improved considerably.[144-149]

Attempts to correlate the antidiuretic potency of analogues (especially AVP and LVP) in vivo with the degree of adenyl cyclase activation in vitro have been made in a variety of species.[148] In the rat, Douša and colleagues[148] found that AVP and LVP had the same intrinsic activity for adenyl cyclase activation, but the affinity of AVP was about six times as high as that of LVP. They suggest that this correlates well with the longer duration of action of AVP. (In terms of the analysis in Section III.B.1.b above, though, the correlation should be with the intensity of the antidiuresis, not its duration, where AVP is perhaps 1.5 times as potent as LVP in molar terms).

In the pig, they found that LVP had two or more times the affinity of AVP,[148] and this is confirmed by other workers:[163] again, they claim that this correlates with the antidiuretic potencies of these analogues in vivo. However, as pointed out by Heller and Spickett,[12] the only in vivo study, carried out on miniature pigs by Munsick et al.,[180] reported the results not in terms of molarities, but of rat pressor units: when correction is made for this, LVP is perhaps slightly less potent than AVP.[12,136] On the basis of their argument with the rat, Douša et al.[148] would presumably expect LVP to have a longer lasting action than AVP, but it is clear that it does not. (My analysis would not necessarily predict a longer antidiuresis for LVP, but whatever interpretation is adopted, it should be internally consistent.) It would be profitable to examine adenyl cyclase activity in the dog, which provides a third sort of situation where the hormones have equal durations of action, but AVP provokes a more intense antidiuresis than LVP.

In the future, in vivo and in vitro studies should preferably be carried out by the same group on the same animals with the same hormone preparations. It might be argued, apart from such methodological problems, that the difference in levels between the whole animal and the renal homogenate is so great that good correlations are not to be expected. If this is true, though, claims that this sort of evidence supports the adenyl cyclase activation theory as the mode of vasopressin action and that it can be used in arguments about the evolution of hormonal receptors and their specificity[148,177] are specious. A demonstration that the same genetic factors affected both systems could overcome some of these objections.

In a genetic study of the activation of renal medullary adenyl cyclase by AVP and LVP, Stewart found that AVP and LVP had the same intrinsic activity and that AVP had a higher affinity than LVP in both CBA/FaCam and Peru mice: the ratio of affinities was higher in Peru mice than in CBA/FaCam mice.[181] Thus, the situation is amenable to genetical investigation. Comparing this with the in vivo results described in Section III.B.1.c above, there is a good correlation for the CBA/FaCam mice, but this breaks down with the Peru animals, where LVP has a low affinity in vitro but a relatively high potency in vivo. As previously indicated, the in vivo studies are not definitive, but it is nevertheless worth considering what a real discrepancy of this sort would mean. There are a number of possible explanations. For example, vasopressin might have some action, apart from that on tubular water permeability, mediated by adenyl cyclase (such as the action on sodium transport in the ascending limb of the loop of Henle as suggested by Morel's group, perhaps related to the natriuretic effect of octapeptides)[106-108,160,182-185] or the antidiuretic effect, like the hepatic actions of vasopressin[140] and the actions of oxytocin on reproductive organs, might not be wholly mediated by cAMP. Alternatively, it may be significant that the levels of vasopressin used to stimulate adenyl cyclase in vitro are usually much higher than endogenous concentrations, so that the activated adenyl cyclase could represent the result of stimulation of relatively low affinity, physiologically insignificant receptors.[136] The unusual ionic conditions in the renal medulla might also be important. Some of these possibilities are physiologically interesting. To the extent that they eventually need to be invoked, however, they may also make the initial circumstantial evidence for cAMP as the second messenger in the antidiuretic effect less compelling.

Douša found that the diabetes insipidus (DI) mice, a strain apparently suffering from true tubular nephrogenic diabetes insipidus (see Section III.B.2 for a description of their origin), show significant deficiencies in their maximal adenyl cyclase activation (of about 23% in DI nonsevere animals and 41% in DI severe animals) as compared with controls.[186,187] There is, thus, a significant correlation between the maximal adenyl cyclase activities and the urine osmolalities, and computer simulation has indicated that the decrease in adenyl cyclase activity could be sufficient to cause the defect in urinary concentrating ability.[71] Further genetic analysis in a segregating generation such as a backcross (or recombinant inbred strains) could provide definitive evidence that it is indeed the same genetic factor in these rather heterogenous strains that leads to both the decrease in maximal adenyl cyclase activity and the defect in urinary concentrating ability. This would come close to proof that cAMP is the second messenger in the antidiuretic action of vasopressin. However, preliminary results indicate that there is *no* correlation between these parameters in the segregating backcross generation.[220] The relevance of these findings to the human syndrome of nephrogenic diabetes insipidus is indicated by the observation of a similar defect in adenyl cyclase activation in man.[188,189]

2. Nephrogenic Diabetes Insipidus

a. The Variety of Defects

As with hypothalamic diabetes insipidus, renal concentrating defects[190] can occur from a wide variety of causes, affecting different aspects of the functioning of the kidney.[63] For example, the ability to create an adequate osmotic gradient into the renal medulla is as important as the ability of the distal tubules and collecting ducts to become water-permeable in response to vasopressin and thus utilize the gradient to produce concentrated urine. The primary effect can even be an obstruction of the urinary tract, leading to kidney damage.[191-193] Inherited nephrogenic diabetes insipidus of various types have been reported; the true form of the disease, apparently characterized by insensitivity of the renal tubule to vasopressin, rare in humans, is probably inherited as a sex-linked disease (for a review, see Grassi).[190] It has been possible to trace the origin of the disease in North America to passengers aboard a single ship, the Hopewell, which landed in Halifax during 1761.[194,195] A concentrating defect in the Gunn strain of rats, inherited as a recessive trait, is a secondary consequence of renal parenchymal damage caused by massive crystalline deposits in the papilla and medulla, in turn associated with the persistent unconjugated hyperbilrubinemia due to congenital absence of hepatic glucuronyl transferase.[196] This is a good example of the manifold pleiotropic effects of a single locus variant.[3] Lyon and Hulse have reported an inherited kidney disease, due to the gene *kd*.[197] This results in a syndrome very similar to nephronopthisis in man and can also result in vasopressin-resistant polydipsia and polyuria. Several examples of nephrogenic diabetes insipidus increasing in severity with age are known in various strains of mice, with females being more severely affected.[198-200] In no case is the primary cause of the defect or the mode of inheritance known; Virgo and Miller ruled out amyloid kidneys, polycycstic kidneys, diabetes mellitus, and nephronophthisis, but suggested hypokalemia, hypercalcemia, or the action of a nephrotoxic substance as possibilities.[200] Autoimmune disease should probably be included in this list.

b. Oligosyndactyly (Os) in the Mouse

The most complex story is that of the nephrogenic diabetes insipidus initially associated with the dominant gene *Os* (oligosyndactyly)[201] in the mouse.[202-204] Stewart and Stewart suggested that this was a secondary consequence of a fivefold reduction in the number of nephrons in the kidneys of affected (*Os*/+) animals compared with normal (+/+) sibs, which was found at[204] and before[48] birth. This would lead to compensatory hypertrophy of the renal tubules, an increased filtration rate in turn causing an increased osmotic load on the tubules, a deficiency in formation of the medullary osmotic gradient, and an inability to respond effectively to vasopressin.[205,206] On this hypothesis, there is no need to invoke a lack of response to vasopressin at the level of the nephron. The hypothesis is supported by later experiments where subtotal nephrectomy of perinatal mice of the same strain resulted in a phenocopy of virtually the entire syndrome.[207] Similar results after nephrectomy have often been reported in man and in experimental animals.[208] A similar renal syndrome has recently been reported in man.[209]

c. The DI Strains

If this were the whole of the matter, this example, like the other animal models described, might be relevant to medical problems, but it would not relate directly to the renal action of vasopressin. However, the severity of the effects of the *Os* gene differed considerably in different genetic backgrounds, ranging from the mild in the original background to the very severe when segregating in the so-called DI strain.[204] Significantly, the +/+ animals of the original DI strain themselves showed a mild concentrating defect. Detailed examination has shown that the DI strain differs from the original heterogeneous strain in a number of renal characteristics, including the reduced length of the loop of Henle, the relative absence of pars recta, and a reduced tubular response to vasopressin.[204,207,210] These effects are the result of different genes segregating and some of these effects are only observed in *Os*/+ animals (i.e., there is an epistatic interaction).[16,207] Stewart, studying the correlation of some of these characters with urinary concentrating ability in a segregating generation, found that the length of the loop of Henle had a large effect, as might be expected, whereas the variation in the presence or absence of the pars recta did not have the functional consequences that might have been predicted.[207] (However, the same might not be true if a different criterion, such as spontaneous drinking, had been chosen.) It therefore seems clear that the really severe diabetes insipidus seen in DI *Os*/+ animals results from the physiological and developmental interaction of a number of different genetic factors. It is rather extraordinary that these genetic factors should all have accumulated in the DI strain; the most probable explanation, especially in the quantitative-genetics laboratory where the defect was first noticed,[202] is that there was selection (whether conscious or unconscious) for increased severity of the trait over several generations in the heterogeneous stock used to maintain the *Os* mutant. Valtin reports that the DI stock is itself heterogeneous and has been selected for mild and severe forms of the syndrome.[71,210] However this may be, the different genetic factors must all have been present in the original and ordinary strains, demonstrating the degree of variation present in them; the *Os* gene merely helped to reveal it in a more critical situation (see Rendel[211] and Fraser et al.[212] for similar examples of the effect of a major disturbance in revealing buffered genetic variation).

The effect on the tubular resonse to vasopressin has naturally attracted particular attention, especially with reference to models of the mode of action of vasopressin (see Section III.B.1.e on adenyl cyclase).

d. *Adenyl Cyclase Variants in Man*

There are possibly two forms of human nephrogenic diabetes insipidus. Some workers find no increase in cAMP production after vasopressin administration,[188] but others[189] do, implying that the defect in the latter form affects the ability to respond to a second messenger. Care must be taken in interpreting results of in vivo experiments, but if two forms of the disease do exist, there must presumably be two loci on the X-chromosome involved in the renal tubular response to vasopressin, one concerned with the production of a second messenger and the other with the response to a second messenger. Since X-linked loci in one mammalian species are frequently X-linked in others, further genetic characterization of the first form of defect, apparently found in the DI strains of mouse (Sections III.B.1.e and III.B.2.c above), will be worthwhile.

IV. EVOLUTIONARY ASPECTS

A. Hormone Structure

1. *General Considerations*

The existence of genetic variation immediately suggests fundamental questions in population genetics: what is the origin of the variation, how is it maintained in natural populations, and what are its evolutionary implications?[13,14] Population genetics has a well-developed mathematical theory; there is now an increasing interest in defining the biochemical and physiological effects of variant genetic loci and considering the selective pressures to which these might or might not lead in different ecological situations. Here, the relationships between the different components of an endocrine system have to be considered. The effect of a particular gene substitution (say, leading to the synthesis of LVP rather than AVP) on the whole animal will depend on the physiological interaction of the gene product with the products of other loci — for example, the alternative forms of the hormonal receptor which might be present in the population. In some circumstances this physiological interaction could lead to nonadditive selective interactions between the two loci.[14,213] Genetic variation in the endocrine system of the posterior pituitary has some potential for experimental studies of this kind.

This discussion is necessarily restricted to what is often called, for the sake of convenience, "normal" variation; that is variation within natural populations or between strains of animals derived from natural populations, as opposed to a variant causing a major defect in the system so great that it seems obvious that natural selection would reduce it to a very low frequency (e.g., the Brattleboro gene and its effect on the mole-ratio of vasopressin to oxytocin). However, the origin of the DI strain of mice (Section III.B.2.c) shows that the distinction is rather arbitrary.

2. The Evolution of Structure

Quite a large number of evolutionary schemes have been constructed for the octapeptide hormones on the basis of their phylogenetic distribution.[9,12,28-32] These have become more complicated with time as detailed knowledge has created problems (for example, the origin of aspartocin).[9] In general, the implications of genetic polymorphism have not been considered except perhaps as a confusing irritant. However, while some schemes may seem more probable than others, if polymorphism is at all common this could mean that it is sometimes theoretically impossible to deduce which hormone is derived from which. For example, AVT, MT, and OT can all be interconverted by single base changes in DNA, so that polymorphism of OT and MT would mean that controversy as to which hormone is the older is pointless.[17] (This dilemma arises with the octapeptide hormones because of their small size and the resultant paucity of alternative biologically active analogues.) Very often the criterion (whether explicit or not)[9] for choosing between alternative evolutionary schemes has been the notion that the simpler scheme must be the more probable. This seems to motivate both Acher's suggestion of a linear progression up the phylogenetic tree from an ancestral molecule through isotocin and mesotocin to oxytocin,[28] as well as the suggestion by Pickering and Heller[32] that the elasmobranchs and the bony fish might have a common evolutionary origin off the main line of vertebrate evolution to account for their common possession of [4-ser]-analogues. Even on the most complicated schemes, though, the rate of evolution of the neutral octapeptides (in terms of amino acid substitutions per codon per unit time) is not unduly high compared with the known rates of evolution of other polypeptides,[14] so there seems little rational basis for this criterion. The main use of evolutionary schemes for these hormones may be to help in the identification of possible evolutionary intermediates, as yet unobserved. There are, however, two interesting features. AVT seems to have remained unchanged throughout the vertebrates (except perhaps the pig), and this represents an unique example of evolutionary stability. Second, gene duplication has apparently occurred, allowing the evolution of the separate neutral and basic octapeptide lines.[9,30,214] Further gene duplication may have occurred in the early mammals, permitting the separate evolution of vasotocins and vasopressins. This argument carries with it the corollary that the possession of two genetic loci rather than one coding for the same octapeptide did not confer a significant evolutionary disadvantage.

The polymorphism of vasopressin in the feral Suina is unusually interesting because it is present in so many quite distinct species that it is clearly very old (like polymorphisms of the blood groups in chimpanzees and man). Although the argument can not be quantified, this clearly implies that the polymorphism is not transient (either in the sense of one allele being replaced by another conferring a selective advantage or in the sense of selectively neutral alleles drifting in the populations), but is maintained by some form of balancing selection such as heterozygous advantage. Further discussion requires a consideration of the restraints operating to determine the selective forces acting on the alleles.

3. Constraints on the Evolution of Structure

The acceptability of an amino acid substitution will depend on a number of factors, such as the effect of the new hormone on the existing target organs and whether or not the new hormone has a different spectrum of effects on the various potential receptors from the old one. The components of the receptor systems may themselves be polymorphic.[30]

This can be illustrated by considering the change from AVP to LVP in the Suina. If the renal receptor system were such that LVP was only weakly antidiuretic, or the reproductive receptor systems were such that they responded to it strongly, there would presumably be effective selection against the new hormone. The lack of such fortuitous preadaptation of the renal-receptor system to LVP in most mammalian groups may explain why LVP is largely restricted to the Suina. If LVP is as effective as AVP in the renal-receptor system, or any deficiency is compensated for by an advantage in another physiological system, there will be no selection against LVP and there may even be selection for it. Under these circumstances the LVP allele could spread through the population. Heller and Spickett[12] pointed out that the potency of a hormone may not be the same as what the author has called its effectiveness. For example, in an aqueous environment (perhaps experienced by the ancestors of the present Suina), a highly potent hormone might cause larger fluctuations in the plasma osmotic pressure via the negative feedback system than a less potent one and, hence, be less effective physiologically. Taking this argument further, some of the feedback characteristics of the system would be affected by variation in k_1, k_2, and k_3 (as defined in Section III.B.1.b above) and by variation in the hypothalamus. It is important to recognize that it is the properties of the target organ system as a whole, together with the feedback characteristics, which are significant, not just the affinity of the collecting duct-hormone receptors for AVP and LVP. In the case of polymorphism maintained by heterozygous advantage, the more common allele is the one which is selectively superior ($p/q = s_2/s_1$ in the terminology of Falconer)[13] so that it may eventually be possible to test these ideas experimentally.

This still leaves undefined the nature of the balancing selection in this situation. There are several possibilities. Taking the case of heterozygous advantage, this could result if both hormones acting together have superior effectiveness to either alone. A synergistic effect on the same set of receptors or each hormone being more effective on one set of receptors (e.g., AVP on tubular antidiuresis, LVP on sodium transport in the ascending limb or even on hepatic metabolism) could cause this. Strangely, I do not know of any studies of the effects of simultaneous administration of physiological doses of AVP and LVP on renal function. These would be particularly valuable in the Suina. It would remain to be demonstrated that physiological synergism resulted in effective selection in the natural population. This task is difficult to achieve by statistical means, as effective selection pressures may be indetectably small even when large numbers of animals can be sampled.[14,60-62] However, a study of the relevant ecological factors could yield a cogent argument. This would be extremely valuable, as there is still a paucity of critically verified examples of heterozygous advantage in natural populations.

With respect to gene duplication, it has been suggested that this mechanism can result in an increase in the complexity of an organism and the flexibility of its homeostatic mechanisms, as two functions that were previously controlled coordinately can now be controlled independently.[30,214] Along with the evolution of a new hormone, this requires the evolution of an independent receptor system in one of the target organs. This process may have occurred with the evolution of vasopressin, which is relatively specific for osmoregulation in mammals, as compared with the reptiles where vasotocin may have embryonic, osmoregulatory, and reproductive functions. However, this example may be more complicated, for it may have to be assumed that oxytocin is free to take over the reproductive functions,[142] leaving vasotocin to the embryonic function (as yet unknown)[33,34] in mammals.

B. Hormone Function

Just as discussion of the constraints on hormone structure demanded a consideration of function, so the converse is true; the selective pressure on a new receptor molecule will be strongly influenced by the chemical structures of the hormones currently elaborated.

Heller and Spickett[12] pointed out that a new hormonal function, such as the milk-ejection reflex mediated by oxytocin in mammals, could evolve in two ways. An existing receptor molecule in one organ (uterus) might become expressed in another organ (mammary gland), resulting in a selective advantage due to the initiation of lactation at the time of parturition. Alternatively, a fortuitous and independent response of the mammary gland to oxytocin could gradually become more specific, with the same effect.[12] It is not yet possible to define receptors chemically, but a genetical approach has been described in Section III.B.1.a above

In the second case, gene duplication of the oxytocin-determining locus could readily result in independent control of the two functions. In the former case, though, independent control could not evolve until duplication of the receptor-determining locus occurred (or a new control system evolved independently) to allow differential responses to the two hormones.

C. Quantitative Aspects

1. The Mole-Ratio of Vasopressin to Oxytocin

In Section II.C.2 above, evidence that a major genetic defect can alter the mole-ratio of vasopressin to oxytocin in the neurohypophysis was presented. Section II. A presented evidence that normal laboratory populations differ genetically both in the individual stores and in their mole-ratio. However, this does not resolve the problem of the adaptive significance or otherwise of the mole-ratio. The observed phylogenetic characteristics of the mole-ratio could result either from selection or from a gradual drift without selection during evolution. Even if (as has been argued) the two stores are to some extent under separate genetic control (perhaps through an effect on the proportions of the two types of neurone which differentiate in the hypothalamus during development),[11] the selective pressures on both stores may sometimes be very similar, as they could be affected by similar factors. For example, a change in the mean circulation time, which is generally correlated with body weight,[215] would be likely to have similar effects on the rate of inactivation of oxytocin and of vasopressin by the liver and might explain the form of the relationship between pituitary stores and body weight. There is no case where the crucial parameter in arguments about the rate of evolutionary change, the extent of genetic variation in the mole-ratio in a natural population, is known. However, if the change in the mole-ratio in Peru mice, as compared with other strains,[15,16] is representative of the natural populations from which these strains are derived, this would suggest that there is indeed sufficient genetic variation in natural populations for reasonably rapid evolutionary change in the mole-ratio to occur. Further data to substantiate this argument that the mole-ratio is of adaptive significance are required. The nature of this adaptive significance is not clear, but it could result from physiological interactions between the vasopressin and oxytocin endocrine systems (such as an effect of oxytocin, which can be released from the pituitary together with vasopressin by some osmotic stimuli, on renal function).[179]

2. Balanced Systems

It seems likely, as suggested by Heller and Spickett,[12] that the adaptive significance of the neurohypophysial store of an octapeptide (orders of magnitude higher than the circulating levels of the hormone) is to allow rapid and flexible response to changes in the environment, using a direct gene product whose complex biosynthesis cannot be so rapidly controlled. This argument is supported by the fact that Brattleboro heterozygotes, with about half the normal store of vasopressin, seem to be under some stress (Section II.C.2). Animals adapted to arid environments may thus have larger stores of vasopressin or perhaps have a high biosynthetic rate (or the ability to increase it rapidly), together with a store comparable to related but nonadapted species.[9,216] The interest of genetic analysis of these parameters has already been mentioned. Similarly, animals in aquatic environments may have unusually low pituitary stores of the osmoregulatory octapeptide.[31] The genetic variation to allow such changes, insofar as they are indeed adaptive, exists in normal laboratory animals and one supposes in natural populations also (Section II.A).

The internal environment is also important. For example, it is tempting to suppose that the increase in the vasopressin store in Peru mice[15,16] (normalized by comparision with oxytocin) is concurrent with the change to LVP, which is less potent than AVP in these mice, thus leaving the total effective store of vasopressin unchanged.[161] Thus, in a balanced genetic system, the same physiological result may be achieved by different mechanisms. This idea is supported to some extent by the observation that the concentrating ability of Peru mice — presumably the character of adaptive significance — is no different from that of the CBA/FaCam mice with which they were compared. Without the use of specific biochemical and physiological techniques, the genetic variation would not have been observed.

The concept of a balanced system is also consistent with the origin of the DI strain of mice. Here again, the normal genetic variation used to derive this strain would not have been observed had it not been for the major disruption caused by the *Os* gene, which then allowed the selection of the unbalanced combination of alleles which characterizes the DI strains. This situation is often a feature of the genetic control of quantitative characters in *Drosophila*[211] as well as mammals.[212]

There are, therefore, several situations where it can clearly be seen that the physiological effect of an allele at one locus will depend on the alleles present at other loci. In population terms, this would correspond with Dobzhansky's concept of the coadapted genotype.[217] It must be stressed that this discussion is inherently selectionist, so that its validity depends on future demonstrations that physiological genetic variation of the type described is indeed of adaptive significance in natural populations.

V. CONCLUSION

This review has described the analysis and experimental use of several examples of genetic variation in the endocrine system of the posterior pituitary. The best authenticated have been cases of pathological variation, where it is obvious that the variation exists. This type of variation (for example, the Brattleboro rat) is now an accepted part of the literature, thanks largely to the work of Valtin and his group.[71] The stage has therefore been reached where there is a need to be critical of the genetical methodology used, in order that the conclusions drawn from such work can be as unequivocal as possible in the future. One difficulty, that of distinguishing direct from indirect effects of the primary lesion, is, however, always likely to remain and constitutes one limitation of this approach. Another limitation is imposed by the fact that a major defect affecting the particular site of interest in the endocrine system may simply not be known.

The use of normal variation together with appropriate genetic techniques (the examination of backcrosses between inbred strains and the use of recombinant inbred strains or of closely related sublines — see volume I, chapter 1) has the potential to overcome these problems to a large extent. The problem here is rather to identify the variation. Variation has usually been found when it has been sought. The development of improved and specific biochemical and physiological techniques will make this increasingly possible and profitable. The discussions of examples of this approach in this chapter have been more speculative than those of the use of pathological variation; however wrong this speculation proves to be, the specific examples given may give an indication of how the potential of this approach may be realized, whether in hypothesis testing, in correlating observations at different levels of organization, or in relation to evolutionary problems.

ACKNOWLEDGMENTS

It is impossible to mention all those who have influenced the development of the ideas presented here, nor can they be blamed for the misconceptions present. I would nevertheless like to acknowledge the help given by former members of the Cambridge group who initiated a program of research in Endocrine Genetics in the 1960s, especially Dr. J. G. M. Shire for his continuing interest; the late Prof. H. Heller and his colleagues at Bristol, who made the initial attempts to teach me something of the endocrinology of octapeptides; and members of the Department of Genetics at the University of Edinburgh.

REFERENCES

1. **Shire, J. G. M.,** The forms, uses and significance of genetic variation in endocrine systems, *Biol. Rev.*, 51, 105, 1976.
2. **Shire, J. G. M.,** Endocrine genetics of the adrenal gland, *J. Endocrinol.*, 62, 173, 1974.
3. **Grüneberg, H.,** An analysis of the "pleiotropic" effects of a new lethal mutation in the rat (*Mus norvegicus*), *Proc. R. Soc. London, Ser. B,* 125, 123, 1938.
4. **Stewart, J.,** Diuretic responses to water-load in four strains of mice, *J. Physiol. (London),* 198, 355, 1968.
5. **Spickett, S. G., Shire, J. G. M., and Stewart, J.,** Genetic variation in adrenal and renal structure and function, *Mem. Soc. Endocrinol.*, 15, 271, 1967.
6. **Stewart, J. and Spickett, S. G.,** Genetic variation in diuretic responses: further and correlated responses to selection, *Genet. Res.*, 10, 95, 1967.
7. **Knobil, E. and Sawyer, W. H., Eds.,** *The Pituitary Gland and Its Neuroendocrine Control, Handbook of Physiology, Section 7: Endocrinology,* Vol. 4 (Part 1), American Physiological Society, Washington, D. C., 1974.
8. **Berde, B., Ed.,** *Neurohypophysial Hormones and Similar Polypeptides, Handbook of Experimental Pharmacology,* Vol. 23, Springer-Verlag, Berlin, 1968.
9. **Valtin, H., Stewart, J., and Sokol, H. W.,** Genetic control of the production of posterior pituitary principles, in *The Pituitary Gland and Its Neuroendocrine Control, Handbook of Physiology, Section 7: Endocrinology,* Vol. 4 (Part 1), Knobil, E. and Sawyer, W. H., Eds., American Physiological Society, Washington, D.C., 1974, 131.
10. **Follett, B. K.,** Mole ratios of the neurohypophysial hormones in the vertebrate neural lobe, *Nature (London),* 198, 693, 1963.
11. **Ferguson, D. R. and Heller, H.,** Distribution of neurohypophysial hormones in mammals, *J. Physiol. (London),* 180, 846, 1965.
12. **Heller, H. and Spickett, S. G.,** The polymorphism of the neurohypophysial hormones, *Mem. Soc. Endocrinol.*, 15, 89, 1967.
13. **Falconer, D. S.,** *Introduction to Quantitative Genetics,* Longmans, London, 1975.
14. **Lewontin, R. C.,** *The Genetic Basis of Evolutionary Change,* Columbia University Press, New York, 1974.
15. **Stewart, A. D.,** Genetic determination of the storage of vasopressin and oxytocin in the neural lobes of mice, *J. Physiol. (London),* 222, 157P, 1972.
16. **Stewart, A. D.,** Genetic Variation in the Metabolism of Neurohypophysial Hormones of Mice, Ph.D. thesis, University of Cambridge, Cambridge, 1969.
17. **Stewart, A. D.,** Genetic variation in the neurohypophysial hormones of the mouse, *Mus musculus, J. Endocrinol.*, 51, 191, 1971.

18. **Waring, H. and Landgrebe, F. W.,** Hormones of the posterior pituitary, in *The Hormones,* Vol. 2, Pincus, G. and Thimann, K. V., Eds., Academic Press, New York, 1950, 427.
19. **Sachs, H., Share, L., Osinchak, J., and Capri, A.,** Capacity of the neurohypophysis to release vasopressin, *Endocrinology,* 81, 755, 1967.
20. **Sachs, H. and Haller, E. W.,** Further studies on the capacity of the neurohypophysis to release vasopressin, *Endocrinology,* 83, 251, 1968.
21. **Norström, A.,** Axonal transport and turnover of neurohypophysial proteins in the rat, *Ann. N.Y. Acad. Sci.,* 248, 46, 1975.
22. **Douglas, W. W.,** Mechanism of release of neurohypophysial hormones: stimulus-secretion coupling, in *The Pituitary Gland and Its Neuroendocrine Control, Handbook of Physiology, Section 7: Endocrinology,* Vol. 4 (Part 1), Knobil, E. and Sawyer, W. H., Eds., American Physiological Society, Washington, D.C., 1974, 191.
23. **Moses, A. M. and Miller, M.,** Osmotic influences on the release of vasopressin, in *The Pituitary Gland and Its Neuroendocrine Control, Handbook of Physiology, Section 7: Endocrinology,* Vol. 4 (Part 1), Knobil, E. and Sawyer, W. H., Eds., American Physiological Society, Washington, D.C., 1974, 225.
24. **Share, L.,** Blood pressure, blood volume, and the release of vasopressin, in *The Pituitary Gland and Its Neuroendocrine Control, Handbook of Physiology, Section 7: Endocrinology,* Vol. 4 (Part 1), Knobil, E. and Swayer, W. H., Eds., American Physiological Society, Washington, D.C., 1974. 243.
25. **Tindale, J. S.,** Stimuli that cause the release of oxytocin, in *The Pituitary Gland and Its Neuroendocrine Control, Handbook of Physiology, Section 7: Endocrinology,* Vol. 4 (Part 1), Knobil, E. and Sayer, W. H., Eds., American Physiological Society, Washington, D.C., 1974, 257.
26. **Ginsburg, M.,** Production, release, transportation and elimination of the neurohypophysial hormones, in *Neurohypophysial Hormones and Similar Polypeptides, Handbook of Experimental Pharmacology,* Vol. 23, Berde, B., Ed., Springer-Verlag, New York, 1968, 286.
27. **Sawyer, W. H.,** Phylogenetic aspects of the neurohypophysial hormones, in *Neurohypophysial Hormones and Similar Polypeptides, Handbook of Experimental Pharmacology,* Vol. 23, Berde, B., Ed., Vol. 23, Springer-Verlag, New York, 1968, 717.
28. **Acher, R.,** Chemistry of the neurohypophysial hormones: an example of molecular evolution, in *The Pituitary Gland and Its Neuroendocrine Control, Handbook of Physiology, Section 7: Endocrinology,* Vol. 4 (Part 1), Knobil, E. and Sawyer, W. H., Eds., American Physiological Society, Washington, D.C., 1974, 119.
29. **Vliegenthart, J. F. G. and Versteeg, D. A. G.,** The evolution of the vertebrate neurohypophysial hormones in relation to the genetic code, *J. Endocrinol.,* 38, 3, 1967.
30. **Wallis, M.,** The molecular evolution of pituitary hormones, *Biol. Rev.,* 50, 35, 1975.
31. **Acher, R., Chauvet, J., and Chauvet, M.-T.,** Phylogeny of the neurohypophysial hormones: two new active peptides isolated from a cartilaginous fish, *Squalus acanthias, Eur. J. Biochem.,* 29, 12, 1972.
32. **Pickering, B. T. and Heller, H.,** Oxytocin as a neurohypophysial hormone in the holocephalian elasmobranch fish, *Hydrolagus collei, J. Endocrinol.,* 45, 597, 1969.
33. **Skowsky, W. R. and Fisher, D. A.,** Immunoreactive arginine vasopressin and arginine vasotocin in the fetal pituitary of man and sheep, *Clin. Res.,* 21, 205, 1973.
34. **Vizsolyi, E. and Perks, A. M.,** New neurohypophysial principle in foetal mammals, *Nature (London),* 223, 1169, 1969.
35. **Cheesman, D. W.,** Structural elucidation of a gonadotrophin-inhibiting substance from the bovine pineal gland, *Biochim. Biophys. Acta,* 207, 247, 1970.
36. **Milcu, S. M., Pavel, S., and Neacsu, C.,** Biological and chromatographic characterization of a polypeptide with pressor and oxytocic activities isolated from bovine pineal gland, *Endocrinology,* 72, 563, 1963.
37. **Pavel, S.,** Endocrine functions of arginine vasotocin from mammalian pineal glands, *Gen. Comp. Endocrinol.,* 9, (Abstr.), 481, 1967.
38. **Pavel, S.,** Evidence for the ependymal origin of arginine vasotocin in the bovine pineal gland, *Endocrinology,* 89, 613, 1971.
39. **Rosenbloom, A. A. and Fisher, D. A.,** Radioimmunoassayable AVT and AVP in adult mammalian brain tissue: comparison of normal and Brattleboro rats, *Neuroendocrinology,* 17, 354, 1975.
40. **Reinharz, A. C., Czernichow, P., and Vallotton, M. B.,** Neurophysin-like protein in bovine pineal gland, *J. Endocrinol.,* 62, 35, 1974.
41. **Rosenbloom, A. A. and Fisher, D. A.,** Arginine vasotocin in rabbit subcommissural organ, *Endocrinology,* 96, 1038, 1975.
42. **Pavel, S.,** Evidence for the presence of lysine vasotocin in the pig pineal gland, *Endocrinology,* 77, 812, 1965.
43. **Sawyer, W. H.,** Comparative physiology and pharmacology of the neurohypophysis, *Recent Prog. Horm. Res.,* 17, 437, 1961.

44. **Ferguson, D. R.**, The genetic distribution of vasopressins in the peccary (*Tayassu angulatus*) and warthog (*Phacochoerus aethiopicus*), *Gen. Comp. Endocrinol.*, 12, 609, 1969.
45. **Ferguson, D. R. and Pickering, B. T.**, Arginine and lysine vasopressins in the hippopotamus neurohypophysis, *Gen. Comp. Endocrinol.*, 13, 425, 1969.
46. **Uttenthal, L. O. and Hope, D. B.**, Neurophysins and posterior pituitary hormones in the Suiformes, *Proc. R. Soc. London, Ser. B*, 182, 73, 1972.
47. **Forsling, M. L. and Stewart, A. D.**, unpublished data, 1972.
48. **Stewart, A. D.**, unpublished data, 1976.
49. **Pickering, B. T.**, The neurohypophysial hormones of a reptile species, the cobra (*Naja naja*), *J. Endocrinol.*, 39, 285, 1967.
50. **Follett, B. K.**, Neurohypophysial hormones of marine turtles and of the grass snake, *J. Endocrinol.*, 39, 293, 1967.
51. **Munsick, R. A.**, Chromatrographic and pharmacologic characterisation of the neurohypophysial hormones of an amphibian and a reptile, *Endocrinology*, 78, 591, 1966.
52. **Acher, R., Chauvet, J., and Chauvet, M-T.**, Evolution of the neurohypophysial hormones, with reference to amphibians, *Nature (London)*, 221, 758, 1969.
53. **Morel, F., Maetz, J., Acher, R., Chauvet, J., and Lenci, M. T.**, A "natriferic" principle other than arginine-vasotocin in the frog neurohypophysis, *Nature (London)*, 190, 828, 1961.
54. **Sawyer, W. H. and van Dyke, H. B.**, Principles resembling oxytocin in neurohypophysis of fishes, *Fed. Proc. Fed. Am. Soc. Exp. Biol.*, 22 (Abstr.), 386, 1963.
55. **Follett, B. K. and Heller, H.**, Pharmacological characteristics of neurohypophysial hormones in lungfish and amphibians, *Nature (London)*, 199, 611, 1963.
56. **Follett, B. K. and Heller, H.**, The neurohypophysial hormones of lungfishes and amphibians, *J. Physiol. (London)*, 172, 92, 1964.
57. **Pickering, B. T. and McWatters, S.**, Neurohypophysial hormones of the South American lungfish, *Lepidosiren paradoxa*, *J. Endocrinol.*, 36, 217, 1966.
58. **Sawyer, W. H.**, The active neurohypophysial principles of two primitive bony fishes, the bichir (*Polypterus senegalis*) and the African lungfish (*Protopterus aethiopicus*), *J. Endocrinol.*, 44, 421, 1969.
59. **Sachs, H.**, Biosynthesis and release of vasopressin, *Am. J. Med.*, 42, 687, 1967.
60. **Lewontin, R. C. and Cockerham, C. C.**, The goodness of fit test for detecting natural selection in random mating populations, *Evolution*, 13, 561, 1959.
61. **Prout, T.**, The estimation of fitnesses from genotypic frequencies, *Evolution*, 19, 546, 1965.
62. **Prout, T.**, The estimation of fitnesses from population data, *Genetics*, 63, 949, 1969.
63. **Randall, R. V., Clark, E. C., and Bahn, R. C.**, Classification of the causes of diabetes insipidus, *Mayo Clin., Proc.*, 34, 299, 1959.
64. **Page, M. M., Asmal, A. C., and Edwards, C. R. W.**, The syndrome of diabetes insipidus, diabetes mellitus, opticatrophy and deafness, *Q. J. Med.*, 45, 505, 1976.
65. **Smith, C.**, Discriminating between different modes of inheritance in genetic disease, *Clin. Genet.*, 2, 303, 1971.
66. **Silverstein, E., Sokoloff, L., Mickelsen, O., and Jay, G. E.**, Primary polydipsia and hydronephrosis in an inbred strain of mice, *Am. J. Pathol.*, 38, 143, 1961.
67. **Dunson, W. A. and Buss, E. G.**, Abnormal water balance in a strain of chickens, *Science*, 161, 167, 1968.
68. **Forssman, H.**, Two different mutations of the X-chromosome causing diabetes insipidus, *Am. J. Hum. Genet.*, 7, 21, 1955.
69. **Martin, F. R.**, Familial diabetes insipidus, *Q. J. Med.*, 28, 573, 1959.
70. **Valtin, H.**, Hereditary hypothalamic diabetes insipidus in rats (Brattleboro strain), *Am. J. Med.*, 42, 814, 1967.
71. **Valtin, H.**, Genetic models in biomedical investigation, *N. Engl. J. Med.*, 290, 670, 1974.
72. **Andersson, K.-E., Arner, B., Fürst, E., and Hedner, P.**, Antidiuretic responses to hypertonic saline infusion, water deprivation, and a synthetic analogue of vasopressin in patients with hereditary, hypothalamic diabetes insipidus, *Acta. Med. Scand.*, 195, 17, 1974.
73. **Braverman, L. E., Mancini, J. P., and McGoldrick, D. M.**, Hereditary idiopathic diabetes insipidus: a case report with autopsy findings, *Ann. Intern. Med.*, 63, 503, 1965.
74. **Raffell, L. J., Buss, E. G., and Clagett, C. O.**, Influence of arginine vasotocin on a genetically determined excessive appetite for water in chickens, *Poult. Sci.*, 55, 1834, 1976.
75. **Mendoza, S. A.**, Syndrome of inappropriate antidiuretic hormone secretion, *Pediatr. Clin. North Am.*, 23, 681, 1976.
76. **Vorherr, H.**, Para-endocrine tumor activity with emphasis on ectopic ADH secretion, *Oncology*, 29, 382, 1974.
77. **Martin, J. E. and Pauerstein, C. J.**, The initiation of labour, *Clin. Anesth.*, 10, 51, 1974.
78. **Chard, T.**, The posterior pituitary in human and animal parturition, *J. Reprod. Fertil. Suppl.*, 16, 121, 1972.

79. **Newton, H. and Newton, M.**, Psychologic aspects of lactation, *N. Engl. J. Med.*, 277, 1179, 1967.
80. **MacVicar, J.**, Acceleration and augmentation of labour, *Scott. Med. J.*, 18, 201, 1973.
81. **Vandesande, F. and Dierickx, K.**, Immuno-cytochemical demonstration of the inability of the homozygous Brattleboro rat to synthesise vasopressin and vasopressin-associated neurophysin, *Cell Tissue Res.*, 165, 307, 1976.
82. **Swaab, D. F., Pool, C. W., and Nijveldt, F,.** Immunofluorescence of vasopressin and oxytocin in the rat hypothalamo-neurohypophyseal system, *J. Neural Trans.*, 36, 195, 1975.
83. **Watkins, W. B.**, Presence of neurophysin and vasopressin in the hypothalamic magnocellular nuclei of rats homozygous and heterozygous for diabetes insipidus (Brattleboro strain) as revealed by immunoperoxidase histology, *Cell Tissue Res.*, 157, 101, 1975.
84. **Livett, B. G,.** Immunochemical studies on the storage and axonal transport of neurophysins in the hypothalamo-neurohypophyseal system, *Ann. N. Y. Acad. Sci.*, 248, 112, 1975.
85. **Cheng, K. W., Friesen, H. G., and Martin, J. B.**, Neurophysin in rats with hereditary hypothalamic diabetes insipidus (Brattleboro strain), *Endocrinology*, 90, 1055, 1972.
86. **Pickering, B. T., Jones, C. W., Burford, G. D., McPherson, M., Swann, R. W., Heap, P. F., and Morris, J. F.**, The role of neurophysin proteins: suggestions from the study of their transport and turnover, *Ann. N.Y. Acad. Sci.*, 248, 15, 1975.
87. **Sunde, D. A. and Sokol, H. W.**, Quantification of rat neurophysins by polyacrylamide gel electrophoresis (PAGE): application to the rat with hereditary hypothalamic diabetes insipidus, *Ann. N.Y. Acad. Sci.*, 248, 345, 1975.
88. **Leclerc, R. and Pelletier, G.**, Electron microscope immunohistochemical localisation of neurophysin in the rat with hereditary diabetes insipidus, *Virchows Arch. B*, 22, 233, 1976.
89. **Kalimo, H. and Rinne, U. K.**, Ultrastructural studies on the hypothalamic neurosecretory neurons of the rat, *Z. Zellforsch. Mikrosk. Anat.*, 134, 205, 1972.
90. **Zimmerman, E. A., Defendini, A., Sokol, H. W., and Robinson, A. G.**, The distribution of neurophysin-secreting pathways in the mammalian brain: light microscopic studies using the immunoperoxidase technique, *Ann. N.Y. Acad. Sci.*, 248, 92, 1975.
91. **Burford, G. D. and Stewart, A. D.**, unpublished data
92. **Burford, G. D., Dyball, R. E. J., Moss, R. L., and Pickering, B. T.**, Synthesis of both neurohypophysial hormones in both the paraventricular and supraoptic nuclei of the rat, *J. Anat.*, 117, 261, 1974.
93. **Moses, A. M. and Miller, M.**, Accumulation and release of pituitary vasopressin in rats heterozygous for hypothalamic diabetes insipidus, *Endocrinology*, 86, 34, 1970.
94. **Möhring, B. and Möhring, J.**, Plasma ADH in normal Long-Evans rats and in Long-Evans rats heterozygous and homozygous for hypothalamic diabetes insipidus, *Life Sci.*, 17, 1307, 1975.
95. **Lauson, H. D.**, Metabolism of the neurohypophysial hormones, in *The Pituitary Gland and Its Neuroendocrine Control, Handbook of Physiology, Section 7: Endocrinology* Vol. 4 (Part 1), Knobil, E. and Sawyer, W. H., Eds., American Physiological Society, Washington, D.C., 1974, 287
96. **Norström, A.**, Biosynthesis of neurohypophysial proteins in rats with hereditary hypothalamic diabetes insipidus, *Brain Res.*, 68, 309, 1974.
97. **Epstein, W. and Beckwith, J. R.**, Regulation of gene expression, *Annu. Rev. Biochem.*, 37, 411, 1968.
98. **Dofuku, R., Tettenborn, V., and Ohno, S.**, Further characterisation of o^s mutation of mouse β-glucuronidase locus, *Nature (London)*, 234, 259, 1971.
99. **Schwartz, D.**, Genetic studies on mutant enzymes in maize. III. Control of gene action in the synthesis of pH 7.5 esterase, *Genetics*, 47, 1609, 1962.
100. **Dickinson, W. J.**, A genetic locus affecting the developmental expression of an enzyme in *Drosophila melanogaster*, *Dev. Biol.*, 42, 131, 1975.
101. **Paigen, K., Meisler, M., Felton, J., and Chapman, V.**, Genetic determination of the β-galactosidase developmental program in mouse liver, *Cell*, 9, 533, 1976.
102. **Tasso, F., Picard, D., and Driefuss, J. J.**, Ultrastructural identification of granules containing oxytocin and vasopressin, *Nature (London)*, 260, 621, 1976.
103. **Driedger, A. A. and Linton, A. L.**, Familial ADH-responsive diabetes insipidus: response to thiazides and chlorpropamide, *Can. Med. Assoc. J.*, 109, 594, 1973.
104. **Berndt, W. O., Miller, M., Kettyle, W. M., and Valtin, H.**, Potentiation of the antidiuretic effect of vasopressin by chlorpropamide, *Endocrinology*, 86, 1028, 1970.
105. **Miller, M. and Moses, A. M.**, Potentiation of vasopressin action by chlorpropamide *in vivo*, *Endocrinology*, 86, 1024, 1970.
106. **Laycock, J. F.**, The Brattleboro rat with hereditary hypothalamic diabetes insipidus as an ideal experimental model, *Lab. Anim.*, 10, 261, 1976.
107. **Harrington, A. R.**, Hyponatraemia due to sodium depletion in the absence of vasopressin, *Am. J. Physiol.*, 221, 911, 1971.

108. **Valtin, H.**, Sequestration of urea and non-urea solutes in renal tissues of rats with hereditary hypothalamic diabetes insipidus: effect of vasopressin and dehydration on the countercurrent mechanism, *J. Clin. Invest.*, 45, 337, 1966.
109. **Tisher, C. C. and Yarger, W. E.**, Lanthanum permeability of tight junctions along the collecting duct of the rat, *Kidney Int.*, 7, 35, 1975.
110. **Balment, R. J., Henderson, I. W., and Chester Jones, I.**, Effects of lithium-supplemented diet on renal and endocrine function in normal Long-Evans and Brattleboro rats, *J. Endocrinol.*, 71, 80P, 1976.
111. **Thomsen, K. and Schou, M.**, The effect of prolonged administration of hydrochlorothiazide on the renal lithium clearance and the urine flow of ordinary rats and rats with diabetes insipidus, *Pharmakopsychiatr. Neuro Psychopharmakol.*, 6, 264, 1973.
112. **Sawyer, W. H. and Valtin, H.**, Antidiuretic responses of rats with hereditary hypothalamic diabetes insipidus to vasopressin, oxytocin and nicotine, *Endocrinology,* 80, 207, 1967.
113. **Vierling, A. F., Little, J. B., and Radford, E. P.**, Antidiuretic hormone bio-assay in rats with hereditary hypothalamic diabetes insipidus (Brattleboro strain), *Endocrinology,* 80, 211, 1967.
114. **Jones, J. J. and Lee, J.**, The value of rats with hereditary diabetes insipidus for the bioassay of vasopressin, *J. Endocrinol.*, 37, 335, 1967.
115. **Schnermann, J., Valtin, H., Thurau, K., Nagel, W., Horster, M., Fischbach, H., Wahl, M., and Liebau, G.**, Micropuncture studies on the influence of antidiuretic hormone on tubular fluid reabsorption in rats with hereditary hypothalamic diabetes insipidus, *Pfluegers Arch. Gesamte Physiol. Menschen Tiere,* 306, 103, 1969.
116. **Möhring, J., Dauda, G., Haack, D., Homsy, E., Kohrs, G., and Möhring, B.**, Increased potassium intake and kaliopenic nephropathy in rats with genetic diabetes insipidus, *Life Sci.*, 11, 679, 1972.
117. **Relman, A. S. and Schwartz, W. B.**, The kidney in potassium depletion, *Am. J. Med.*, 24, 764, 1958.
118. **Welt, L. G., Hollander, W., and Blythe, W. B.**, The consequences of potassium depletion, *J. Chronic Dis.*, 11, 213, 1960.
119. **Green, H., Harrington, A. R., and Valtin, H.**, On the role of antidiuretic hormone in the inhibition of acute water diuresis in adrenal insufficiency and the effect of gluco- and mineralo corticoids in reversing the inhibition, *J. Clin. Invest.*, 49, 1724, 1970.
120. **Balment, R. J., Chester Jones, I., Henderson, I. W., and Oliver, J. A.**, Effects of adrenalectomy and hypophysectomy on water and electrolyte metabolism in male and female rats with inherited diabetes insipidus (Brattleboro strain), *J. Endocrinol.*, 71, 193, 1976.
121. **Schleiffer, R., Koch, B., and Mialhe, C.**, Depletion in ACTH content of the posterior pituitary in vasopressin-deficient (Brattleboro) rats after adrenalectomy, *Horm. Metab. Res.*, 8, 495, 1976.
122. **Oliver, J. A., Balment, R. J., and Henderson, I. W.**, Sex differences in vasopressin-induced changes in plasma renin activity of Brattleboro and Long-Evans rats, *J. Endocrinol.*, 71, 79, 1976.
123. **Hunt, N. H., Perris, A. D., and Sandford, P. A.**, Role of vasopressin in the mitotic response of rat bone marrow cells to haemorrhage, *J. Endocrinol.*, 72, 5, 1977.
124. **Share, L.**, Role of cardiovascular receptors in the control of ADH release, *Cardiology,* 61 (Suppl. 1), 54, 1976.
125. **Linden, R. J.**, Reflexes from receptors in the heart, *Cardiology,* 61 (Suppl. 1), 7, 1976.
126. **Wooten, G., Hanson, T., and Lamprecht, F.**, Elevated serum dopamine β-hydroxylase activity in rats with inherited diabetes insipidus, *J. Neurol Transm.*, 36, 107, 1975.
127. **Bohs, B., van Wimersma Greidanus, T. J. B., and de Wied, D.**, Behavioural and endocrine responses of rats with hereditary hypothalamic diabetes insipidus (Brattleboro strain), *Physiol. Behav.*, 14, 609, 1975.
128. **Urban, I. and de Wied, D.**, Inferior quality of RSA during paradoxical sleep in rats with hereditary diabetes insipidus, *Brain Res.*, 97, 362, 1975.
129. **De Wied, D., Bohus, B., and van Wimersma Griedanus, T. J. B.**, Memory deficit in rats with hereditary diabetes insipidus, *Brain Res.*, 85, 152, 1975.
130. **Robinson, A. G. and Zimmerman, E. A.**, Cerebrospinal fluid and ependymal neurophysin, *J. Clin. Invest.*, 52, 1260, 1973.
131. **Coculescu, M. and Pavel, S.**, Arginine vasotocin-like activity of cerebrospinal fluid in diabetes insipidus, *J. Clin. Edocrinol. Metab.*, 36, 1031, 1973.
132. **Pavel, S.**, Arginine vasotocin release into cerebrospinal fluid of cats induced by melatonin, *Nature (London) New Biol.*, 246, 183, 1973.
133. **Pavel, S. and Coculescu, M.**, Arginine vasotocin-like activity of cerebrospinal fluid induced by injection of hypertonic saline into the third cerebral ventricle of cats, *Endocrinology,* 91, 825, 1972.
134. **Marshall, J. M.**, Effects of neurohypophysial hormones on the myometricum, in *The Pituitary Gland and Its Neuroendocrine Control, Handbook of Physiology, Section 7: Endocrinology,* Vol. 4 (Part 1), Knobil, E. and Sawyer, W. H., Eds., American Physiological Society, Washington, D.C., 1974, 469.

135. **Bissett, G. W.**, Milk ejection, in *The Pituitary Gland and Its Neuroendocrine Control, Handbook of Physiology, Section 7: Endocrinology,* Vol. 4 (Part 1), Knobil, E., and Sawyer, W. H., Eds., American Physiological Society, Washington, D.C., 1974, 493.
136. **Sawyer, W. H.**, The mammalian antidiuretic response, in *The Pituitary Gland and Its Neuroendocrine Control, Handbook of Physiology, Section 7: Endocrinology,* Vol. 4 (Part 1), Knobil, E. and Sawyer, W. H., Eds., American Physiological Society, Washington, D.C., 1974, 443.
137. **Robertson, G. L.**, Vasopressin in osmotic regulation in man, *Annu. Rev. Med.*, 25, 315, 1974.
138. **Bentley, P.L.J.**, Actions of neurohypophysial peptides in amphibians, reptiles and birds, in *The Pituitary Gland and Its Neuroendocrine Control, Handbook of Physiology, Section 7: Endocrinology,* Vol. 4 (Part 1), Knobil, E. and Sawyer, W. H., Eds., American Physiological Society, Washington, D.C., 1974, 565.
139. **Nakano, J.**, Cardiovascular responses to neurohypophysial hormones, in *The Pituitary Gland and Its Neuroendocrine Control, Handbook of Physiology, Section 7: Endocrinology,* Vol. 4 (Part 1), Knobil, E. and Sawyer, W. H., Eds., American Physiological Society, Washington, D.C., 1974, 395.
140. **Hems, D. A. and Ma, G. Y.**, Resistance to hepatic action of vasopressin in genetically obese (*ob/ob*) mice, *Biochem. J.*, 160, 23, 1976.
141. **Maetz, J. and Lahlou, B.**, Actions of neurohypophysial hormones in fishes, in *The Pituitary Gland and Its Neuroendocrine Control, Handbook of Physiology, Section 7: Endocrinology,* Vol 4 (Part 1), Knobil, E. and Sawyer, W. H., Eds., American Physiological Society, Washington, D.C., 1974, 521.
142. **La Pointe, J. L.**, Effect of ovarian steroids and neurohypophysial hormones on the oviduct of the viviparous lizard, *Klauberina riversiana*, J. Endocrinol., 43, 197, 1969.
143. **Kar, K., Sur, R. N., and Dhawan, B. N.**, Sensitivity of male rats of different strains to vasopressin, *Indian J. Exp. Biol.*, 8, 194, 1970.
144. **Roy, C., Rajerison, R., Bockaert, J., and Jard, S.**, Solubilisation of (8-lysine)-vasopressin receptor and adenylate cyclase from pig kidney plasma-membranes, *J. Biol. Chem.*, 250, 7885, 1975.
145. **Jard, S., Bockaert, J., Roy, C., and Rajerison, R.**, Vasopressin receptors, in *Methods in Receptor Research, Part II, Methods in Molecular Biology Series,* Vol. 9, Blecher, M., Ed., Marcel Dekker, Basel, 1977, chap. 11.
146. **Bockaert, J., Roy, C., Rajerison, R., and Jard, S.**, Application of theory of occupation of renal receptors of lysine vasopressin connected to adenyl cyclase-study using tritiated vasopressin, *C. R. Acad. Sci.*, 276, 649, 1973.
147. **Bockaert, J., Roy, C., Rajerison, R., and Jard, S.**, Specific binding of ^{3}H-lysine-vasopressin to pig kidney plasma membranes, *J. Biol. Chem.*, 248, 5922, 1973.
148. **Douša, T., Hechter, O., Schwartz, I. L., and Walter, R.**, Neurohypophyseal hormone-responsive adenylate cyclase from mammalian kidney, *Proc. Natl. Acad. Sci. U.S.A.*, 68, 1693, 1971.
149. **Grantham, J. J. and Burg, M.**, Effect of vasopressin and cyclic AMP on permeability of isolated collecting tubules, *Am. J. Physiol.*, 211, 255, 1966.
150. **Rado, J. P., Marosi, J., Borbély, L., and Tako, J.**, Individual differences in the antidiuretic response induced by single doses of 1-deamino-8-D-arginine-vasopressin (DDAVP) in patients with pituitary diabetes insipidus, *Int. J. Clin. Pharmacol. Ther. Toxicol.*, 14, 259, 1976.
151. **Kushner, Kh. F., Velitok, I. G., Sebryakov, E. V., and Sergienko, N. A.**, Phenotypic and genetic parameters of functional characteristics of the udder quarters in cows: communication. V. Genetic parameters of the functional characteristics of the cow udder, *Sov. Genet.*, 7, 1148, 1974.
152. **Mackay, D.**, A new method for the analysis of drug-receptor interactions, *Adv. Drug. Res.*, 3, 1, 1966.
153. **Soloff, M. S.**, Oxytocin receptors in the mammary gland and uterus, in *Methods in Receptor Research, Part II, Methods in Molecular Biology Series,* Vol. 9, Blecher, M., Ed., Marcel Dekker, Basel, 1977, chap. 5.
154. **Polaček, I., Krejči, I., and Rudinger, J.**, The action of oxytocin and synthetic analogues on the isolated mammary-gland myopeithlium of the lactating rat; effect of some ions, *J. Endocrinol.*, 38, 13, 1967.
155. **Sturmer, E.**, Bioassay procedures for neurohypophysial hormones and similar polypeptides, in *Neurohypophysial Hormones and Similar Polypeptides, Handbook of Experimental Pharmacology,* Vol. 23, Berde, B., Ed., Springer-Verlag, New York, 1968, 130
156. **Sawyer, W. H., Chan, W. Y., and van Dyke, H. B.**, Antidiuretic responses to neurohypophysial hormones and some of their synthetic analogues in dogs and rats, *Endocrinology,* 71, 536, 1962.
157. **Orloff, J. and Handler, J.**, The role of adenosine 3′5′-phosphate in the action of antidiuretic hormone, *Am. J. Med.*, 42, 757, 1967.
158. **DeHaven, J. C. and Shapiro, N. Z.**, Simulation of the renal effects of antidiuretic hormone (ADH) in man, *J. Theor. Biol.*, 28, 261, 1970.
159. **Barth, T., Rajerison, M. R., Roy, C., and Jard, S,.** Activation of rat kidney adenylate cyclase by vasopressin analogues: lack of correlation with antidiuretic activity, *Mol. Cell. Endocrinol.*, 2, 81, 1975.

160. **Morel, F.**, Action of neurohypophyseal hormones on the active transport of sodium, in *Water and Electrolyte Metabolism,* De Graeff, J. and Leijnse, B., Eds., Elsevier, Amsterdam, 1964, 91.
161. **Stewart, A. D.**, Sensitivity of mice to (8-arginine)- and (8-lysine)-vasopressins as antidiuretic hormones, *J. Endocrinol.,* 59, 195, 1973.
162. **Smith, M. W.**, The effect of hyaluronidase and cortisol on the inactivation of vasopressins by rat kidney slices, *J. Endocrinol.,* 24, 415, 1962.
163. **Jard, S., Roy, C., Rajerison, R., Barth, T., and Bockaert, J.**, Caractérisation du récepteur rénal de l'hormone antidiurétique, *J. Urol. Nephrol.,* 12, 961, 1974.
164. **Thorn, N. A. and Willumsen, N. B. S.**, Inactivation of arginine and lysine vasopressin by slices from different zones of the rat kidney and by rat liver slices, *Acta Endocrinol. (Copenhagen),* 44, 545, 1963.
165. **Dicker, S. E. and Eggleton, G.**, Hyaluronidase and antidiuretic activity in urine of man, *J. Physiol. (London).,* 154, 378, 1960.
166. **Dicker, S. E. and Greenbaum, A. L.**, The degree of inactivation of very small amounts of antidiuretic activity of vasopressin by the kidneys and the livers of rats, *J. Physiol. (London),* 126, 116, 1954.
167. **Schwartz, I. L., Rasmussen, H., Schoessler, M. A., Silver, L., and Tong, C. T. O.**, Relation of chemical attachment to physiological action of vasopressin, *Proc. Natl. Acad. Sci. U.S.A.,* 46, 1288, 1960.
168. **Smith, M. W. and Sachs, H.**, Inactivation of arginine vasopressin by rat kidney slices, *Biochem. J.,* 79, 663, 1961.
169. **Smith, M. W. and Ginsburg, M.**, Fate of synthetic oxytocin analogues in the rat, *Br. J. Pharmacol.,* 16, 244, 1961.
170. **Ginsburg, M. and Smith, M. W.**, The fate of oxytocin in male and female rats, *Br. J. Pharmacol.,* 14, 327, 1959.
171. **Levi, J., Rosenfeld, S., and Kleeman, C. R.**, Inactivation of arginine-vasopressin by the isolated perfused rabbit kidney, *J. Endocrinol.,* 62, 1, 1974.
172. **Douša, T. P.**, Possible role of microtubules in the cellular action of ADH in mammalian kidney, *Clin. Res.,* 22, 206A, 1974.
173. **Taylor, A., Maffly, R., Wilson, L., and Reaven, E.**, Evidence for involvement of microtubules in the action of vasopressin, *Ann. N.Y. Acad. Sci.,* 253, 723, 1975.
174. **Handler, J. S. and Orloff, J.**, in *Handbook of Physiology, Section 8: Renal Physiology,* Orloff, J. and Berliner, R. W., Eds., American Physiological Society, Washington, D.C., 1973, 791.
175. **Jard, S., Butler, D., Rajerison, R., and Roy, C.**, The vasopressin-sensitive adenylate cyclase from mammalian kidney: mechanisms of activation and regulation of hormonal responsiveness, in *Hormones and Cell Regulation,* Vol. 1, Dumont, J. and Nunez, J., Eds., Elsevier, Amsterdam, 1977, chap. 2.
176. **Douša, T. P.**, Role of cyclic AMP in the action of antidiuretic hormone in kidney, *Life Sci.,* 13, 1033, 1973.
177. **Roy, C., Barth, T., and Jard, S.**, Vasopressin-sensitive kidney adenylate cyclase-structural requirements for attachment to receptor and enzyme activation-studies with vasopressin analogues, *J. Biol. Chem.,* 250, 3149, 1975.
178. **Douša, T. P., Walter, R. W., Sands, H., Schwartz, I. L., and Hechter, O.**, Role of cyclic AMP in the action of neurohypophyseal hormones on the kidney, *Adv. Cyclic Nucleotide Res.,* 1, 121, 1972.
179. **Thorn, N. A.**, Influence of the neurohypophysial hormones and similar polypeptides on the kidneys, in *Neurohypophysial Hormones and Similar Polypeptides, Handbook of Experimental Pharmacology,* Vol. 23, Berde, B., Ed., Springer-Verlag, New York, 1968, 372.
180. **Munsick, R. A., Sawyer, W. H., and van Dyke, H. B.**, The antidiuretic potency of arginine and lysine vasopressins in the pig with observations on porcine renal function, *Endocrinology,* 63, 688, 1958.
181. **Stewart, A. D.**, Genetic study of the effects of (8-arginine)- and (8-lysine)-vasopressins on adenyl cyclase activity of mouse kidney, *J. Endocrinol.,* 61, 447, 1974.
182. **Imbert, M., Chabardis, D., Montegut, M., Clique, A., and Morel, F.**, Vasopressin dependent adenylate cyclase in single segments of rabbit kidney tubule, *Pfluegers Arch. Gesamte Physiol. Menschen Tiere,* 357, 173, 1975.
183. **Fourman, J. and Kennedy, G. C.**, An effect of antidiuretic hormone on the flow of blood through the vasa recta of the rat kidney, *J. Endocrinol.,* 35, 173, 1966.
184. **Atherton, J. C., Green, R., and Thomas, S.**, Influence of lysine-vasopressin dosage on the time course of changes in renal tissue and urinary composition in the conscious rat, *J. Physiol. (London),* 213, 291, 1971.
185. **Antoniou, L. D., Burke, T. J., Robinson, R. R. and Clapp, R. J.**, Vasopressin related alterations of sodium reabsorption in the loop of Henle, *Kidney Int.,* 3, 6, 1975.
186. **Douša, T. P. and Valtin, H.**, Cellular action of antidiuretic hormone in mice with inherited vasopressin-resistant urinary concentrating defects, *J. Clin. Invest.,* 54, 753, 1974.

187. **Douša, T. P.**, Cellular action of antidiuretic hormone in nephrogenic diabetes insipidus, *Mayo Clin. Proc.*, 49, 188, 1974.
188. **Bell, H. H., Clark, C. M., Avery, S., Sinha, T., Trygstad, C. W., and Allen, D. O.**, Demonstration of a defect in the formation of adenosine 3′,5′-monophosphate in vasopressin-resistant diabetes insipidus, *Pediatr. Res.*, 8, 223, 1974.
189. **Zimmerman, D. and Green, O. C.**, Nephrogenic diabetes insipidus type II: defect distal to the adenylate cyclase step, *Am. J. Hum. Genet.*, 26, 97a, 1974.
190. **Grassi, A.** Diabete nefrogeno, *Minerva Pediatr.*, 27, 1155, 1973.
191. **Hoffmann, L.**, Die Bedentung der Harnwegsveränderungen beim Diabetes insipidus für den Urologen, *Z. Urol. Bed.*, 66, 889, 1973.
192. **Ramsey, E. W., Morrin, P. A. F., and Bruce, A. W.**, Nephrogenic diabetes insipidus associated with massive hydronephrosis and bladder neck obstruction, *J. Urol.*, 111, 225, 1974.
193. **Wiggelinkhuizen, J., Wolff, B., and Cremin, B. J.**, Nephrogenic diabetes insipidus and obstructive uropathy, *Am. J. Dis. Child.*, 126, 398, 1973.
194. **Bode, H. H. and Crawford, J. D.**, Nephrogenic diabetes insipidus in North America — the Hopewell hypothesis, *N. Engl. J. Med.*, 280, 750, 1969.
195. **Schrager, G. O., Josephson, B. H., Fine, B. F., and Berger, G.**, Nephrogenic diabetes insipidus presenting as fever of unknown origin in the neonatal period, *Clin. Pediatr. (Philadelphia)*, 15, 1070, 1976.
196. **Call, N. B. and Tisher, C. C.**, The urinary concentrating defect in the Gunn strain of rat, *J. Clin. Invest.*, 55, 319, 1975.
197. **Lyon, M. F. and Hulse, E. V.**, An inherited kidney disease of mice resembling nephronophthisis, *J. Med. Genet.*, 8, 41, 1971.
198. **Szalay, G. and Moll, J.**, Note on the polydipsia-polyuria syndrome in aged inbred mice, *Exp. Gerontol.*, 2, 47, 1966.
199. **Kutscher, C. L., Miller, M., and Schmalbach, N. L.**, Renal deficiency associated with diabetes insipidus in the SWR/J mouse, *Physiol. Behav.*, 14, 815, 1975.
200. **Virgo, N. S. and Miller, J. R.**, Hereditary vasopressin-resistant diabetes insipidus in SWV mice, *Can. J. Physiol. Pharmacol.*, 52, 995, 1974.
201. **Grüneberg, H.**, Genetical studies on the skeleton of the mouse. XXVII. The development of oligosyndactylism, *Genet. Res.*, 2, 33, 1961.
202. **Falconer, D. S., Latyszewski, M., and Isaacson, J. H.**, Diabetes insipidus associated with oligosyndactyly in the mouse, *Genet. Res.*, 5, 473, 1964.
203. **Naik, D. V. and Valtin, H.**, Hereditary vasopressin-resistant urinary concentrating defects in mice, *Am. J. Physiol.*, 217, 1183, 1969.
204. **Stewart, A. D. and Stewart, J.**, Studies on the syndrome of diabetes insipidus associated with oligosyndactyly in mice, *Am. J. Physiol.*, 217, 1191, 1969.
205. **Naik, D. V.**, Influence of neurosecretion on the activity of median eminence and pars intermedia in hereditary nephrogenic diabetes insipidus mice with bilateral supraoptic lesions, *Z. Zellforsch. Mikrosk. Anat.*, 125, 460, 1972.
206. **Naik, D. V.**, Salt and water metabolism and neurohypophyseal vasopressor activity in mice with hereditary nephrogenic diabetes insipidus, *Acta Endocrinol. (Copenhagen)*, 69, 434, 1972.
207. **Stewart, J.**, Renal concentrating ability in mice: a model for the use of genetic variation in elucidating relationships between structure and function, *Pfluegers Arch. Gesamte Physiol. Menschen Tiere*, 327, 1, 1971.
208. **Kaufman, J. M., Siegel, N., Lytton, B., and Hayslett, J. P.**, Compensatory renal adaptation after progressive renal ablation, *Invest. Urol.*, 13, 441, 1976.
209. **Royer, P., Habib, R., Courtecuisse, V., and Leclerc, F.**, L'hypoplasie rénale bilatérale avec oligonephronie, *Arch. Fr. Paediatr.*, 24, 249, 1967.
210. **Kettyle, W. M. and Valtin, H.**, Chemical and dimensional characterization of the renal countercurrent system in mice, *Kidney Int.*, 1, 135, 1972.
211. **Rendel, J. M.**, *Canalisation and Gene Control*, Logos, London, 1967.
212. **Fraser, A. S. and Kindred, B. M.**, Selection for an invariant character, vibrissae number, in the house mouse, *Aust. J. Biol. Sci.*, 13, 48, 1960.
213. **Arunachalam, V. and Owen, A. R. G.**, *Polymorphisms with Linked Loci*, Chapman and Hall, London, 1971.
214. **Adelson, J. W.**, Enterosecretory proteins, *Nature (London)*, 229, 321, 1971.
215. **Heller, H. and Ginsburg, M.**, Secretion, Metabolism and fate of the posterior pituitary hormones, in *The Pituitary Gland*, Vol. 3, Harris, G. W. and Donovan, B. T., Eds., Butterworths, London, 1966, 330.
216. **Buchanan, J. G. and Stewart, A. D.**, Neurohypophysial store of vasopressin in the normal and dehydrated gerbil (*Meriones unguiculatus*), with a note on kidney structure, *J. Endocrinol.*, 60, 381, 1974.

217. **Dobzhansky, T.**, *Genetics and the Origin of Species,* 3rd ed., Columbia University, New York, 1951.
218. **Brownstein, M. J. and Gainer, H.**, Neurophysin biosynthesis in normal rats and rats with hereditary diabetes insipidus, *Proc. Natl. Acad. Sci. U.S.A.*, 74, 4046, 1977.
219. **Moore, G. J., Swann, R. W., and Lederis, K.**, Failure of neurohypophysial neurosecretory granule lysate to liberate arginine-vasopressin from synthetic model prohormones simulating covalent attachment of arginine-vasopressin to neurophysin, *J. Endocrinol.*, 75, 341, 1977.
220. **Valtin, H.**, unpublished data, 1977.

INDEX

A

B

C

D

E

F

G

H

I

N

O

P

R

S

T

U

V

W

X

Y

Z